CW01372709

COVER

What Public Health Won't Tell You

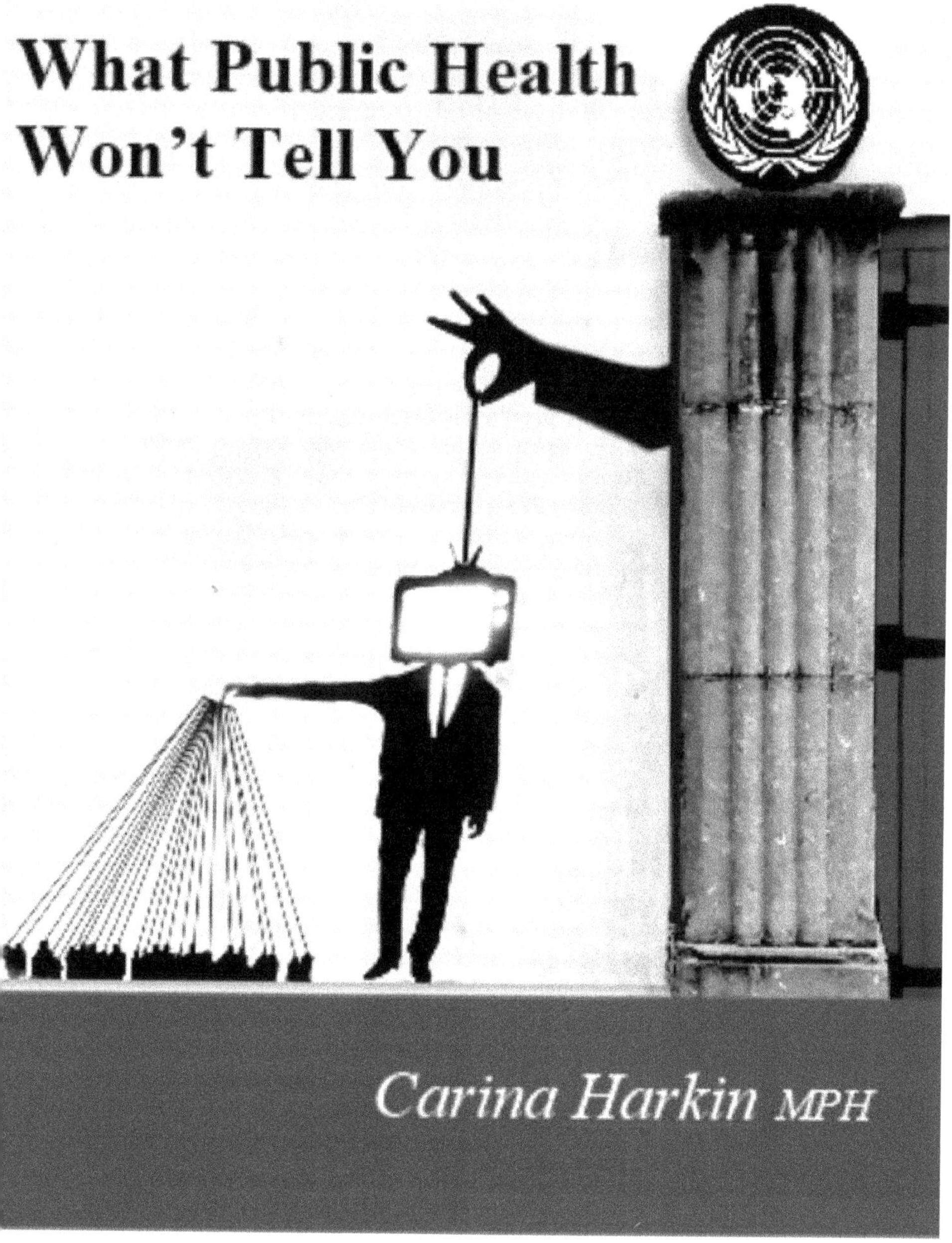

Carina Harkin MPH

Copyright © 2021 by Carina Harkin.

All rights reserved. This book may be ordered via contracted vendors in the UK / USA / Europe / Asia / Australia / South America / Canada / China and/or other locations worldwide. No part of this publication may be reproduced, stored in a retrieval system, or transmitted in any form or by any means, electronic, mechanical, photocopying, recording, digital or otherwise, without the prior written permission of the publisher and/or the author (as per CheckPoint Press contract terms); except in the case of journalists or commentators who may quote brief passages in a review.

COVERT-19: WHAT PUBLIC HEALTH WON'T TELL YOU
No 1 in the series: 'What Public Health Won't Tell You'

ISBN: 978-1-906628-796

Published by CheckPoint Press, Ireland.

CheckPoint Press
Books With Something to Say..

www.checkpointpress.com

Table of Contents

List of Tables

'Irish Banksy' Art: *(included with kind permission of the artist)*

*　　*　　*

ACKNOWLEDGEMENTS

To my father Gerry, for introducing me to my roots and Republic and lighting the fire. To Jeremy my one and only, for feeding, watering and standing by me. To my kids for (whether they like to admit it or not) being on the same page. Straight talking Dr Kimberly Hughes for steering me in the right direction. My best friend and confidant Elena Lenz who I bounced it all off. My guru Andrew Worley for blowing my mind. My rambling ear on the ground and cyber DJ Shane O'Donnell. My hero superspreader, fine eye and the cover designer Judyth Satyn. Irish Banksy for his political art that I captured before it was censored by the Thought Police. Friends Neill Bairéad and Joe Ferri for helping proofread. My hairdresser-come-psychologist Maria Dunican for her encouragement and support. My fellow comrades of Galway Rise up Unite the Tribes, in particular, young Dannan Gaughan and Roisin Higgins for their sheer Irishness and for giving me hope in the youth. And the rebels, revolutionaries and freedom fighters everywhere, you know who you are.

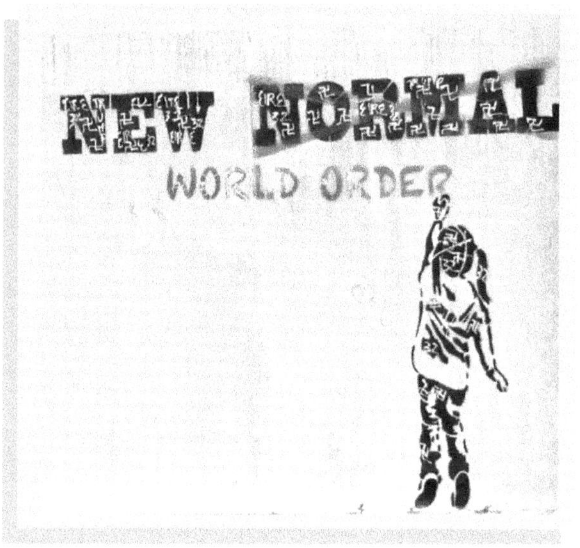

DEDICATION

For my descendants, I need you to know that I could see straight through propaganda and cared so deeply and madly that I had to stand.

PREFACE

"The ultimate tragedy is not the oppression and cruelty by the bad people but the silence over that by the good people".

Martin Luther King, Jr. [(1)]

With this book, I hope to provide the evidence needed to make informed health choices and to protect individual freedoms. My motivations are the truth, freedom and the environment. I have been protesting since I was 10 years old, first attending commemorations of Irish hunger strikers defending Irish civil rights and fighting for freedom from British tyranny. Aged 14, I campaigned against ozone layer damaging chlorofluorocarbons. Aged 16, during the Gulf War, I lived outside the US embassy to protest the New World Order. Aged 17, I lived at a blockade in Canberra that successfully shut down the Australia International Defence Exhibition (AIDEX). Aged 20, I lived in the forests of Kuranda in Far North Queensland, protesting the building of Skyrail in Word Heritage National Park. In 2008 we set up camp in Eyre Square Galway to protest the bank bailouts. I stood against war and nuclear armaments. I stood against the Group of Seven global agenda. I stood to protect the forests, the Great Barrier Reef, Australian Aboriginal land rights, women's rights, the right to asylum, the right to same-sex marriage and the right to choose. I have stood against apartheid. Vaccines are not green! The pharmaceutical industry destroys our environment. I stand for our continued right to protest to protect our environment. I ask you all to stand for our collective freedom.

When you Google 'government cover-ups', Google throws out 'government conspiracies'. I never trusted my government. We've had the Watergate scandal, the Pentagon Papers, Operation Northwoods to overthrow Castro, the MKUltra human LSD experiments, and weapons of mass destruction. I never trusted public health. We've seen a thalidomide cover-up, tobacco industry cover-up, the ethically abusive Tuskegee syphilis study, the Primodos pregnancy test causing miscarriages and congenital anomalies, and the contaminated blood scandal. More recently, we've seen Purdue's opioid epidemic, toxic PIP breast implants, damaging vaginal mesh implants and sodium valproate significantly increasing the risk of autism. DuPont and the EPA covered up the Teflon toxin for decades. The Global Fund to Fight AIDS, TB and Malaria partnered with beer company Heineken. The WHO's Pan American branch took cash handouts from Coca-Cola. Big Sugar sponsored the so-called 'Sugar Research Foundation' to pin heart disease on saturated fats, then Big Sugar bought the Heart Healthy Tick. Healthcare industry pension funds invest in Big Tobacco! The latest scandal; the French pharmaceutical firm Servier prescribed amphetamines to diabetics and were found guilty of deception and the manslaughter of 2,000 people. Many of us will have been personally affected by or is close to someone who has been affected by a public health scandal. Government and public health scandals should be taught in school.

As a Naturopath, Acupuncturist and Homeopath I have a large armament to support natural immunity. 2020 was the year natural immunity ceased to exist. As a mother who has raised seven children without drugs, I advocate natural immunity. I make no apologies for my family and I having robust immune systems because we have been exposed to, and not protected from, infectious disease. Every piece of public health advice being dished out now, bar washing your hands with soap and water, weakens our immune system and makes us more susceptible to all diseases, including COVID-19. Our sickness is their wealth. I thought I called it back in March 2020 when I wrote an article entitled 'COVID-19; How Long will Lockdown Last' that described how we would remain in lockdown until we have a vaccine. I was wrong. It's far, far worse! Seemingly intent on destroying our very raison d'être, our governments keep moving the goalposts. Their aim is to achieve a 'critical mass' of vaccination, which is when enough people take the vaccine, thereby creating a need to continue to take the vaccine every year. Then there'll be booster shots and new vaccines coming online for each and every new variant and emerging disease. Those of us who won't comply will be segregated by vaccine status in our new dystopian future where discrimination has been signed into law, and where we live among transhumans.

I recently spent two years completing a Masters in Public Health; the three words I repeatedly heard during the course were vaccines, mandates and taxes. I debated these and other public health policies, including the current COVID-19 nanny state approach, and advocated the 'night watchman' approach we saw used in Sweden. Little did I realise that when the highly anticipated pandemic hit, not only would people readily accept the loss of their personal freedoms, they would actually beg to be locked down harder. People begged for freedom from decision making and responsibility. As someone who speaks public health, I tell you what public health won't. Public health knows the truth is more contagious than COVID.

Living a quiet life is no longer a choice. We are under biological attack, and now our children are under attack. The battle for our freedom will be fought in parliament and the courts, and if that fails, we, the free people, will voice our grievances on the streets. My grievances are not against doctors and nurses; they are against public health. I stand with doctors and nurses threatened with mandatory vaccines. Polymerase chain reaction (PCR) tests are meaningless, COVID fatality and death rates are inflated, and now the boffins are rolling out the saviour, experimental biological agent to every man, woman, person and child on the planet every year. People are receiving this 'vaccine', testing positive for COVID, then dying 'with COVID', and the narrative is, as the narrative was, to blame 'vaccine failure' on 'failure to vaccinate'. The daily propaganda has already coined the phrase 'the pandemic of the unvaccinated'. Worse still, people are being maimed and killed in droves after receiving this experimental shot, and there is a complete media blackout. The narrative is, as the narrative was, 'the benefits outweigh the risk'.

This is the age of censorship. The COVID-19 'cure' prescribed by our governments is killing many, yet rational debate on the subject of the COVID-19 response is censored, and those opposing lockdowns are demonised. The indoctrination is complete. People are so woke their eyes are wide shut. Our wombs have been privatised and our opinions homogenised. The human race has lost its ability to critically analyse, and the universities are satisfied. Public Health Police Powers sit within constitutional law. Public health is our oppressor! Article 5 of the Humans Rights Act states, "Everyone has the right to liberty and security of person, and no one shall be deprived of his liberty...except for the lawful detention of persons for the prevention of the spreading of infectious diseases". Human rights are our oppressor! We need to amend the constitution and redefine our human rights.

This is a return to the Burning Times. I know that by writing this book and by sticking my head above the parapet, I will be personally denigrated and publicly vilified. I have already been targeted for speaking out by the Irish Health Products Regulatory Authority and the Advertisisng Standards Authority. I was interviewed by an undercover 'investigative journalist' from *The Sunday Times*, posing as a parent of a newborn concerned about vaccines. The 'father' kept pushing me on the Wakefield study. Wakefield is a smokescreen to detract from the study that has not been done. Said 'journalist' quoted me on the front page, saying, "I would never stick a vaccine in my children!" and painted me as a baby killer for practising my profession. At the beginning of the pandemonium, I upset Newspeak by using the terms 'natural immunity' and 'herd immunity' in an article I wrote on herbal medicine targets for past coronaviruses and influenza viruses. As a result, under the order of then-president Trump, the FDA sent me a threatening letter and posted six pages of warnings on Google painting me as a snake-oil peddler.

This is a civil rights movement. I am a civil rights activist and *COVERT-19 What Public Health Won't Tell You* challenges inequality and discrimination against people who do not vaccinate. I speak because I know and I am compelled to do so. Our descendants need to know that we could see through the propaganda and that we cared deeply enough to fight for their freedom. We, with open eyes, need to get informed, get involved and create positive change. In the words of Mel in Braveheart;

> *"Aye, fight, and you may die. Run, and you'll live at least a while, and dying in your beds many years from now, would you be willing to trade all the days from this day to that for one chance, just one chance to come back here and tell our enemies that they may take our lives, but they'll never take our freedom!"* [2]

We will not shut up! We will not obey! We will never comply! Join up! Rise up! Dúisigh!

Carina Harkin: MPH, BHSc Nat, BHSc Hom, BHSc Acu, Cert IV TAE

* * *

INTRODUCTION

"If you are neutral in situations of injustice,
you have chosen the side of the oppressor".

Desmond Tutu (3)

I started writing an article for the website back in March 2020. Originally I wanted to create an A5 flyer to share with people that highlighted the central arguments against authoritarian emergency COVID measures to encourage people to stand to demand our autonomy and freedom be reinstated. 350 plus pages, 1500 references later; I still have to do that flyer. This book is a culmination of 15 years study, 20 years experience and 17 months work. Being qualified in public health, it is unacceptable that opinions such as my own have no voice in mainstream media and that there is no healthy debate. *COVERT-19 What Public Health Won't Tell You* expresses my professional opinion on how public health has handled the pandemic. Whilst this is not a research article aimed for publication in a scientific journal, it is a book of scientific evidence refuting the current public health approach. Scientific language is designed to bamboozle us. Whilst I try and demystify the language of science, this book is very sciencey. If some chapters make your head explode, that's OK. I have difficulty understanding the branches and fields of the science involved. Read, digest, absorb then stand. The subheadings provide the gist which is all we need to form our argument. Science is ever-evolving and continually improving. Where I can, I use their science against 'the science'. To the best of my ability, I have provided an accurate account of what is occurring and encourage you to look at the evidence and draw your own conclusions. I hope that presenting the evidence in a practical and tangible form helps provide you with the confidence to have the conversations that need to be had in our workplaces, in our parks, in our pubs, and on the streets. Whilst we may live in the age of censorship, and they may be successful in controlling the conversation online, we will not be silenced. These are the tools I use to defend my freedom. I aim to present you with the tools you need to support your argument, defend your right to bodily autonomy and your freedom to choose.

I have attempted to document the majority of COVID-19 propaganda we have been indoctrinated with since March 2020 and compare and contrast this with the untold alternative paradigm. I begin by describing the global order and their global agenda from the financial sector down, and the coercive control techniques used by them. I show how Bill Gates and his cronies at the World Economic Forum set the Global Health Security Agenda which is not in our interest. I outline the crux of our problems; Big Oil Rockefeller setting up public health and the global push for public health police powers, and Big Bank Rothschild setting up Big Media Reuters, the global propaganda machine. Banks profit from arms dealers and drug pushers, and the media profits from driving a fear campaign. Pharmaceutical companies lobby our government to allow the daily bombardment of advertisements for multiple maladies and the magic 'cure', which makes us sicker. Meanwhile, the criminals have zero liability and laugh all the way to the bank. I outline the ruling class agenda, the push for radio-frequency biometric identification and on-person vaccine records, and the steps that are being taken to secure their vision of an authoritarian state. I explain the law surrounding the authority of the state to enforce compulsory vaccination. *COVERT-19 What Public Health Won't Tell You* contains the evidence I would use as points of law to defend my right to personal autonomy and informed consent.

I continue by explaining the nuts and bolts used by the ruling class to perpetuate the pandemonium, including meaningless PCR tests and masks, and inflated case and fatality rates. I ask the question, does SARS-CoV-2 even exist? I review the trial protocols and describe what they reveal regarding safety and efficacy, and explain the pitfalls in COVID-19 vaccine trial design. I discuss flaws in all vaccine trials and vaccine safety and efficacy in general. I outline pharmaceutical company zero liability and no-fault compensation, criminality and litigation. I describe how they trained us on measles, another innocuous disease in healthy children, that laid the ground for mandatory COVID-19 vaccines when we accepted measles vaccine mandates. I explain how natural immunity works, what the herd immunity level for SARS-CoV-2 is, and natural medicine and medical COVID-19 treatments and prophylactics. I highlight how the pharmaceutical industry destroys our environment. I lay out the dystopian health future intended by the ruling class. I stand with healthcare workers and all workers against mandatory vaccination by providing valid reasons for vaccine refusal, which I hope will encourage workers to speak out. I speak for the billions worldwide without a voice suffering from the devastating effects of lockdown and stand for the billions who chose traditional medicine as their primary healthcare. I describe how I believe COVID is a smokescreen for the two concurrent pandemics, the 'obesity pandemic' and the 'antibiotic apocalypse', both of which were already predicted to crash the global economy. Importantly I provide near 1500 references so that you have the evidence, including links to newspaper articles, journals and videos. Regarding the videos, I have transcribed the video to text and included the main supporting points. Some links may be broken; no surprise there.

Finally, I provide what I see as solutions to our current dilemma. Vaccinations and healthy ageing is an oxymoron. With the challenges we face, a robust immune system is the only thing we can rely upon. We must get healthy and stop depending on public health. As a CAM practitioner, I teach you about the power of your immune system and provide natural medicine prevention and treatment options that boost natural immunity. Emergency COVID laws are disproportionate, discriminatory, unethical and against our fundamental rights. Emergency COVID laws have been shown to be illegal and are being challenged in the courts. I describe how I believe we should fight our case in court to overturn the precedent for mandatory vaccine laws. The only divide the human race faces is rich and poor. I call on us all to stand for those without a voice and to protect our right to freedom of assembly and speech. The ruling class want order; it is our responsibility to create disorder. History will judge us on our action or inaction now. Only a return to the truth and the restoration of self-belief will set us free.

*　　*　　*

REFERENCES & ABBREVIATIONS

COVERT-19 contains approximately 1500 fully-referenced quotes from qualified sources – as indicated. To keep production costs down in this paperback version, those references can be found in a free searchable online document on the CheckPoint Press website. The academic hardcover version of COVERT-19 contains all 80+ pages of references in full print format. Many organisations, institutions and scientifc formulae are referred to in this book. At their first mention, and ocassionally interspersed, the full-format description will be used. A full list of alphabetically-sorted abbreviations can be found at the rear of the book.

CHAPTER ONE

NEW NORMAL / NEW WORLD ORDER

"If you're not careful, the newspapers will have you hating the people who are being oppressed and loving the people who are doing the oppressing".

Malcolm X[4]

This is no conspiracy. It's a global health security agenda for population control. Far from care about us, the ruling class exploit us under the guise of health. We are great apes in their global experiment. Their agenda is population control. The Global Health Security Agenda (GHSA) was launched in February 2014. The GHSA is a group of 70 countries, international organisations, non-governmental organisations (NGOs), and private sector companies. The GHSA's purpose is to keep us safe and secure from global health threats posed by infectious diseases (whether we like it or not). The GHSA is set by the World Economic Forum (WEF), World Trade Organisation (WTO), World Bank Group (WBG), International Monetary Fund (IMF), United Nations (UN), World Health Organisation (WHO), Centres for Disease Control and Prevention (CDC), Food and Drug Administration (FDA), WHO member states and private sector companies including Bill Gates and his cronies [5]. The IMF, WBG, WHO and WTO launched a joint vaccine information website in July 2021 to serve as a platform for information on access to the COVID-19 vaccine [6]. The GHSA is universal vaccination; vaccinating every man, woman, person and child on the planet every year to achieve 'healthy ageing'. Next on their agenda are digital currency, biometric ID and on-person vaccine records on an implantable chip.

Besides securing all of our 'health', their security agenda is to "take out anti-vaxxers". The United Kingdom's (UK's) intelligence and security agency, the Government Communications Headquarters (GCHQ), has been told to "take out anti-vaxxers" online and on social media. The GCHQ have begun an offensive cyber operation to tackle online 'anti-vaccine propaganda' by 'hostile states' doublespeak for 'intelligent parents'. The GCHQ has a relationship with other eavesdropping agencies in the US,

Australia, Canada and New Zealand in an intelligence alliance known as the Five Eyes. The Five Eyes are on us, looking to take us out. The GCHQ is part of the global censorship mechanism and the clampdown on natural medicine as described in Chapter 4, Vaccine Refusal and the Age of Censorship'. Now for the GHSA players.

World Economic Forum, Agenda 2021 and the Great Reset: Is it just me, or does everyone decimating our civil liberties resemble Hollywood balding, bad guy movie villains or stereotypical evil nerds? Take our supreme leader Klaus Schwab, founder and chairman of the old boy network, The WEF. The WEF is a conglomeration of the world's filthy rich consisting of 1,000 leading companies that want to 'shape a better future'; doublespeak for 'shape a better future for them' (7). The old boy network of the WEF never learnt to share as children. Satan Klaus, as I call him, authored two books, *The Fourth Industrial Revolution* and my top pick for a bedtime story for the children, *The Great Reset,* co-written by 'global strategist' Thierry Malleret. The Great Reset is not a conspiracy theory; it is a plan. The Great Reset was announced on June 20th 2020, at the Davos Agenda 2021 event at the 51st WEF annual meeting.

The Great Reset is the 'great reset' of capitalism, doublespeak for 'transfer all the wealth from the poor to the rich'. Their agenda is total control via digital currency, biometric ID and on-person vaccine records. The coronavirus disease 2019 (COVID-19) pandemonium accelerated the shift to contactless cards and digital wallets to hold digital or cryptocurrency. In 2021, the WEF describes the main issue that needs to be resolved before becoming a cashless society as the "disabled and disadvantaged", some of which have no bank accounts. The WEF old boy network describes these people as unbanked or underbanked. In 2021 the WEF discussed how a central bank digital currency in the form of electronic cash can be directly issued from central banks to consumers and can reduce costs and reach the vulnerable. India's unified payments interface (UPI) and its Aadhaar biometric identity systems have shown that a government utility for digital payments can reach a large population quickly. In the UK, a country going cashless faster than other countries, the government says it is committed to keeping the infrastructure for polymer notes and metal coins from collapsing (8). The UK government also purports to hold a libertarian view and treat its citizens like responsible adults.

Global domination: Another name for global domination is cosmocracy. How cosmocrazy. The following is priceless. Here are the ruling class blatantly announcing they're already global dominators, so put up, shut up and obey. A video on You-will-obey-Tube entitled 'What is the Great Reset? / Davos Agenda 2021' says, "All we really want to say is...", then flash...! at 1 minute 12 seconds, OBEY! This propaganda continues to boast how the WEF and their cronies have benefited from our misfortune. "At the start of 2020, 1% of the world's population owned 44% of the wealth. Since the start of the pandemic, billionaires have increased their wealth by 25% whilst 150 million people fell back into extreme poverty" (9). The WEF were correct about one thing. History will judge this consortium of criminals for direct violations of the Nuremberg Code by their indiscriminate use of experimental biological agents in the biological warfare they are waging on us. Greta and Bono make the front page, all smiles. I call it the 'Greta Reset'. Greta needs to be educated in how vaccines, personal protective equipment (PPE), and electric vehicles destroy our planet.

You'll own nothing; we'll own everything: Another excellent box office smash brought to us peasants by the ruling class is the fabulous, 'You'll own nothing, and we'll own everything' video. In the video, the WEF says by 2030, "you'll own nothing, and you'll be happy". The themes are whatever you want, you'll rent it, and it will be delivered by drone. We won't transplant organs; we'll print new ones instead. You'll eat much less meat for the good of the environment (and inject many more vaccines that decimate the environment, as explained in Chapter 22, 'Vaccines are not Green'). Polluters will pay for emissions, which will make fossil fuels history [while the non-renewable, fossil fuel-based personal protective equipment (PPE) industry will thrive]. Meanwhile, the Greta Reset will be rewarded with a trip on a big rocket ship to inner space with Branson's Virgin Galactic, Bezo's Blue Origin and Musk's SpaceX (10). The whole shebang is completely nonsensical. The ruling class have not taken into account the 'antibiotic apocalypse' and the return to a pre-antibiotic era where routine surgery relying on antibiotics will no longer be possible. A mother would say, let's address the obesity crisis, so we don't need organ transplants, not promote sitting on your derrière getting everything you need delivered, however the state has rendered mothers superfluous.

Whilst the daily propaganda says, 'the Great Reset is a conspiracy', the

Rockefeller Foundation (RF), an American private foundation described later in this chapter, is "rebuilding towards the Great Reset". The off-their-rocker-fellas believed that prior to the COVID-19 pandemonium, "policymakers have long been accustomed to incremental processes and solutions that push gradually against the boundaries of popular and political will". How convenient then, that fear created by the daily propaganda has pushed the boundaries of popular and political will to new lows. The foundation plans to commit US$1 billion to ensure wider access to COVID-19 tests and vaccines and in delivering more science-based tools to address the pandemic, doublespeak for 'control us' (11).

Event 201; the Novel Coronavirus Simulation: Event 201 is not to be confused with Agenda 2021, which launched the Great Reset in Davos on June 20th 2020. The Johns Hopkins Centre for Health Security partnered with the WEF and the Bill & Melinda Gates Foundation to host Event 201 on October 18th 2019. Event 201 simulated a novel (new) zoonotic coronavirus outbreak that transmits from bats to pigs to people, eventually becoming efficiently transmissible from person to person and leading to a severe pandemic. Event 201 covered many objectives we have become familiar with, particularly in Ireland, where our children are still paying promissory notes to bail out the banks after the 2008 crash. These included identifying critical nodes of the banking system and global and national economies that are "too essential to fail" and directing emergency international financial support towards these. Other objectives included the Coalition for Epidemic Preparedness Innovations (CEPI), Gavi, the Vaccine Alliance (Gavi), and the WHO creating an experimental vaccine stockpile for WHO Research and Development (R&D) blueprint pathogens that could be deployed during outbreaks.

Additionally, governments were to direct more resources towards the development and surge manufacturing of vaccines. This simulated scenario ended at 18 months and resulted in 65 million deaths. The authors say, "The pandemic is beginning to slow due to the decreasing number of susceptible people. The pandemic will continue at some rate until there is an effective vaccine or until 80-90% of the global population has been exposed", and then say it will become an endemic circulating coronavirus childhood disease (12). This simulated scenario is an improvement on the actual scenario being played out now, as it recognises a decrease in the susceptibility of people who have been exposed to the disease and achieved natural immunity. Whilst Event 201 acknowledges natural immunity; Event 2021 says shut up! Obey! Take your shot!

Event Cyber Polygon: Just when you thought it was safe to go back into the water, enter Cyber Polygon. On June 9th 2020, the WEF old boy network partnered with the Russian government and world banks to run a high-profile cyber attack simulation named Cyber Polygon. Cyber Polygon targeted financial institutions in what they describe as an "actual event" that would pave the way for a (Greta) "reset" of the global economy. This cybersecurity event featured an online conference with senior officials from the world's largest organisations and corporations and offered technical training for corporate teams. Cyber Polygon is part of the WEF's Centre for Cybersecurity Platform and, just like the Rocky saga, it goes on and on and on, with tickets selling fast for Cyber Polygon project 2021 (13). We need a good screenwriter. The second Cyber Polygon event was on June 9th, 2021.

In his welcome video, our supreme leader Satan Klaus firstly acknowledges his friend and fellow old boy, CEO and chairman Herman Gref of the WEF. Klaus goes on to say (Have a listen and you will hear Klaus actually sounds like this):

> *"Ze forum has built an excellent rrrelationship wiz ze Rrussian federrrations and Prresident Putin. 2020, the year that has changed ze vorld and it iz sanks to technology zat ve are able to join ze cyber polygon entirrrely rrremotely".* Satan Klaus goes on to describe, *"Ze crisis"* and, *"ze strructural shortcomings...vich impede social cohesion, fairness and inclusion and equality. Our existing architecture is not fit for purpose in ze 21st century. It's high time for a grrreat rrrreset! In zis post corrrona vorld ve must use our time to rrreimagine our vorld and build a new. Ve need a grrreat rrreset that vil shape a much more rrresilient system for ze post corrrona errra".* Klaus continues, *"Utilise innovation of ze fourth industrrrial rrrevolution. Technology and zybersecurrity are of crrucial imporrtance in zis post corrrona errra".* Then Satan Klaus tucks us in with a bed-time story of a, *"Frrightening scenarrio of a comprehensive cyber attack vich vud bring to a complete halt to ze power supply, transportation, hospitals ...our society as a whole".* He warns us, *"ze COVID-19 crrrisis vil be seen as a small disturrbance in comparrison to a major cyberr attack"* (14).

Agenda 2030: "Leave no one behind"; doublespeak for 'leave no one unvaccinated': The future is bright; the future is adult vaccines. The WHO, member states and partners for Sustainable Development Goals (SDGs) created a Global Strategy and Action Plan for Ageing and Health for 2016-2020 in continuance with the WHO's Decade of Healthy Ageing 2020-2030 [15]. The WHO definition of healthy ageing is described as the process of maintaining functional ability to enable wellbeing in older age, doublespeak for 'maintaining the financial wellbeing of Big Pharmaceutical Research and Manufacturers of America (PhRMA)'. The Immunisation Agenda 2030 is an extension of the UN SDGs, which are 17 pie-in-the-sky goals with 169 targets that 191 UN member states have agreed to achieve by 2030, but will fail to meet. The SDGs build on the Millennium Development Goals (MDGs), which were eight goals, made of unicorns and rainbows to end hunger, halve extreme poverty rates and disease, halt the spread of infectious disease and educate the world (in their agenda). The Immunisation Agenda 2030 aims to, *"Achieve universal health coverage ...access to safe, effective, quality, and affordable, essential medicines and vaccines for all"* (whether we like it or not). Immunisation Agenda 2030 states that there is, *"a global opportunity to develop and seek ways to promote healthy ageing, including adult vaccinations".* The agenda is to vaccinate every person, of every age, every year [16]. I can think of better ways to improve health and increase longevity.

The WEF's 2030 Vision, under the umbrella of the 2030 Agenda for Sustainable Development and the 17 SDGs, also encompass how emerging technologies can help address the environmental, economic and social challenges of our time. The Fourth Industrial Revolution's technological innovations are network technology, Big Data, 3D printing, Artificial Intelligence (AI) & robotics. These technologies change the nature of work, negatively affecting the social determinants of health to widen health inequities. Additionally, massive unemployment and income loss resulting from the COVID-19 restrictions further erode social cohesion [17]. The SDG's are a pipe dream, as explained shortly; the WEF old boy network's wet dream is 'population control'; doublespeak for 'depopulation'.

The World Bank Group and the International Monetary Fund: The WBG shares a unique partnership with the WEF. The WBG comprises five constituent institutions: the International Bank for Reconstruction and Development (IBRD), the International Development Association (IDA), the

International Finance Corporation (IFC), the Multilateral Investment Guarantee Agency (MIGA), and the International Centre for Settlement of Investment Disputes (ICSID). The WBG and the IMF collaborate routinely to assist member countries. The IMF oversees the stability of the global monetary system, while the World Bank's goal is purported to be to 'reduce poverty' by offering assistance to middle-income and low-income countries. Gerald Celente of the *Trends Journal* calls the International Monetary Fund (IMF) the International Mafia Fund. Very apt [(18)].

The WBG, IMF and WTO (World Trade Organisation) and have been in cahoots since 1994 when WTO members added a declaration to the WTO agreement on achieving greater coherence in global economic policymaking known as the Marrakesh Mandate on Coherence declaration. The declaration called on the WTO to cooperate with the IMF and the World Bank and stated that achieving a more coherent global economic policymaking is one of the five main functions of the WTO [(19)]. Managing Director of the IMF Kristalina Georgieva made a plea to the WEF for "The Great Reset" rather than the "Great Reversal" and how the future is going to be greener, smarter and fairer [(20)]. Obey proletariat! Oui Oui, bourgeoisie, I'll take my 'green' vaccine for the common good. A journal article published in 2021 in the *Journal of World Trade* asked can the WEF re-connect the WTO to the global business community and called on the WTO to take advantage of the WEF's expertise and for an institutionalised system enabling repeated, systematic cooperation and accountability between the WTO and the WEF. The authors asked for a 'holistic' representation of business community views [(21)]. Their 'holistic' is perhaps more *whoristic.*

The World Bank and the International Bank for Reconstruction and Development (IBRD) ..is the largest development bank in the world and was created in 1944 to help Europe rebuild after World War II. Deconstruct: Reconstruct. Blow it up, then send in the contractors. The IBRD see COVID as an opportunity to crash the global economy, steal all the cash and then hit reset. In April 2020, the World Bank devised their COVID-19 Strategic Preparedness and Response Programme (SPRP). The strategy is entitled *International Bank for Reconstruction and Development and International Association Project Appraisal Document on a COVID-19 Strategic Preparedness and Response Programme*. The SPRP proposes 25 Projects under Phase 1 using the Multiphase Programmatic

Approach (MPA) to establish an overall financing envelope of up to US$6 billion, consisting of US$4 billion for health financing, US$1.3 billion for the International Development Association (IDA), and US$2.7 billion for the IBRD. Below I summarise the main unsavoury catchphrases from some of the 25 proposals. These proposals basically relate to emerging disease, rolling lockdowns and new vaccines. The rest is fear on steroids and reiterates how the ruling class are going to steal our money and give it to their rich cronies whilst saving the environment (they destroy), feeding the poor (they create) and creating equality (after driving division).

SPRP Proposal Summaries

These are some of those 25 proposals, as numbered in their project:

5. 'Global public goods and externalities' refers to their product range and pipelines for emerging and reemerging infectious disease.

8. 'COVID-19 is one of several emerging infectious diseases (EID) outbreaks in recent decades', mentions zoonotic diseases (diseases transferred between animals and people), including Hendra virus (1994), Nipah (1998), severe acute respiratory syndrome coronavirus (SARS-CoV) (2003), H5N1 avian influenza (2005), Middle East respiratory syndrome coronavirus (MERS-CoV) (2012), Ebola (2014 and 2018), Lassa fever and other such zoonotic diseases and new vaccines for each.

9. 'Older adults with coexisting chronic health conditions' mentions ***"air pollution"***. Step in the orchestrators of the new era of deep sea mining, Greta Reset and Elon Musk to flatten and vacuum the seafloor for minerals for electric vehicles in the new era of seabed mining.

10. 'Containment and mitigation response' refers to mitigating us using social distancing measures including cancelling public gatherings, school closures, remote working, no craic Irish for enjoyable social activity), no life, we're 'saving lives'.

12. 'The risk of resurgence or new wave of infections' warns of intense resurgence or a new wave of infection.

13. 'Impact of COVID-19' refers to mandating school closures. Breathe parents, breathe.

14. 'Protecting the poor' shows the blatant hypocrisy of a document that admits to an additional 20 million people being forced into poverty due to their restrictions. Additionally, the document mentions that East Africa, the Horn of Africa, and South Asia are struggling to deal with the historic locust infestation, and COVID-19 is putting such countries and the poorest at an extremely high risk of imminent food shortages. It is apparent the only lives worth saving are those in high-income countries with obese, ageing populations dependent on pharmaceutical drugs.

15. *'The imperative of healthy populations'* involves ***"health taxes"*** to increase what public health calls 'the old faithful', taxes on tobacco which is mentioned twice. According to this document, smokers in China had higher rates of COVID-19 complications; however, the document does not mention that in France, it emerged that tobacco (nicotine) had a protective factor they called the "smokers paradox and COVID-19" (22).

16. *'Critical steps for the COVID-19 response'* refers to a suppression strategy of social distancing, home isolation, and household quarantine of family members and measures including school and university closures to suppress transmission. More school and university closures!

19. *'Relevance to higher-level objectives'* refers to the aforementioned COVID-19 Strategic Preparedness and Response Plan (SPRP). The SPRP refers to the crony capitalist ideals of the World Bank Group (WBG), World Health Organisation's (WHO's) International Health Regulations (IHR) (2005), Integrated Disease Surveillance and Response (IDSR), Universal Health Coverage, WTO's World Organisation for Animal Health (OIE), Global Health Security Agenda (GHSA), the Paris Climate Agreement, Universal Health Coverage, and the Sustainable Development Goals (SDGs). The higher-level objective of the Paris Climate Agreement is to create a climate of fear and to increase taxes on the little guy. 'Universal' refers to universal vaccines.

25. *'Critical interventions'* is the final proposal that again supports anti-social distancing.

The expected project closing date is March 31st 2025 (23). However, when the ruling class realised they didn't grab enough money and power from crooked agenda number 1, they devised crooked agenda number 2. On October 13th 2020, a new proposal much like the old one entitled, *International Bank for Reconstruction and Development and International Association Projection Paper on a Proposed Additional Financing to the COVID-19 Strategic Preparedness and Response Programme (SPRP) using the Multiphase Programmatic Approach*, describes an additional IBRD and IDA financing of up to US$12 billion from the IDA and up to US$6 billion from the IBRD. The expected project closing date for the latest money grab is December 31st 2025 (24). The fact is there is no end date until we stand up to our oppressive governments.

World Health Organisation and dubious donors: The World Health Assembly (WHA) is the world's highest health policy setting body and makes all the decisions for the WHO's 194 Member States regarding the Global Health and Security Agenda (GHSA). The WHO (who is subject to the WHA) is the specialised agency of the UN responsible for directing and coordinating international health within the UN. The WHO has been bought out hence I refer to them as the World Wealth Organisation. The corruption is top-down. WHO Director-General Dr Tedros Ghebreyesus, I refer to him as 'Dr scare-the-bejesus-out-of-us', is friends with ex-President Robert Mugabe. Dr scare-the-bejesus-out-of-us was such good friends with ex-President likes-a-good-massacre Mugabe that he made Mugabe the WHO Goodwill Ambassador for non-communicable disease (NCD) in Africa [25]. This appointment caused a huge uproar, and so Mugabe rescinded the appoint-ment and was eventually removed. It goes without saying that Mugabe's administration consistently denies reports of mass massacres and killings. Tell that to the thousands of opposition insurgents killed and tortured in Matabeleland by his Fifth Brigade, or the tens of thousands who died after Mugabe ordered the Gukurahundi killings to maintain a one-party state [26, 27]. A person with free will may question if the World Wealth Organisation approves of psychopaths.

According to the World Wealth Organisation, they only receive funding from government agencies, non-governmental organisations (NGOs), foundations and scientific institutions or professional organisations. This is a blatant lie. The WHO has been repeatedly caught breaking its own rules. Back in 2007, The WHO was caught in the act of attempting to secure a US$10,000 donation from Britain's biggest pharmaceutical company, GlaxoSmithKline (GSK). The WHO asked the European Parkinson's Disease Association (EPDA) patients' group to act as a covert channel for the funds, as accepting money from a drug company breaks the WHO's own rules. Emails between Benedetto Saraceno, the WHO's Director of the Department of Mental Health and Substance Abuse Management and the EPDA suggested that the WHO was willing to take US$10,000 from GSK to help pay for the preparation of a report on neurological disorders, for which GSK makes pharmaceutical therapeutics for [28]. This is likely the tip of the iceberg.

WHO's Geneva headquarters and five regional offices have only recently stopped accepting financial donations from Big Food and Big Soda [29]. In

2014 the sugar industry blocked a policy proposal relating to WHO guidelines on sugar and changes to the nutrition facts panel on packaged food proposed by the United States (US) FDA [30]. The WHO's impartiality was also brought into question when it emerged that the WHO regional office for the Americas, the Pan American office (PAHO), accepted US$50,000 from Coca-Cola, US$150,000 from Nestlé and US$150,000 from Unilever. The steering group for WHO's Pan American Forum for Action on NCDs, a group helping to determine strategies to combat obesity in Mexico, included International Food and Beverage Alliance representatives. Financial supporters included Kraft Foods, Pepsi-Cola, Grupo Bimbo, Pfizer, GSK, Humana, Merck, Medtronic, Sanofi, and Johnson & Johnson [31]. The WHO excused this association (with Big Food and Big Soda only), saying PAHO are unique in that they contain two separate legal entities with different policies, PAHO and the WHO Regional Office for the Americas (AMRO) [32]. The World *Wealth* Organisation is too close to all Big Industries; Tobacco, Alcohol, Agriculture, Sugar, Soda, PhRMA, Data etc. Needless to say, there is no Big Traditional Medicine (TM) even though, according to the WHO, they are the biggest providers, with 65-80% of the world's primary healthcare practices using traditional medicines [33].

Even our own 'health' services make unethical investments. You may believe Big Tobacco has lost favour, yet public money still supports it. According to Credit Suisse, tobacco stocks are the best performers [34]. In the UK, millions are invested in tobacco brands to fund university superannuation schemes. Healthcare providers, fire authorities and schools support the tobacco industry through council pension funds [35]. The Ireland Strategic Investment Fund and Courts Services of Ireland also invest millions in the tobacco industry [36, 37].

The WHO's obsession with supporting vaccine manufacturers: The main link in this chain of accepting unethical funding sources is the International Federation of Pharmaceutical Manufacturers Association (IFPMA). The IFPMA is the main communication medium for industry exchanges between the WHO, World Bank, WTO and World Intellectual Property Organisation (WIPO). Relationships also exist between the WHO and NGO status with the Council of Europe. The IFPMA's first recommendations are to encourage more public-private partnerships to develop and distribute medicines and vaccines, i.e. Gate's Gavi.[38] IFPMA representatives have one seat on the Gavi board. The IFPMA represents more than 55 national industry associations, including Johnson & Johnson, GSK, Merck & Co., Novartis, Sanofi Pasteur, the vaccines division of Sanofi-Aventis and Pfizer [39]. These are quite literally the names of the companies that are benefitting from the current COVID-19 vaccine rollout. The WHO is overly focused on delivering vaccines and therapeutics that make pharmaceutical companies rich instead of building resilient health systems to prepare for and effectively respond to crises. If the WHO had done their job, including enforcing laboratory biosafety and biosecurity standards, perhaps we wouldn't be in the circumstance we find ourselves in.

The WHO's coronavirus origins cover-up: The WHO's credibility has been called into question several times during the pandemic. In January 2021, WHO coordinator and official Francesco Zambon, accused the WHO of censoring a report into Italy's response to the coronavirus pandemic. There is currently an ongoing internal dispute over Zambon's allegations. Zambon alleged that the WHO pulled the study at the request of a top Italian official, as its content would attract international condemnation and cause the Italian government embarrassment. It goes without saying that the WHO and the officials denied any wrongdoing, however Zambon was concerned that this had been brushed under the carpet and called for the WHO to be free of any external influences before its mission in China [40].

In January 2021, the WHO team investigating the coronavirus origins was denied entry into China. WHO Director-General Dr scare-the-bejesus-out-of-us said he was, "very disappointed" [41]. Far from being a 'reliable source of information', the World Wealth Organisation is not transparent and far from trustworthy. In January 2021, after spending four weeks in Wuhan investigating the coronavirus pandemic's origins, a WHO team of scientists concluded, whilst all hypotheses remain open, it was highly unlikely that the virus had come from a laboratory. The team maintained that severe acute respiratory syndrome coronavirus 2 (SARS-CoV-2) most likely transferred from bats to humans through an unidentified intermediary host. The Chinese government used the same investigation to promote the theory that the virus had arrived in Wuhan on frozen food packaging! In March 2021, a team of scientists responded by publishing an open letter calling for a new investigation into the coronavirus pandemic origins amid concerns that Beijing exercised political influence over the WHO team leading the investigation. Twenty-six virology, zoology and microbiology experts claimed the WHO mission did not "constitute a thorough, credible and transparent investigation". The open letter went on to say, "*We believe it essential that all hypotheses about the origins of the pandemic be thoroughly examined and full access to all necessary resources be provided without regard to political or other sensitivities*" [42].

Trump's 'Chinacentric' WHO: Not going into potential election fraud, Trump had to go for two reasons. Firstly, he pulled the US out of the WHO and secondly, he pulled the US out of COVID-19 Vaccines Global Access (COVAX), the no-fault compensation for vaccine injury mechanism. This was not part of the WEF old boy network agenda. COVAX is discussed in Chapter 16, 'Criminality, Litigation and Zero Liability'. Whilst the world may purport it no longer wants to accept Uighur forced labour cotton, the World Wealth Organisation is more than happy to accept money from China [43]. China's contributions to the World Wealth Organisation have risen by 52% since 2014 to approximately US$86 million. Beijing voluntary contributions also increased from US$8.7 million in 2014 to approximately US$10.2 million in 2019. Compare that to the organisation's largest donor, the US, which contributed US$893 million to the WHO in 2018/19. This donation from China represents 14.6% of all voluntary contributions given globally in 2018/19 [44]. Rather suspiciously, the WHO fails to mention China is a donor on their 'How WHO is funded' webpage [45]. When Trump suspended funding to the WHO and accused the organisation of promoting Chinese 'disinformation' about the virus, which emerged in the central city of Wuhan, China pledged to donate a further US$30 million to the WHO [46]. The China Population Welfare Foundation (CPWF) is a national public welfare foundation based in Beijing. The CPWF channels donations from Chinese companies, charities and individuals towards the COVID-19 Solidarity Response Fund for the World Health Organisation [47].

Wuhan Virology Institute connections to America's NIH and EcoHealth Alliance: The WHO experts' narrative is that the virus arrived in Wuhan on food packaging. Conveniently, as mentioned, live coronavirus was found on frozen food packaging in China in October 2020 [48]. However, before the pandemonium, the Wuhan Institute of Virology (WIV) experimented on bats from the area already known to be the source of COVID-19 bat coronaviruses [49]. Additionally, US officials had previously expressed safety concerns regarding Chinese biosafety laboratory safety breaches. Two years before the COVID pandemonium, *The Washington Post* reported on two State Department cables warning of safety issues at the WIV. These warnings were made after two American embassy officials in Beijing made several visits to the WIV and were concerned about inadequate safety measures. At the time, WIV researchers were conducting studies on bat coronaviruses. Regarding this novel coronavirus, the US intelligence community was originally examining whether coronavirus had emerged accidentally or whether 'patient zero' worked there [(50)]. Then Trump called it "the Chinese virus", and the idea the virus came from a Chinese laboratory was discounted.

Washington and Beijing are thick as thieves. The further revelation that the WIV was using American money to experiment on bats already known to be the source of COVID-19 caused political uproar. China's WIV names on their website as a 'partner', Fauci's National Institute of Health (NIH), the US (!), EcoHealth Alliance and several other American academic institutions [(51)]. America's NIH is the primary agency of the US government responsible for biomedical and public health research. EcoHealth Alliance is an NGO that claims to protect people, animals and the environment from emerging infectious diseases and focuses on finding unknown viruses in nature. In April 2020, the NIH cancelled a grant to the EcoHealth Alliance after President Trump complained that the US was funding China's WIV. Then in August 2020, the NIH reinstated an award of US$7.5 million grant to EcoHealth Alliance [(52)]. A total of all awards equalling US$3,748,715 of NIH funding was directed from the US government to the EcoHealth Alliance project "to understand what factors allow coronaviruses, including close relatives to SARS, to evolve and jump into the human population". The project yielded 20 scientific reports on how zoonotic diseases may transfer from bats to humans [(53)].

Fauci Gate: Given the Fauci's NIH funds the WIV, the recent email leak known as Faucigate came as no surprise. In June 2021, over 3000 pages of Fauci's work emails during the COVID-19 pandemic were leaked. One email, in particular, boosted the theory of origin that the SARS-CoV-2 was man-made and had been leaked from the WIV, a statement that ex-President Trump often made that was, according to CNN, refuted because Trump had said it. Professor of Immunology at Scripps Research Institute in California, Kristian Andersen, had previously explained to Fauci in an email that the virus causing the COVID-19 pandemic showed signs of having been manipulated in a laboratory [(54)]. Andersen's email to Fauci supported the theory that the disease began after a leak from the WIV.

Both Andersen and Fauci later disputed that theory. Fauci actively downplayed the possibility of a lab leak with other scientists and pushed the theory and the WHO conclusion that the virus had animal origins or arrived in Wuhan on frozen food packaging. At the time of this reveal, Fauci faced calls to resign under a barrage of criticism. Meanwhile, the indoctrinated are still donning 'I Love Fauci' masks.

In June 2021, Tucker Carlson interviewed Chinese virologist Dr Li-Meng Yan, who investigated the origin of the COVID-19 virus during the initial outbreak in Wuhan and had previously accused Beijing of a cover-up regarding the coronavirus origins.

> Yan says, *"This virus COVID-19* SARS-CoV-2 *actually is not from nature. It is a man-made virus created in a lab-based on the Chinese military discovery and their own very unique bat virus, which can not affect people, but after the modification becomes a very harmful virus like now"*.
>
> Tucker Carlson, *"You're saying the Chinese government manufactured this virus if I'm hearing you correctly, that's what you're saying?"*
>
> Yan answers, *"Based on the virus genome, which is basically like the fingerprint, you can see the very unusual character in their genome, which clearly based on the other evidence they left using the modification, this comes from their own special bat coronavirus that can then target humans"*.
>
> Tucker Carlson, *"This genome is in the possession of many researchers around the world. Why is this information being suppressed?"*
>
> Yan replies, *"Nobody is saying it because of big suppression come from Chinese communist party government and also their friends in the scientific world"* (55).

CHAPER ONE – PART II

UNITED NATIONS & PHILANTHROLATERALISM

Dubious donors are under-mining democratic global governance. Philanthrolateralism describes the private funding and corporate influence in the UN. Philanthrolateralism pushes up the price of vaccines. Private funding from corporations and 'philanthropic' foundations such as Gates Foundation for UN activities is rising steadily. Private funding has turned UN agencies into contractors for bilateral or public-private projects, eroded the multilateral character of the system, and undermined democratic global governance [(56)]. UNICEF's Vaccine Independence Initiative (VII), a mechanism that supports lower and middle-income countries to become self-reliant in vaccine acquisition, receives funding from Gavi. In December 2017, UNICEF announced that funding for its VII increased from US$15 million to US$35 million. The increase was made possible again by a US$15 million financial guarantee from the Gates Foundation [(57)].

Gates is neither the first nor the last power-hungry megalomaniac. Many billionaire 'philanthropists' and their foundations have ever-increasing influence and are overriding governments to set global health and agriculture agendas. The world's largest 'philanthropic' foundations aside from the Gates Foundation are the Wellcome Trust, Howard Hughes Medical Institute, Garfield Foundation, Weston Foundation, Ford Foundation, Kamehameha Schools, the Church Commissioners for England, Robert Wood Johnson Foundation, J. Paul Getty Trust and Lilly Endowment. A report by the independent Global Policy Forum, a policy watchdog which monitors the work of UN bodies and their role in global policymaking, says that the Gates and Rockefeller Foundations are playing an increasingly active role in agenda-setting and funding priorities of governments and international organisations, which potentially undermines the UN bodies. The report provides the following example; Médecins Sans Frontières (MSF) states that while Gate's Gavi subsidises vaccines, the cost to fully immunise a child has increased by over 68 times between 2001 and 2014 [(58)]. Gates is Big Farmer. Gates is now officially America's largest owner of farmland. Gates is working on his recipe for those appetising, nutritious protein bars we'll all be begging for when we all own nothing and are happy, while Bill Gates owns 240,000 acres of American soil [(59)].

Bill Gates wants to control our fertility with his big remote control: Gates is a textbook megalomaniac. One only needs to watch Gate's weird hands and smirk at impending disasters combined with his uncomfortable squirming at the difficult questions. Bill Gates gets treated like a statesman, yet he is not an elected representative. Mr 'I-identify-as-a-doctor' is a medical school dropout. Gate's wet dream is Microsoft microchips in medicine and depopulation. I am a child of the 70s. The world has been predicting the next Armageddon since the last Armageddon. Mystic Gates predicted the pandemic in October 2019 at Event 201. For decades Gates has been working on global political strategies of depopulation and dictatorial control, aiming to control agriculture, technology and energy. Whilst industry-sponsored 'fact-wreckers' have debunked this fact, Gate's Ted Talk delivered back in 2010, entitled, 'Innovating to Zero', confirms it to be true. At 4 minutes 21 seconds, Mr Smirk says,

> *"First, we've got population. The world today has 6.8 billion people. That's headed up to about nine billion. Now, if we do a really great job on new vaccines, health care, reproductive health services, we could lower that by, perhaps, 10 or 15%"* (60).

The WEF old boy network; the WHO, UN Population Fund, UN Development Programme, World Bank, Population Council, Rockefeller Foundation, US National Institute of Child Health and Human Development, All India Institute of Medical Sciences, and Uppsala, Helsinki, and Ohio State universities, are all involved in the development of anti-fertility vaccines using human chorionic gonadotropin (hCG) (61). By 1998 there were already six anti-fertility vaccines that had entered phase I clinical trials (62). The potential impact of COVID-19 vaccines on fertility is discussed in Chapter 15, 'COVID-19 Vaccines and Pregnancy Safety Concerns'. Gates' desire to control our fertility is discussed in Chapter 21, 'Chips, Dots and Bots'.

Gates bought the UN: Most billionaires buy an island; Bill Gates bought the UN. Gates is the largest donor to the UN. The Gates Foundation originally endowed US$39.6 billion to the UN and has an annual spend of US$4.2 billion. The money is spent on areas dedicated to global health and global agriculture (56). The UN includes the United Nations Conference on Trade and Development (UNCTAD), United Nations Economic and Social Council (ECOSOC), United Nations International Children's Emergency Fund (UNICEF), United Nations Industrial Development Organisation (UNIDO), United Nations Educational, Scientific and Cultural Organisation (UNESCO),

United Nations High Commissioner for Refugees (UNHCR), the Joint United Nations Programme on HIV and AIDS (UNAIDS), World Intellectual Property Organisation (WIPO) and the United Nations Population Fund (UNFPA). Big PhRMA make pledges to (buys) UN agencies.

Gates bought the WHO: The Gates Foundation is the major investor in the WHO, the UN agency responsible for global public health. In 2017, the Gates Foundation gave US$3.3 billion to the WHO, equalling donations by the UK and surpassing US donations. Being the largest donor, the Gates Foundation has the largest influence in setting the Global Health Security Agenda (GHSA). The Gates Foundation now controls global health data and how this data is disseminated and uptaken by the WHO and the World Bank. The Gates Foundation finances the Institute for Health Metrics and Evaluation (IHME) which produces the global burden of disease data. The power of one institute to define health data is unprecedented. The global burden of disease studies data is published exclusively in *The Lancet*, and the Gates Foundation pays for these studies to be open access [(63)]. It goes without saying that the IHME describe themselves as 'independent'. Gates' Kingpin is Heidi Larson of the Vaccine Confidence Project, the global Thought Police, covered in Chapter 4, 'Vaccine Refusal in the Age of Censorship'.

The CDC, FDA and WHO financial conflicts of interests and lack of impartiality: Whilst the World Wealth Organisation and the CDC are separate agencies, they are both the global health police. The CDC is the national public health agency in the US and is described as a health protection agency. The CDC and FDA are sister agencies within the US Department of Health and Human Services. The CDC and FDA act as global health agencies and set the GHSA. Whilst the CDC and the WHO don't always read off the same page, they work in partnership on pandemic preparedness through the Collaborating Centre for Surveillance, Epidemiology and Control of Influenza. This collaboration works to improve vaccine development. The CDC and WHO also work closely to coordinate epidemiologic and virologic surveillance through the WHO's Global Influenza Surveillance and Response System (GISRS) [(64)]. The CDC is sponsored by earth pillaging multinationals that seek to destroy human health, then benefit from our misfortune. The following are a few prime examples of their sponsors. The full list is available on the website entitled, *CDC Foundation; Our Partners: Corporations*. Some of the socially responsible, environmentally sustainable, pro-health and pro-natural immunity sponsors include; Abbot Ireland, AstraZeneca, Bayer, Bill & Melinda Gates Foundation, Coca-Cola, CNN, Exxonmobile, Facebook, General Motors, Google, Johnson & Johnson, McDonald's, Merck, Microsoft, Nike, NorthAmerican Vaccine Inc, Novavax, Oxford University, PayPal, Pfizer, Roche, Starbucks, UPS etc. (65). Agains, these are literally the names of the companies benefitting from the pandemonium. The CDC will always say what their sponsors tell them to say; that is, the benefits of vaccination outweigh the risks.

Rockefeller and Rothschild; Public Health and Big Media: As previously mentioned, the Rockefeller Foundation (RF) is another 'philanthropic' organisation. An article examining the WHO-RF relationship from the 1940s to the 1960s stated that the RF profoundly shaped the WHO and have maintained a long and complex relationship with it over time (66). The RF is in bed with the UK banking magnates Rothschild, and have granted each other non-executive directorships (dictatorships). In 2012 Lord Jacob Rothschild's RIT Capital Partners plc, formerly Rothschild Investment Trust, and Rockefeller Financial Services, formed a strategic partnership to commandeer investment funds, joint acquisitions and asset managers (67). Rockefeller set up Public Health and the global push for public health police powers. Rothschild set up Reuters, the global propaganda machine. In 1913 the RF set up the International Health Commission, which launched the foundation into international public health activities. Following a grant from the RF in 1916, the commission established and endowed the world's first School of Hygiene and Public Health at Johns Hopkins University, later at Harvard, then spent more than US$25 million in developing other public health schools in the US and in 21 foreign countries (68). I have a Masters in RF indoctrination. In 1850 Paul Reuter approached Rothschild in London to ask if they would be his client for the first telegraphic codes. Reuter was offering Rothschild a service he developed to speed information (propaganda) across Europe. Big Media had arrived (69).

Rockefeller's Operation Lockstep pandemic simulation: Operation lock us up, I mean Operation Lockstep is included in a RF report entitled *Scenarios for the Future of Technology and International Development* published in 2010. The report describes a series of scenarios, one including a pandemic, in which technology comes to the rescue to save humanity. The 'Lockstep' section outlines a scenario of authoritarian control in the wake of a hypothetical novel influenza pandemic similar to COVID-19. On page 18 of the report, lockstep envisions *"a world of tighter top-down government control and more authoritarian leadership, with limited innovation and growing citizen pushback"*. According to the report, in this scenario, within seven months, 20% of the global population was infected with the novel virus, and eight million people died.

Whilst never linking to this report, the fact-wreckers say the novel coronavirus is not mentioned anywhere in the Rockefeller Foundation's report. They also apply Jedi magic on us by cherry-picking parts of the transcript they think we will find acceptable whilst selectively omitting other parts that would send chills down our spine. Beginning on page 19:

> *"China's government was not the only one that took extreme measures to protect its citizens from risk and exposure. During the pandemic, national leaders around the world flexed their authority and imposed airtight rules and restrictions, from the mandatory wearing of face masks to body-temperature checks at the entries to communal spaces like train stations and supermarkets. Even after the pandemic faded, this more authoritarian control and oversight of citizens and their activities stuck and even intensified. In order to protect themselves from the spread of increasingly global problems, from pandemics and transnational terrorism to environmental crises and rising poverty, leaders around the world took a firmer grip on power.*
>
> *At first, the notion of a more controlled world gained wide acceptance and approval. Citizens willingly gave up some of their sovereignty and their privacy to more paternalistic states in exchange for greater safety and stability. Citizens were more tolerant and even eager for top-down direction and oversight, and national leaders had more latitude to impose order in the ways they saw fit. In developed countries, this heightened oversight took many forms: biometric IDs for all citizens, for example, and tighter regulation of key industries whose stability was deemed vital to national interests.*
>
> *In India, for example, air quality drastically improved after 2016, when the government outlawed high-emitting vehicles...there were other downsides, as the rise of virulent nationalism created new hazards: spectators at the 2018 World Cup, for example, wore bulletproof vests*

that sported a patch of their national flag...By 2025, people seemed to be growing weary of so much top-down control and letting leaders and authorities make choices for them...Wherever national interests clashed with individual interests, there was conflict. Sporadic pushback became increasingly organised and coordinated, as disaffected youth and people who had seen their status and opportunities slip away, largely in developing countries, incited civil unrest...

Even those who liked the greater stability and predictability of this world began to grow uncomfortable and constrained by so many tight rules and by the strictness of national boundaries. The feeling lingered that sooner or later, something would inevitably upset the neat order that the world's governments had worked so hard to establish" [(70)].

So whilst 'Lockstep' may not mention COVID-19, in particular, it is clear the ruling class are off their rocker-fellas and deserve bottom-up disorder. The Rothschild patent for a COVID-19 test and other dubious patents are discussed in Chapter 21, 'Chips, Dots and Bots'.

Dark winter exercise; Bioterrorism exercise: This is another fine example of the ruling class boasting about their plans whilst labelling them as 'conspiracy theories'. Coincidentally, in December 2020, Biden warned, in relation to COVID-19, of the "the dark winter". The Dark Winter Scenario and Bioterrorism exercise was held at Andrews Air Force Base, Washington, DC. On June 22-23rd, 2001. The Dark Winter exercise portrayed a fictional scenario whereby 3000 people were infected with smallpox in a covert attack on US citizens. The scenario was set in three successive National Security Council (NSC) meetings and occurred over two weeks, and was an exercise wherein senior former officials responded to a bioterrorist induced national security crisis.

Media representatives observed the mock NSC meetings. The Dark Winter exercise was a collaboration between the Centre for Strategic and International Studies (CSIS), Johns Hopkins Centre for Civilian Biodefense Strategies (CCBS) and the Johns Hopkins Centre for Civilian Biodefense Studies and Analytic Services Inc. (ANSER). General Dennis Reimer of the Memorial Institute for the Prevention of Terrorism (MIPT) provided funding [(71)]. The word 'vaccine' is mentioned 64 times in the report.

Kissinger Report; Population control and the US must cover up this disturbing truth: *The Kissinger Report*, also known as the *National Security Study Memorandum* (NSSM), was Henry Kissinger's baby. Kissinger must be Gates' idol. *The Kissinger Report* is essentially about depopulation strategies focused on the young, particularly to preserve US resources. The report says, "The United States needs widespread access to the mineral resources of less-developed nations". The report focuses on rapid population growth in developing countries, which hampers economic development and social progress and results in instability. This instability undermines the US requirements for expanded output and a sustainable flow of non-renewable resources, including world food supplies, minerals and fuel, and focuses on resource-rich African countries. The rapid population growth is seen as a political national security threat for the US and a risk to the world economy and political stability. The primary sources of these US imports during the period 1969-1972 were commodities or raw materials, or agricultural products. The report describes the solution to the "population situation" as being less amenable to voluntary measures and suggests mandatory programmes and tight control of our food resources. The report states, "We cannot wait for overall modernisation and development to produce lower fertility rates".

The report mentions contraception methods, including improved methods for ovulation prediction for couples wishing to practice the rhythm method, sterilisation of men and women, injectable contraceptives for women, and legal abortion. The report encourages the use of financial incentives to increase abortion, sterilisation and contraception. The report suggests concentrating on "indoctrinating" the children of least developed countries (LDCs) with anti-nationalist propaganda (don't have lots of children, which is your tradition). While investigating the desirability of mandatory population control programmes, the report says that the "smooth flow of resources to the US could be jeopardised by LDC government action, labour conflicts, sabotage, or civil disturbance, which are much more likely if population pressure is a factor.

Young populations are said to be much more likely to challenge imperialism and the world's power structures, so their numbers should be kept down if possible. The report says that the US must develop a commitment to population control among key LDC leaders while "bypassing the will of their people". Do you hear that, young people?

The report goes on to say,

> *"The US must hide its tracks and disguise its programmes as altruistic otherwise there could be a serious backlash. The US must convince the leaders and people of LDCs that population reduction is in their own best interests, hiding the fact that the United States wants access to their natural resources. The US also must cover up, or distract attention from, this disturbing truth"* [72].

An actual example of these policies in action; between 1996 and 2000, more than 200,000 women in Peru were sterilised without giving free, prior and informed consent [73].

Not another ruddy coronavirus simulation! It was only recently disclosed under a freedom of information (FOI) request in 2016 that the UK government conducted a secret planning exercise modelling the impact of a simulated MERS outbreak in the UK. The previously unpublicised Exercise Alice involved officials from Public Health England (PHE) and the Department of Health and Social Care (DHSC). MERS-CoV is a coronavirus. Exercise Alice was in fact one of ten previously unpublicised pandemic planning exercises that occurred in the five years before COVID-19. The other exercises included three on the Ebola virus, four on pandemic influenza, two on the Lassa virus, one on acute viral haemorrhagic illness, three on avian influenza and Exercise Cerberus, a simulated radiation incident. PHE previously refused to reveal details of these exercises, citing the need to safeguard national security [74]. That old chestnut. According to these exercises, we still have a few years to go before people start growing restless of such tight restrictions. On a positive note, the ruling class literally told us that we can, "challenge imperialism and the world's power structures", so it is our responsibility to fulfil their predictions.

CHAPTER TWO

MONEY, POWER AND CONTROL

"If you want to preserve your power indefinitely, you have to get the consent of the ruled".

Aldous Huxley [75]

Our governments and Big PhRMA are in cahoots to keep us dependent on public health and under control. In a nutshell, pharmaceutical companies lobby governments to legislate direct-to-consumer pharmaceutical advertising (DTCPA) that allows us to be bombarded with daily advertisements for countless maladies. This normalises obscure disorders and turns us into drug-dependent hypochondriacs [76]. If I may put things in perspective, at the height of the pandemic, COVID-19 killed one American every minute [77]. Diabetes kills one American every six seconds, every day [78]. Yet public health's 'scientific' response is to impose lockdowns that encourage a sedentary lifestyle, more time spent in front of a screen, more food shopping, more takeaways and more alcohol intake to prevent an illness that is ten times less deadly than obesity. Public health policies have created a new pandemic called 'covibesity' [79]. The 'cure' for obesity is bariatric surgery which costs US$25,000 to US$30,000 [80]. That's how much public health care about our health.

Keeping people in poverty keeps people down and out. Poverty changes our mindset. Poor people suffer from more physical disease and mental health problems, and this cycle of poverty can persist across generations. Socioeconomic status (how wealthy you are) is an effect modifier of alcohol consumption and harm. The poorest in society do not necessarily drink more alcohol, however they are at greater risk of alcohol's harmful impacts on health [81]. Socioeconomic status is a determinant risk factor for several cancers [82]. Socioeconomic factors increase COVID-19 mortality and related health outcomes [83]. Fortunately for us though, poverty decreases compliance. When you have nothing, you have nothing to lose.

The Five Horsemen of the Apocalypse: This is the largest transfer of wealth the world has ever witnessed. A new Oxfam report entitled, *The Inequality Virus*, found the rich get richer, the poor get the picture (Midnight Oil). In 2020, fat cat billionaires gained $3.9 trillion while workers globally lost $3.7 trillion. Oxfam declared that history will "likely remember the pandemic as the first time since records began that inequality rose in virtually every country on Earth at the same time" (84). A World Bank report entitled, *Global Economic Outlook During the COVID-19 Pandemic: A Changed World*, says that public health's COVID-19 response exacerbated humanitarian crises; famine, war and pestilence (85).

The Millennium Development Goals (MDGs) and Sustainable Development Goals (SDGs) to end hunger, halve extreme poverty, halt the spread of HIV/AIDS and provide universal primary education, all by the target date of 2015, were already proof that the ruling class were off their rocker fellas (86). The swift and massive shock of the coronavirus pandemonium and forced shutdown of the economy plunged the global economy into a severe contraction. According to World Bank forecasts in its June 2020 *Global Economic Prospects*, the global economy is set to shrink by 5.2% in 2021. This figure represents the deepest recession since the Second World War, with the largest fraction of economies experiencing declines in per capita output since 1870 (87).

The consequences of the COVID-19 lockdown continue to widen global socioeconomic inequalities, with the world's wealthiest five billionaires enjoying a 59% rise in their combined wealth between March and September 2020, while 47 million people were pushed into poverty (88). Amid an unprecedented increase in unemployment, and with half a billion people around the world being pushed into poverty, there has been an unprecedented rise of stock market wealth for a few individuals, with the American billionaires alone worth increasing by US$434 billion from March to May 2020 (89). American billionaire's wealth increased again to US$637 billion, and the pandemic is not over. The names of the Five Horsemen of the Apocalypse who profited most from our misery should come as no surprise. Amazon's CEO Jeff Bezos' net worth increased by US$48 billion, Zoom founder Eric Yuan's net worth increased by US$2.5 billion, former Microsoft CEO Steve Ballmer's net worth increased by US$15.7 billion, casino magnate Sheldon Adelson's net worth increased by US$5 billion and

Elon Musk's net worth increased by US$17.2 billion [90]. The ruling class are modern-day Hood Robins.

Jedi mind trick; the World Wealth Organisation cares about health equity. A World Wealth Organisation report entitled *Closing the Gap in a Generation* called for health equity through action on the social determinants of health (SDH). The SDH are the non-medical factors influencing health outcomes, such as economic stability, neighbourhood and community, education and health, all of which have suffered immensely in lockdown. COVID-19 lockdowns have widened the socioeconomic gap, caused irreparable damage to education, made us afraid of our neighbours and physical environment, decimated our employment, ripped apart social support networks, and prevented us from accessing health care. The call to close the gap and promote health equity in this "COVID generation" by the people responsible for widening the gap is disingenuous [91]. Before COVID (BC), an Oxfam report entitled *Reward work, not wealth*, described that eight billionaires had as much net worth as, "half the human race" [92]. As previously described, the World Economic Forum (WEF) old boy network members never learned to share as children.

The NHS is for profit: I'd like to use the United Kingdom's (UK's) National Health Service (NHS) as an example of how taxpayer money is transferred to the pharmaceutical and healthcare industry under the guise of 'Save the NHS' (and let the rest of us go down the pan). Society wouldn't be so keen to save the NHS if society wasn't so dependent on it. Again I am not referring to the people working in the NHS. I stand with healthcare workers (HCWs) against mandatory COVID-19 vaccines. I stand with HCWs for fairer pay. The NHS may be the publicly funded healthcare system in the UK, however the NHS is not the noble enterprise the daily propaganda would have us believe.

Both NHS Trusts and Foundation Trusts have been able to set up companies called organisations. Just like a commercial company, these 'trusts' have long-term commercial business plans that put profit before people. Grant Thornton, the sixth largest accounting and advisory organisation in the United States (US) say NHS companies offer trusts the opportunity to work in partnership with the commercial sector to develop new income sources, to "increase efficiency while maintaining the same quality, values and ethos as the NHS" [93]. This is not the reality however, with the trust model having been described as, "death by a thousand cuts". Operating margins in English NHS trusts progressively worsened during 2011-2016, and this change was associated with more unsatisfactory performance on several process measures [94]. A Freedom of Information (FOI) request by UNISON, one of the UK's largest trade unions, revealed that NHS trusts are frittering away millions in taxpayer funds by outsourcing staff to private companies, in particular, to pay consultants. This private company model appeals to the NHS trusts because they are arms length, reduce their value-added tax (VAT) liability and cut pay and pensions for new staff [95]. Additionally, NHS Trusts and NHS Foundation Trusts offer private healthcare services.

The start of the NHS in the UK marked the end of preventative medicine and the push towards a pharmaceutical 'cure'. If you are not in the pay packet of a pharmaceutical company, health promotion and preventative medicine (naturopathy) is a no brainer. The Peckham Experiment, as it was called, was conducted in the Pioneer Health Centre, South London, after the Second World War. In contrast with treating those already ill with western medical drugs, which they described as a 'curative' approach, the Peckham Experiment advocated health promotion by concentrating on disease prevention. Adopting this approach, the nearly 1000 families who signed up for this experiment got to relax in a club-like atmosphere, participate in physical exercise, games, workshops, and learn how to relax.

After the establishment of the NHS, the Peckham Experiment ceased in 1950 due to a lack of funding. The Pioneer Health Centre's experimental ethos did not fit the new NHS's 'curative' approach [96]. The 'cure' was a pharmaceutical drug whose adverse effects can be worse than the disease. Pharmaceutical drugs, for example, are an ignored cause of weight gain and obesity. Drugs including, antidiabetics, antidepressants, antiepileptics, antihypertensives. antipsychotics, steroids, hormone replacement therapy (HRT), and the oral contraceptive pill (OCP) all have weight gain as a side effect [97]. But have no fear; there is a drug for obesity too!

Additionally, the problem is not lack of spending! The US spend a disproportionate amount on health yet have the worst health outcomes, coming last on the health tables [98, 99]. I won't clap for the demise of preventative medicine, the transfer of taxpayer money to private companies and the grinding down of the public health system.

Big PhRMA, crony capitalism and spend on lobbying: Big PhRMA sit at the top of WEF founder Satan Klaus' Christmas tree. To use the term Big Pharma does not indicate I wear a tinfoil hat. Big Pharma is the actual name for the trade group in the US that is the Pharmaceutical Research and Manufacturers of America (PhRMA) [(100)]. Big PhRMA describes the consortium of the world's largest pharmaceutical companies and represents leading biopharmaceutical researchers and biotechnology. Pharmaceutical companies are not knights in shining armour. Big PhRMA is a trillion-dollar industry that is highly influential, and its hold is vast.

George Merck said, "We try never to forget that medicine is for the people. It is not for the profits". Yeah right. By 2020, the European Pharmaceutical Market was projected to be worth US$43.7 billion per year, and the African Pharmaceuticals Market forecast for 2020 was projected to be even greater at US$45 billion [(101, 102)]. Big PhRMA is *the* crony capitalist industry. The pharmaceutical giants work for the uber-wealthy one per cent. Big PhRMA shareholders are the activist managers of hedge funds and private equity firms that are major stakeholders in American pharmaceutical companies. Activist investors save underperforming companies and increase shareholder value to help fellow shareholders achieve even greater wealth [(103)]. Activist managers hire doctors to comb the federal research terrain for the most promising inventions and then invest in the companies that own the monopoly licenses to those inventions. Then they profit squeeze them and repeat. When an unfair price-gouging scandal erupts amid howls of public outrage, the CEOs endure a day of public reprimand on Capitol Hill and explain that inflated drug prices are an unfortunate cost of innovation [(104)].

Our governments receive large sums of money that the pharmaceutical industry spends on lobbying and campaign contributions. An observational study analysing publicly available data on US federal government lobbying and campaign contributions from 1999 to 2018 found that the pharmaceutical and health product market spent US$4.7 billion, an average of US$233 million annually. Contributions included US$414 million to presidential and congressional electoral candidates, national party committees, and outside spending groups and US$877 million to state candidates and committees. Contributions were targeted at senior Congress legislators involved in drafting health care laws and state committees either opposing or supporting drug pricing and regulation referenda [105]. This, in turn, 'informs' (buys) government.

In addition to Big PhRMA, as previously mentioned, there is also Big Media, Big Oil, Big Alcohol, Big Soda, Big Tobacco, Big Data etc., all WEF members. Major stakeholders in the healthcare system are patients, physicians, employers, insurance companies, pharmaceutical firms and government, the latter two being joined at the hip [106]. PhRMA and the Biotechnology Innovation Organisation (BIO), the world largest biotech trade association, make connections between the lawmakers and the drug companies they regulate. In 2020 in the US, the companies' political action committees (PACs) donated US$8.62 million to individual political candidates or their affiliated committees. Another US$2.59 million was directed to broader political groups such as the Moderate Democrats PAC, the National Republican Senatorial Committee, and other drug industry PACs, including Big PhRMA's [107].

A report entitled *Divide and Conquer: A look behind the scenes of the EU pharmaceutical industry lobby*, authored by the Corporate Europe Observatory (CEO) and Health Action International (HAI), revealed that the pharmaceutical lobby spends more than €40 million annually to, 'influence decision making in the European Union (EU)', doublespeak for 'mandate vaccines in the EU'. Pharmaceutical manufacturers spend approximately €20 million on in-house lobbyists. A large share of the industry doesn't declare spending, and calls have been made for greater transparency [108]. An article appearing in *The BMJ* in 2012 had higher estimates, reporting that the pharmaceutical industry may be spending €91m a year on lobbying in the EU [109].

Google is a PHARMA biased search engine: In 2016 Google parent Alphabet's life sciences (formerly Google Life Sciences) and GlaxoSmithKline (GSK) created a new US$715 million Bioelectronics medicines firm called Galvani. GSK own 55%, and Alphabet's Verily Life Sciences own 45%. Bioelectronics is a new field of medicine focused on fighting diseases by targeting electrical signals in the body [110]. Bioelectronic medicines include microanalytical devices such as microchips, gene chips and bioelectronic chips [111]. Google's role in the global censorship mechanism is to tell us that Google Life Sciences wanting to inject microchips in us is a conspiracy. I refer to Google as GSKoogle.

Pharmaceutical companies are chemical companies: Merck is the world's oldest operating chemical and pharmaceu-tical company [112]. In the years of the Nazi rule, the company was led by Karl Emanuel Merck, who became a member of the Nazi Party in 1933, receiving the title of 'Wehrwirtschaftsführer'. The Wehrwirtschaftsführer were company executives of, or the bosses of factories key to war materials production known as 'rüstungswichtiger Betrieb' [113]. The German chemical company called IG Farben made Zyklon-bthe cyanide-based pesticide used in the gas chambers. Merck recently departed from generic drugs and spent €10 billion building a presence in highly specialised chemicals [114]. Ethics exist around dual-use research of concern (DURC) chemicals manufactured by pharmaceutical companies. The risk is so significant that the World Health Organisation (WHO) has been called on to develop global guidelines on integrating DURC training into undergraduate and postgraduate medical curricula [115]. Soon to be ex-chancellor Angela Merck-hell's government has a list containing the names of German companies believed to have assisted Syrian dictator Bashar al-Assad and his father's build-up of Syria's chemical weapons arsenal. The Organisation for the Prohibition of Chemical Weapons (OPCW) provided this list to the German government. The OPCW received the Nobel Peace Prize in 2013 for its "extensive efforts to eliminate chemical weapons". Merkel's government however, failed to investigate the German company's involvement with the Bundestag and immediately classified the list, stating that releasing the names would "significantly impair foreign policy interests and thus the welfare of the Federal Republic of Germany", and that it would be akin to releasing "trade secrets" and would violate the German constitution. That old chestnut again.

Foreign ministry files however, make it clear that the Bundestag was fully aware that German companies had potentially been involved in chemical weapons manufacture long before the OPCW delivered its list. According to the OPCW, several German companies are thought to have helped Syrian dictator Bashar al-Assad build up Syria's chemical weapons arsenal. The German government-funded Institute for Contemporary History, known as the Institut für Zeitgeschichte, publishes documents after the standard 30 year embargo expiration date. The most recently published inventory stems from 1984 and includes a document that the German government may have accidentally released containing the names of companies suspected of supplying the Syrian chemical weapons programme, including, among others, the pharmaceutical company Merck [116]. Another example of a noble effort to stave off food shortages by a pharmaceutical partner is Bayer Monsanto producing glyphosate-resistant 'round-up ready' crops. Carcinogenic and mutagenic glyphosate was considered an advantageous herbicide until its overuse led to glyphosate-resistant weeds. Bayer Monsanto responded by producing glyphosate-resistant genetically modified (GM) crops [117].

In sickness and in power: Pharmaceutical companies drive drug resistance which takes lives. Public health has succeeded in reducing deaths from communicable infectious disease, but those days are over. While antibiotics were hugely successful in treating bacterial infections, their overprescription has led to the rise in antibiotic resistance, which currently threatens global health, global security and the global economy [118]. Overprescribing drugs is the main driver of drug resistance. The WHO describes drug resistance as, "a catalogue of 12 families of bacteria that pose the greatest threat to human health" [119]. Drug resistance is not exclusive to overprescribing antibiotics. Antiviral drug resistance also exists. The current practice of treating neglected tropical diseases (NTDs) in Africa uses substantial drug-donation programmes that have resulted in both emergent disease and a variety of drug resistance [120]. All influenza A viruses are resistant to one category of antiviral drugs. Whilst the WHO's Global Influenza Surveillance and Response System (GISRS) report resistance to the antiviral medication Oseltamivir, trade name Tamiflu, is low, other sources confirm 100% of circulating influenza A virus is resistant to Oseltamivir [121, 122].

Prior to COVID-19, human immunodeficiency virus (HIV), malaria and tuberculosis (TB) were already some of the human race's deadliest diseases, however, progress to combat the Big Three has now peaked due to drug resistance. Antimalarial drug resistance to all classes of antimalarial drugs exists and now includes artemisinins-resistance in five countries [121, 123]. Widespread insecticide resistance stops insecticide-treated mosquito nets from protecting against malaria [124]. Multidrug-resistant tuberculosis (MDR-TB) , extensively drug-resistant TB (XDR TB) (resistant to four anti-TB drugs) and totally drug-resistant TB (TDR-TB) exists [121, 125]. According to the WHO, there are about 10.4 million new cases and 1.8 million deaths from 'vaccine-preventable' TB per year [126]. The WHO admits their HIV prescribing recommendations have resulted in antiretroviral therapy (ART) resistance in 7% of people in developing countries and 10-20% in developed countries [121, 127]. Other MDR diseases include Methicillin-resistant *Staphylococcus aureus* (MRSA), MDR *Chlamydia trachomatis*, MDR *Neisseria gonorrhoeae*, MDR *Helicobacter pylori*, MDR *Streptococcus pneumonia* and MDR *Haemophilus influenza*, MDR *Candida albicans*, to name a few. Emergent infections for which new vaccines will be manufactured include Ebola and Lyme neuroborreliosis. By contrast, noncommunicable diseases (NCDs) such as diabetes, cancer and heart disease are now responsible for 71% of all deaths globally [128]. That suits Big PhRMA and public health's agenda down to a tee. Public health's response when the drugs don't work is, the dose is not high enough so increase the dose. The antibiotic apocalypse and the obesity pandemic as an undocumented cause of death in COVID-19 is discussed further in 'Chapter 9, Inflated Deaths'.

War, Famine and Pestilence… are used by the ruling class to increase their money, power and control. Warlords and arms dealers are having a great time of it all together during the pandemic. Poverty is the root cause of violent conflict in developing countries. Lockdowns drive further political, social unrest and economic inequalities between groups, predisposing them to conflict [129, 130]. It's a win-win for the Davos warlords and the military-industrial complex arms dealers. In addition to the pandemonium exacerbating social and economic inequalities, lockdown policies complicate conflict resolution efforts as warmongers capitalise on others misfortune. Additionally, the economic effects weaken state institutions, undermine proper governance and hit poverty affected conflict zones, particularly in Colombia, Libya, Sudan, Ukraine and Yemen [131].

The US already saw deaths on the scale of war every year on its home ground. 100,000 Americans are killed or injured each year as a result of guns [132]. The CDC states that the rate of gun death in the US is now 40,000 a year [133]. COVID-19 lockdowns saw an increase of an estimated 4,000 extra murders in 2020 [134]. As of December 2020, *Forbes* reported 10.9 million Americans were still unemployed. At the peak of lockdown, 22 million Americans lost their jobs during the pandemic [135]. According to criminologists, spikes in gun crime are due to "too much idle time and pent up frustrations". Additionally, US citizens bought more guns for self-protection (I now understand it's to provide protection from their government).

War on us: Security bills to quash protests: They can film us, but we can't film them. Around the world, countries are seeing the introduction of new security bills allowing broad sweeping new police powers. These bills have the sole purpose to quash protests. Advocates say the bills will protect police from harassment and targeting on social media. Critics of these bills say media freedom and citizens' right to film police action must not be impeded, particularly in light of Climate Protests, Black Lives Matter and Reclaim the Streets. Enter the narrative, only protesters wearing masks are legitimate protesters; freedom protesters are illegitimate. On April 27th 2021, the *Irish Examiner* reported an outline of the Garda Síochána (Digital Recording) Bill 2021, introduced to the Cabinet by Justice-Monster Helen McEntee. The bill related to reports that the public's filming of Gardaí (Irish police) leads to serious threats to officers' safety as these images are shared online, and the Garda's addresses are published. McEntee wants to allow the Gardaí to be able to record the public with body cameras and drones; however, the public will face massive fines or imprisonment should they film the Gardaí. The changes in the law again serve to give the police more power and more powers of public surveillance to discourage people from attending protests [(136)]. The French have been protesting Article 24 of the new French police security bill, which makes it a criminal offence to publish images of police officers with the intent to harm their "physical or psychological integrity". Offenders could be fined €45,000 or face up to a year in prison [(137)]. The UK National Security and Investment Bill is a landmark government crime bill and groups together a range of changes to enforcement and sentencing in England and Wales to curtail protests. The bill was met with massive backlash and protests in Bristol, UK. The bill will come into force on January 4th 2022 [(138)].

COVID laws are an extension of terrorism laws: In March 2020, the UK Parliament passed a Coronavirus Act to provide various emergency measures to help deal with the COVID-19 pandemic. Section 24 of the Coronavirus Act 2020 enabled the Secretary of State to make regulations that allowed the police to keep fingerprints and DNA for six months on national security grounds, even when there was no other statutory basis for keeping this biometric data. Counter-Terrorism Policing in the UK made a formal request for a six-month extension of section 24 [(139)]. Additionally, COVID-19 is considered a 'biological agent'. This means that an individual can be charged with terroristic threats for using a biological agent (sneezing, coughing or spitting). Prosecutors in Maryland charged such individuals with simple assault, Connecticut prosecutors charged these individuals with a breach of peace, prosecutors in South Africa charged these individuals with attempted murder. The basis for federal prosecutions is the Rosen memorandum, which lists several relevant federal statutes. The most important of these statutes is 18 USC § 2332a, which criminalises the use of weapons of mass destruction against persons within the United States (US). Section 2332a(c)(2) states, "weapon of mass destruction" are classified as;

> *"Any weapon involving a biological agent, toxin, or vector".* Under *"weapon of mass destruction"* is *"biological agents"*, which includes viruses *"capable of causing death, disease, or other biological malfunction in a human"*, thereby constituting a federal offence.

However, unlike many other federal terrorism statutes, Section 2332a does not require the government to prove that the offence contains a transnational or foreign element, such as a connection with a terrorist group. Thus an infected individual who maliciously coughs on another person need not have the specific intent to kill to be found guilty. An individual found guilty of violating section 2332a faces imprisonment for any term of years or life. If the offence causes death (from any cause within 28 days of a positive COVID-19 test), the person could face the death penalty (140). They are currently employing vicious anti-terrorism police in my hometown of Melbourne, Australia against unarmed citizens.

Famine: The COVID-19 response exacerbates food insecurity. A new UN report has warned global hunger and population displacement was already at record levels prior to COVID-19 and that this is a worsening situation as remittances dry up. David Beasley, Executive Director of the World Food Programme (WFP), said that the socioeconomic effects of the pandemic are more devastating than the disease itself (141). BC, we also saw the scale of international migration increase in line with recent trends. Before the latest refugee crisis in Afghanistan, the number of international migrants was estimated to be 272 million globally, with nearly two-thirds being migrant workers (142). Of the estimated one billion migrant workers in total, 270 million worked outside their home countries, and 760 million were internal migrants. The 270 million migrants workers sent home a staggering US$689 billion per year to help feed, clothe and shelter up to three people back home (143). According to the World Bank, migrant wages sent home dropped by almost 20% to US$142 billion in 2020. This figure is four times greater than during the 2009 financial crisis [144]. Oxfam estimated that COVID-19 linked hunger would kill 12,000 people each day [145]. Thus, lockdowns have potentially caused 4,380,000 deaths in 2020 from starvation! This COVID effect is not at all limited to developing countries. Hundreds of thousands of taxpayers in Australia on skilled worker visas are out of work, not entitled to benefits and in desperate need of aid [146]. Food insecurity in the US has doubled since 2019 and is at the greatest level since 1998 [147]. The latest Oxfam report entitled *The Hunger Virus Multiplies*, published in July 2021, warns 11 people are dying from hunger a minute as the pandemic (restrictions) drives a starvation crisis. Oxfam continues to say a further 20 million people had been pushed to "extreme levels of food insecurity" in 2021, taking the total to 155 million in 55 countries [148]. At the peak of the pandemic, one person died every minute from COVID-19, yet 11 people per minute currently die from lockdown-related hunger.

Despite World Wealth Organisation guidance that countries remove all healthcare user fees for the duration of the pandemic, 89% of the World Bank's country projects didn't commit to that. Moreover, out of the eight that committed to removing healthcare user fees during the pandemic, none explicitly stated that the waivers covered all health services and, in three of those eight, the measure only covered treatment relating to COVID-19. *"Let's make no mistake, user fees for health (services) kill and are pushing millions of people into poverty"*, said Oxfam's health policy adviser Anna Marriott [149].

Worse still, the money to help the poorest countries respond quickly to the outbreak is difficult to access because of bureaucracy and red tape and can only be accessed after the disease has spread extensively. Senior fellow at Harvard Global Health Institute and former economist at the World Bank, Olga Jonas, described the World Bank and Gates Foundation's US$500m pandemic scheme as;

> *"So convoluted, it is not at all clear whether they will payout at all. It is too little, too late, and in this case, maybe never"*. Jonas said, *"What's obscene is that the World Bank set it up this way, to wait for people to die!"* [150].

As mentioned in Chapter 1, 'New Normal Slash World Order' the World Bank Group describe themselves as being committed to fighting poverty.

Pestilence: As previously mentioned, non-communicable diseases (NCDs) are the real killer, killing 41 million people each year globally equating to 71% of all deaths. Infectious diseases such as severe acute respiratory syndrome coronavirus 2 (SARS-CoV-2) are generally a leading cause of death in low-income countries and account for only 29% of global deaths [(128)]. Yet here we are, crashing the global economy, enslaving citizens and creating a covibesity pandemic that, low and behold, leads to more of us becoming eternally dependent on 'life-saving' medications. COVID-19 lockdowns have resulted in increased deaths from other causes as lockdowns have significantly impacted health services for NCDs, including cardiovascular disease, cancers, respiratory diseases and diabetes. Additionally, fewer people have been seeking treatment, and there is less funding and treatment available for other diseases. The pandemic however, may also result in fewer deaths from other causes, including road accidents and influenza [(151)].

The total impact of the COVID-19 pandemic includes deaths resulting from COVID-19 and deaths caused by the consequences of lockdowns, predominantly due to disruption to health services and starvation in poorer countries. The CDC states that between January 31st and October 3rd 2020, an estimated 299,028 excess deaths occurred in the US. 66% of these excess deaths were, according to their definition, COVID-19 deaths, i.e. 'deaths from any cause within 28 days of a positive test', 'suspected', 'probable' and 'possible'. This figure equates to 44% of all excess deaths having been caused by the COVID-19 lockdowns [(152)]. This extrapolates to 197,358 COVID-19 deaths by their definition and 101,670 deaths due to the consequences of lockdown. 101,670 people have been sacrificial lambs in the US lockdown experiment.

The UK's Scientific Advisory Group for Emergencies (SAGE), in collaboration with the Office for National Statistics (ONS) and analysts from several government departments, estimated that there were 38,500 excess deaths in England connected to COVID-19 between March and May 1st 2021, but that 41% of these deaths resulted from missed medical care rather than the virus. In other words, for every three COVID-19 deaths by their definition, the lockdown has caused another two [(153)]. Many will likely know that the effect of the public health measures causes physical isolation and that this isolation seriously threatens our mental health and well-being [(154)]. According to the International COVID-19 Suicide Prevention Research

Collaboration, it is still too early to measure the ultimate effect of the pandemic on suicide rates [(155)]. Divorce lawyers in the UK and the US report significant increases in enquiries, with one Washington DC law firm recording a 70% increase in calls in October 2020 compared to the previous year [(156)].

Cancer pandemic: On May 10th 2021, reports in Europe emerged of a "cancer epidemic", with an expected one million cancer cases going undiagnosed due to disruptions to primary care and screening programmes caused by COVID-19 lockdowns [(157)]. In Ireland, in November 2020, reports emerged that up to 2,000 cancers might be undiagnosed because of disruptions to screening programmes due to COVID-19 lockdowns [(158)]. A European Cancer Organisation report entitled *Time to Act:1 million undiagnosed cancer*, notes that restrictions to cancer services as a result of COVID-19 lockdowns resulted in one in two cancer patients not receiving surgical or chemotherapy treatment, with one in five is still not receiving cancer treatment. A total of 100 million cancer screening tests were not performed. Additionally, four in ten HCWs working in the sector have shown signs of burnout, with three in ten being clinically depressed [(159)].

Maternal and child death pandemic: Indirect mortality due to COVID-19 lockdowns is vast and unacceptable. While the COVID-19 pandemic increased mortality due to the virus, indirect mortality increased substantially. A *Lancet Global Health* study across the 118 countries calculated two scenarios. The first conservative estimate resulted in 253,500 additional child deaths and 12,200 additional maternal deaths over six months (531,400 in one year total). The more severe scenario estimated 1,157 000 additional child deaths and 56,700 additional maternal deaths over the course of a year (1,213,700 in total). The additional deaths represent an increase of between 9.8-44.7% in under-5 child deaths and an 8.3-38.6% increase in maternal deaths per month during the COVID-19 lockdowns due to restrictions to maternal and child health services [(160)]. A systematic review and meta-analysis entitled 'Effects of the COVID-19 Pandemic on Maternal and Perinatal Outcomes' published in *The Lancet Global Health* on March 31st 2021, analysed data on more than six million pregnancies and found that the disruption to services due to nationwide lockdowns resulted in an increase in maternal deaths, stillbirths, ruptured ectopic pregnancies and maternal depression. The study concluded that stillbirth and maternal mortality rates increased by about one-third, while ectopic pregnancy surgeries increased by almost sixfold [(161)]. More than 3.2 million stillbirths occur globally each year [(162)]. Thus COVID-19 restrictions to maternal and child services have resulted in approximately one million more child deaths in 2020. The WHO estimated that in 2015, there were 302,680 maternal deaths globally [(163)]. That equates to an extra 100,000 maternal deaths in 2020. The World Wealth Organisation chose to sacrifice the lives of poor mothers and babies to 'save lives' in affluent, ageing, high-income countries more likely to be dependent on pharmaceutical drugs.

Depriving children of their right to be educated: Our children's human right to education has been violated. I had five children at home during 2020. The public health czars making these rules are far removed from the reality of a parent's role in the home and the value of in school face-to-face teaching. In Ireland, schools were closed from March 2020 (we were told two weeks to flatten the curve) until September 2020. Then again, from December 2020 (again, we were told two weeks) until April 2021. There is no evidence whatsoever of secondary transmission of COVID-19 from children in schools [(164)]. A *Lancet* article referred to a report entitled *Global Girlhood Report 2020*, stated that school closures during lockdown would lead to 2.5 million more child marriages, 500,000 additional girls being at risk of child and forced marriage and one million additional girls expected to become pregnant in 2020. The author of the report, Gabrielle Szabo, senior gender policy adviser at Save the Children UK, says the school closures and economic destitution caused by the pandemic threatened to reverse 25 years of progress on child marriage [(165)]. So much for #generationequality.

COVID lockdowns have thrown global progress into reverse. Frankly, anyone that supports lockdowns supports widening the socioeconomic gap, driving conflict and disease, increasing deaths from starvation and reversing gender equality progress to save their own necks. The irony is that, far from saving their own necks, lockdown supporters are complicit in their own perpetual imprisonment, the destruction of their children's futures and the demise of democracy globally.

CHAPTER THREE

COERCIVE CONTROL

"The enemy is fear. We think it is hate, but it is really fear". Gandhi [166]

One of the central emotional responses during a pandemic is fear. Functional fear helps people develop coping strategies, and the 'right' amount of anxiety can help us perform better and stimulate action. However, the fear created during this pandemic is completely disproportionate and irrational [167]. The COVID-19 pandemonium is associated with highly significant levels of anxiety, depression, post-traumatic stress disorder and psychological distress [168]. The ruling class say functional fear predicts our compliance in the coronavirus disease 2019 (COVID-19) pandemic [169]. The more anxious we are, the more we comply. Eastern religion philosopher Alan Watts wrote, *"If we look deeply into such ways of life as Buddhism, we do not find either philosophy or religion as these are understood in the West. We find something more nearly resembling psychotherapy"* [168]. Psychotherapy, or talk therapy, helps eliminate or alleviate disturbing symptoms to enable one to encourage personal well-being and encourage healing. Our controllers know this hence they apply behavioural science techniques on us that discourage well-being and healing, the intention to increase compliance [170].

'Project Fear' is a 21st century term used in British politics that entered British politics in the 2014 Scottish independence referendum and again during the 2016 United Kingdom (UK) Brexit referendum [171]. Our elected representatives call it the "fear appeal". Fear appeal is a means of persuasion that threatens us with a negative, physical, psychological, and/or social consequence that will likely happen if we behave a certain way or engage in certain behaviour [172]. Hardly appealing. In the case of the COVID-19 pandemonium, policymakers are supposedly 'guided by the science'. However the science is, in many cases, preliminary and very often conflicting. It is apparent that our policymakers are being guided by a perceived 'public clamour' for draconian measures to tackle the pandemic, or, at the very least are using this so as to *appear* as if they're actually doing something. What our policy makers may 'perceive' however, is often filtered by a media skewed toward hyping the fear factor.

Human rights are our oppressor! Article 5 of the Human Rights Act supersedes all human rights and is the power the ruling class use to coercively control us. Article 5 of the Human Rights Act is entitled 'Right to Liberty' and states that; *"everyone has the right to liberty and security of person. No one shall be deprived of their liberty save in the following cases and in accordance with a procedure prescribed by law: The lawful detention of persons for the prevention of the spreading of infectious diseases, of persons of unsound mind, alcoholics or drug addicts or vagrants"* (173). Article 5 is doublespeak for; 'If you're infected, crazy, an alcoholic or a drug addict we have the right to lock you up indefinitely without trial'. Human rights are our oppressor! We must stop citing Gatesist human rights! The United Nations (UN) Convention on the Rights of the Child takes away our rights as a parent and allows our 14 year olds to the right to choose the Gardasil human papillomavirus (HPV) vaccine, or to block their pubertal development (174)! They can't vote, drive, drink or have sex but they can choose to irrevocably change their lives. If our children get narcolepsy, a lifelong, debilitating 'incurable' disability, it is the parents, not the state, who will be burdened with the duty of care. Natural medicine can treat narcolepsy.

Public health is our oppressor! Have no doubt, public health can plunge a needle in our arm. Vaccine passports and mandatory vaccines are the least of our worries when it comes to the power of public health. A video on You-will-obey-Tube entitled 'Alan Dershowitz Says Mandatory, FORCED Vaccines For Everyone!', at 2 minutes shows American constitutional law scholar and former Harvard Law Professor Alan Dershowitz explaining how we have no right to endanger the public and spread disease and no right not to be vaccinated. Dershowitz describes that in United States (US) constitutional law, public health police power of the constitution means "the state has the power to literally take you to a doctor's office and plunge a needle into your arm" (175). Public health police powers are the powers of a state government to make and enforce all laws necessary to preserve public health, safety, and general welfare, including mandatory quarantine, mandatory social distancing, mandatory masking, mandatory vaccines, mandatory inspections and removals, mandatory blood tests, mandatory urine tests, mandatory whatever they deem (176). Public health police power is the power to coercively control us. Not that mandates are acceptable, however public health would never mandate pure drinking water, nourishing food, exercise and relaxation.

"Az long az not everybody iz vaxzinated, nobody vill be safe".

Klaus Schwab

Public health's seven-step recipe for project fear: The recipe is entitled the 'Seven-Step Recipe for Generating Interest in, and Demand for, Flu (or any other) Vaccination'. The recipe aimed to foster public interest and high vaccine demand was discussed at the National Influenza Vaccine Summit 2004, sponsored by the Centres for Disease Control and Prevention (CDC) and the American Medical Association (AMA) and devised by Glen Nowak Acting Director of Media Relations, CDC. The recipe includes;

- Statements of alarm in the media by medical experts and public health authorities.
- Prediction of dire outcomes from influenza (or other infectious disease).
- Continued reports by the media of influenza (or other infectious disease) causing severe illness affecting lots of people.
- Repeated urging of influenza (or other infectious disease) vaccination.
- Roll out the celebrity or past president to get the 'vaccine' on national media [(177)].

We have all witnessed how public health employ the daily propaganda to apply the seven-step recipe to generate interest in and increase demand for the measles-mumps-rubella (MMR) vaccines by increasing insecurity, anxiety, and uncertainty surrounding measles outbreaks. Public health wilfully omits that these outbreaks most often occur in vaccinated communities due to vaccine waning immunity, as explained in Chapter 23, 'Measles Shmeezles and the Great Autism Cover-up'.

Public health says ridicule is man's most powerful weapon: Public health promotion campaigns are designed to elicit fear [(178)]. As mentioned, 'fear appeal' appeals to our oppressors as a means of persuasion to threatens us with negative, physical, psychological, and/or social consequences should we not comply [(172)]. Irish tyrannical member of the Independent Scientific Advocacy Group (ISAG), Dr Gabriel Scallywag, was the person who originally called for a zero-COVID approach in Ireland, placing the Irish in indefinite imprisonment if the vaccines didn't work for the variants [(179)]. At the time of writing ironically, in June 2021, UK Monster-of-Health, double-jabbed Savid Javid had COVID [(180)]. There has since been a raft of doubled-jabbed celebrities with COVID. Enter the narrative 'no vaccine is 100% effective', blame the unvaccinated and recommend a booster shot.

Back to Ireland's ISAG, I have not personally seen the leaked reports however a webpage called 'Gript' reported that hundreds of emails, draft documents, and ISAG internal communications were leaked to Gript. ISAG members were instructed to "review and internalise" instructions to "look for ways to increase insecurity, anxiety, and uncertainty" and to "go after people and not institutions" because "people hurt faster than institutions". The instructions were shared to the group by Professor Anthony Staines, one of the founders of ISAG, in a note titled, 'Notes from 2020-02-08 ISAG meeting' (the note's title contains a typo, it was actually posted on February 8th 2021). The note reminded ISAG members of the importance of ridicule as, "man's most powerful weapon". ISAG members, many of whom are regular guests in Irish media, were told that they could count on "imagination" to "dream up many more consequences" as "the threat of a thing is usually more terrifying than the thing itself" [181].

Social engineering and psychosis: Social engineering is taking advantage of a potential victim's natural tendencies and emotional reactions. Fear is a powerful social-engineering technique. One study sampled a large international community to evaluate factors associated with compliance, including self-perceived risk, fear of the virus, moral and ethical principles, political orientation, and behaviour changes in response to the pandemic and found that the only predictor of positive behaviour change (compliance) was fear of COVID-19 [182]. Three billion people globally were living under lockdown during the spring of 2020. The World Economic Forum (WEF) themselves admit that this is the largest psychological experiment ever and will result in a secondary epidemic of burnouts and stress-related absenteeism in the latter half of 2020. How hypocritical that the authors of the Greta Reset purport to care about our mental health and are calling on a two-tier approach; one for the wounded and one to treat the invisible, psychological wounds of trauma [183]. A *Lancet* review of 245 studies exploring the psychological effects of lockdowns concluded that those quarantined experienced psychological stress disorders such as depressed mood, insomnia, stress, anxiety, anger, irritability, emotional exhaustion, depression and post-traumatic stress symptoms [184]. Public health lockdowns have driven anxiety, fear and phobias and exacerbated feelings of social isolation. The severe stress of lockdowns has resulted in three newly documented COVID-19 related neuropsychiatric disorders; COVID-19-associated brief psychotic disorder, COVID-19-induced psychosis and suicidal behaviour and COVID-19 psychosis [185-187].

A cross-sectional online survey among the general population in France explored attitudes regarding COVID-19 lockdown. Whilst the survey found overall that consensus in favour of the national lockdown had been maintained and that excessive politicisation of public health had been avoided, 35% of low-income respondents compared to only 10% of high-income respondents agreed with the statement 'lockdown was disproportionate considering the real gravity of the epidemic'. The authors acknowledged that financial support during lockdown was significantly lower among low-income respondents and that preexisting social inequality meant that consensus remained fragile. During the 2009 influenza A(H1N1) pandemic, only 8% of adults complied with the mass vaccination campaigns indicating that French people's social acceptability of public health authorities is not as strong [188]. The French give us hope.

Stoke the fear factor by exaggerating children's risks: PIMS anyone? Yes, thanks I'll have a Pimm's and lemonade. To generate interest in and increase uptake of vaccines, the daily propaganda indoctrinates us with repeated stories of paediatric inflammatory multisystem syndrome (PIMS), a COVID-related illness found in children [189]. With the aim to baffle us with science jargon, PIMS is also known as multisystem inflammatory syndrome in children (MIS-C). PIMS is a serious health issue that requires prompt medical attention, however the vast majority of children affected by it survive. Because PIMS has only recently been identified, the medical community is still trying to understand the exact causes, including understanding why it only appears in children. Whilst there is mounting evidence that it is linked to COVID-19, the relationship between the two is not yet established. Severe COVID-19 disease is rare in children, with children having a one in a million chance of serious illness from COVID-19 [190]. An article published in *The New England Journal of Medicine* entitled 'COVID-19, and Child and Teacher Morbidity in Sweden' discussing Swedish statistics, found that between March and June 2020, one child in 130,000 confirmed COVID-19 positive children were treated in an intensive care unit due to COVID-19. Schools in Sweden were open during the pandemic. Social distancing was encouraged in Sweden, but wearing a face mask was not [191]. A University College London (UCL), Imperial College London and the universities of

Bristol, York and Liverpool study published in July 2021, found that children with confirmed COVID-19 had a roughly one in 50,000 chance of being admitted to intensive care with COVID and a two in a million chance of dying [192].

Long COVID: Public health named their fear porn 'Long COVID'. On the 12th October 2020, World Wealth Organisation Director-General Dr scare-the-bejesus-out-of-us announced that he had met with patient groups experiencing long-term health impacts of COVID-19, a term he said is now described as "Long COVID". Dr scare-the-bejesus-out-of-us used this opportunity to say, *"allowing a dangerous virus that we don't fully understand to run free is simply unethical"* [193]. Long COVID is neither new nor a surprise. Post-viral fatigue syndrome, also known as chronic fatigue syndrome (CFS) or myalgic encephalomyelitis (ME), is a relatively common disorder. These post-viral fatigue syndromes have been common since I began practising back in 1999. Complementary and Alternative Medicine (CAM) practitioners help people recover from 'never been well since' syndromes, where western medicine has no recourse. Adult population-based studies in the US have estimated the prevalence of ME or CFS diagnosis is 519-1,038 per 100,000 with a 3:1 female-to-male ratio [194].

The UK Office for National Statistics (ONS) is still working on estimating the prevalence of long COVID [195]. The daily propaganda is now using Long COVID in children to generate interest in and increase uptake of COVID-19 vaccines in that group. On March 3rd 2021, *The Irish Times* reported that up to one in seven UK children under 17 reported at least one symptom five weeks after COVID-19 [196]. Promoting fear is a win-win to generate interest in and increase uptake of vaccines. Fear manifests on a physical level and suppresses the immune system, and anxiety about COVID-19 increases the risk of infection [197].

Roll out the celebrity: There are too many to mention. A report on the Moderna vaccine published in *The New England Journal of Medicine* credits Dolly Parton and others for a donation to Vanderbilt University Medical Centre. Biggest heart breakers for me; Willy Nelson, Mick Jagger and Sean Penn. On December 3rd 2021, then US President-elect Joe Biden-his-time-until-Kamala-takes-over said he would publicly take a COVID-19 vaccine to demonstrate its safety to the public and increase public confidence in the vaccine [198]. Then roll out, roll out former Presidents, Obama, Bush and Clinton pledging to publicly take a COVID-19 vaccine [199].

That part of the seven-step recipe doesn't always go as planned: Katie Price appeared in a documentary entitled *Harvey and Me,* about her disabled son Harvey turning 18 in which Katie campaigned for vulnerable people to be prioritised in the COVID-19 vaccine rollout. After Harvey's first dose of the Oxford-AstraZeneca COVID-19 vaccine, Harvey was rushed to hospital after a reaction to the vaccine. Harvey "was shaking uncontrollably" and had a temperature of 39.9°C. Doctors confirmed his reaction was caused by the vaccine. Katie's friend said, "Harvey only had the jab yesterday, and she's convinced it's some sort of allergic reaction. She can't think what else it could be" [200]. Thankfully Harvey received his second dose without incident. Iconic American baseball player and Hall of Famer Hank Aaron said how proud he was after being publically injected with the COVID-19 vaccination. Hank had hoped that his willingness to be vaccinated would decrease vaccine hesitancy in Black Americans. Aaron said, "(Getting vaccinated) makes me feel wonderful", and "I don't have any qualms about it at all, you know. I feel quite proud of myself for doing something like this...It's just a small thing that can help zillions of people in this country" [201].

Three weeks later, Hank Aaron was dead. Whether or not Hank's death is attributable to the vaccination, why on God's green earth would a feeble octogenarian want to take an unlicensed medical product under emergency use authorisation (EUA), using completely new technology that is known to cause more severe side effects than standard vaccines [202]? The extent of vaccine injuries and deaths, including how to search for them, are outlined in Chapter 13, 'COVID-19 Vaccines are Safe for Two Months'.

Apply doublethink: The use of doublethink is a political indoctrination technique described by George Orwell in *1984* that forces us to accept contrary opinions or beliefs at the same time. Some examples;

- *'We are all in this together'*- but there is no solidarity between the rich and the poor.
- *'Staying apart keeps us together'*- the Victoria, Australian saying. Are you fair dinkum?

- *'New normal'*- more 'strange future' than normal.
- *'Stay home, stay safe'*- there were more domestic accidents, specifically paediatric domestic accidents during lockdown.
- *'Freedom bracelets'*- Israel's security jewellery.
- *'Immunity passports'*- provides a pass to spread infection.
- *'Green pass'*- As discussed in Chapter 22, 'Vaccines are not Green'.
- *'Breakthrough infections means the vaccine is working'*- that's a new one.
- *'Freedom day'*- our day will come.

Lack of medical ethics regarding financial coercion in COVID-19 vaccine trials: In their book, *Principles of Biomedical Ethics*, Beauchamp and Childress describe the four principles of medical ethics as autonomy, nonmaleficence, beneficence and justice [(203)]. There are more medical ethics, however with increasing calls for mandates, practising according to these four principles already seems impossible. Financial coercion violates respect for autonomy primarily, and financial coercion is unjust as it targets low socioeconomic status groups. The Nuffield Council on Bioethics has created the 'Nuffield Ladder', an intervention ladder that is used to assess the acceptability and justification of public health policies. The Nuffield Council recognises in its Intervention Ladder 29 that people may legitimately be incentivised to take on risks [(204)]. According to public health 'ethicists' all mandatory vaccination, including vaccination for COVID-19, can be ethically justified if the threat to public health is 'grave'. It does not matter to these ethicists that the threat to public health from COVID-19 is gravely overstated. There is absolutely no sense or logic being applied to weigh up the pros and cons of the effects of lockdown on all health services and mortality from all causes. The only global health problem that is acknowledged at present is COVID-19. Other approaches these ethicists deem acceptable is penalties including the withholding of benefits, costs including the imposition of fines, the allocation of community service or loss of personal freedoms. Payment in kind for risk for vaccination use under Emergency Use Authorisation (EUA) is also an option [(205)]. Roll on 'no jab no jobseekers', 'no jab no jive' and 'no jab no joining in society'.

Financial coercion to participate in vaccine trials: Payment for research participation is ethically questionable. Certain payments are more justifiable than others, even in the context of a 'global pandemic'. The three types of research payments are reimbursement, compensation and incentive. Reimbursement is straightforward and pays the participant back for research-related expenses such as travel expenses, including mileage, lodging and food whilst travelling. Compensation is for time and effort, discomfort and inconvenience. Incentives, on the other hand, are ethically dubious and are offered to increase trial enrolment. Reimbursement and compensation payments are deemed ethically correct. It is argued however, that given the extreme psychological distress and fear experienced by people in pandemic times, that there is an increased risk of undue influence, and that incentive payments should be avoided unless absolutely essential to recruit and retain patients in trials where the social value is deemed to outweigh this risks [206, 207].

Incidentally, In January 2019, financial coercion in a domestic relationship was classified as abuse [208]. The law states that coercion is a 'duress crime', which means that (theoretically) we have the lawful right to defend ourselves from our coercive controllers [209].

Financial coercion to participate in human challenge trials: Human challenge trials using SARS-CoV-2 are deemed controversial. Human challenge trials involve intentionally infecting research participants to improve and accelerate vaccine development by rapidly providing estimates of safety and efficacy. 'Scientific ethicists' weigh up the potential benefits to public health and to participants, the risks and uncertainty involved for trial participants, and third-party risks to research staff and the community as a whole. 'Scientific ethicists' put forward the argument that these human challenge trials could reasonably be considered as ethically acceptable as long as such trials were accepted by the international communities in which they are conducted, could be realistically expected to accelerate vaccine development, have the potential to have a direct benefit to participants, that trial designs limit risk to participants, and that strict infection control procedures are in place to limit and reduce third-party risks [210]. It goes without saying that the 'scientific ethicists' deemed that the threat to global public health outweighed the risks of deliberately infecting people with the 'deadly' virus. The same 'scientific ethicists' did not however think that it was ethical to allow infected individuals to infect another individual with SAR-COV-2 in order to satisfy Koch's postulate and to prove that SARS-CoV-2 causes COVID-19, as is covered in Chapter 7, 'Does SARS-CoV-2 Exist?'.

On December 7th 2021, the World Health Organisation's (WHO) Working Group for Guidance on Human Challenge Studies in COVID-19 meeting reviewed existing plans for human challenge trials and discussed concerns. 1Day Sooner is a nonprofit organisation advocating for human challenge trial volunteers [211]. An article published in *The BMJ* entitled 'COVID-19 vaccines: Should we allow human challenge studies to infect healthy volunteers with SARS-CoV-2?', by a number of spokespersons for 1Day Sooner reflected that much of our current understanding of coronaviruses comes from human challenge trials conducted in the 1960s, and that efficacy data from these had helped the cholera vaccine achieve licensure.

The authors say that over 38,000 people had registered their interest to participate in COVID-19 human challenge trials through 1Day Sooner and that the UK government had invested £33.6million to support these trials. The main arguments put forward by 1Day Sooner were that human challenge trials may prove valuable towards accelerating second and third-generation vaccines, which will allow greater access to poorer countries.

A member of the WHO's Working Group for Guidance on Human Challenge Studies in COVID-19 argued the opposite, that's SARS-CoV-2 challenge trials proposed including people who were at high risk of the disease and that this could unfairly target certain communities and violate justice, and as uncertainly exists around the long-term effect of COVID-19, it would be dangerous and unjustified [212]. 'Listen to the expert'; unless the expert isn't listening to the expert that the experts have told them to listen to.

On March 8th 2020, it was reported that iHvivo, a world leader in the testing of vaccines and antivirals using human challenge trial models were to conduct an experiment at the Queen Mary BioEnterprises Innovation Centre in Whitechapel, UK. The experiment involved deliberately infecting 24 volunteers with laboratory manufactured 0C43 and 229E strains of the coronavirus. The UK boffins openly admit to manufacturing coronaviruses in a laboratory. These volunteers were paid £3,500 to be deliberately infected with what was described as a less harmful form of the coronavirus. Queen Mary University Virologist Professor John Oxford described it as, *"our little virus..."* How Professor John Oxford's little virus can accurately reflect a vaccine's effectiveness against the real McCoy I do not know [213].

An article published in the *Journal of Medical Ethics* argued that underpayment is of more concern than overpayment in COVID-19 challenge trials. The study referred to Rimwade et als' survey of investigators who studied 25 human challenge trials for diseases other than COVID-19 and found that whilst the maximum payment amount was US$4446 and the average payment amount was US$1770. These figures equated to an average payment of US$13.77 per hour. While this figure was greater than the US current federal minimum wage of US$7.25 per hour, it was less than the recommended fair minimum wage of US$15 per hour and failed to account for hazard pay for the extra risks to participants of COVID-19, which for exposure to a virulent biological agent, is recommended to be an extra 25%. In summary, the data raised significant questions about underpayment, exploitation and unfair treatment of human challenge trial participants [(214)].

Paying us to take our shot: Former US congressman John Delaney proposed paying people a US$1,500 stimulus cheque to receive the COVID-19 vaccine with the goal to achieve a vaccination coverage of 75% vaccination faster [(215)]. 75% isn't good enough anymore; the boffins want to 'vaccinate the world'.

Coercion through medical apartheid: Even though the COVID-19 vaccine is still under EUA and currently in a continuing global experiment, the ruling class have now championed an International Certificate of Vaccination or Prophylaxis (ICVP). The ruling class use yellow fever vaccination mandates in certain countries as an example. The yellow fever vaccination is associated with a rare multisystem organ failure syndrome, which is why I made an informed choice not to take it [(216)]. Additionally, the daily propaganda won't tell you that many countries requiring this vaccine only require it if you are travelling from an area where a yellow fever outbreak is occurring. The daily propaganda will also not tell you that the P in ICVP stands for prophylaxis [(217)].

I am a homeopath and prescribe homeoprohylaxis against yellow fever. Why do we need to take a vaccine when we can take a cheap, safe and effective alternative? Because the WEF old boy network would not increase their wealth. Prophylaxis is covered in Chapter 19, 'COVID Medical & Natural Medicine Prevention & Treatment'.

Double-jabbed get greater privileges: 'Fully vaccinated global citizens', doublespeak for 'citizens who obey', are being given greater freedoms than unvaccinated citizens. There is no question that increasing freedoms for the vaccinated is medical apartheid; segregation by vaccine status. The CDC's interim clinical considerations for the use of mRNA COVID-19 vaccines currently authorised in the US was updated on February 10th 2020. Updated quarantine recommendations included that fully vaccinated people will no longer be required to quarantine following exposure to COVID-19 [218]. The vaccine that does not stop the spread of infection now gets you a get out of quarantine free card! Additionally, even though the COVID-19 vaccines have not been shown to reduce infection, the CDC said fully vaccinated Americans can gather indoors without masks [219]. All hail our supreme leader! Vaccinated grandparents can now see their healthy children and grandchildren [220]. All hail our supreme leader! Meanwhile, the new sub-class of unvaccinated people must continue to wear fashion masks, avoid large gatherings and physically distance themselves from their fellow human beings. Greater freedoms for vaccinated equate to discrimination and I will never be a global citizen.

European Parliament said it will not mandate COVID-19 vaccines: The daily propaganda uses threats of mandates under orders of the public health seven-step recipe to generate interest in and increase uptake of vaccines. On January 27th 2021, the European parliamentary assembly said it would not mandate COVID-19 vaccines. Resolution 2361 (2021) says explicitly, *"7.3.1 ensure that citizens are informed that the vaccination is not mandatory and that no one is politically, socially, or otherwise pressured to get themselves vaccinated if they do not wish to do so themselves. 7.3.2 ensure that no one is discriminated against for not having been vaccinated, due to possible health risks or not wanting to be vaccinated"* [221]. No one is politically, socially, or otherwise pressured to get themselves vaccinated! In another European U-turn, they call them 'near mandates' also known as the 'green pass'.

CHAPTER THREE – PART II

NATION-SPECIFIC EXAMPLES OF COERCIVE ABUSE

Coercive abuse against Galicians: On February 23rd 2021, dictators in Galicia, an autonomous community in northwestern Spain, mandated COVID-19 vaccines and introduced fines for vaccine refusers who "don't follow the rules". Fines ranged from €1,000 to €60,000. The regional government announced that the COVID-19 vaccine will be compulsory for all 2.7 million inhabitants. According to a survey by the Centre for Social Research in Spain in December, originally more than 40% of Spaniards preferred not to be vaccinated with approved drugs. Another survey in early February 2021 by Spanish consumer rights group Organisation of Consumers and Users found more than half of Spaniards wanted to get the COVID-19 vaccine as soon as possible, leaving half that would refuse a COVID-19 vaccine [(222)].

Coercive abuse against the Spanish: On December 29th 2020, Spain said it is going to keep a COVID vaccine registry of those who refuse the vaccine and share this information with its European partners whilst adhering to European General Data Protection Regulation (GDPR) to which they have a lawful obligation. The privacy implications of linking biometric information such as fingerprints, facial patterns and voice recognition to COVID-19 vaccination are immense [(223)].

Coercive abuse against the French: In December 2020, after the French government repeated they would not make the COVID-19 vaccine mandatory, the French parliament still debated how they would make it as mandatory as possible with the introduction of a new 'health passport'. The health passport would allow the French Prime Minister the authority to require COVID-19 vaccination for activities during a 'health crisis'. The proposal presented to French Ministers on December 21st 2021, put forward the idea that people's movements, activities and use of public transport could become conditional upon COVID-19 vaccination or proof of a negative test. The new rules were intended to come into force from April 1st 2021 [(224)]. Macron recently officially announced it, but it was always on the cards. Hours after Emmanuel Macron announced that the unvaccinated would be banned from cafés, restaurants, shopping malls, and trains, many French rushed to get their shot [(225)]. Many other French rushed to the streets to stand. The idea of allocating a potentially unhealthy person who has received a vaccine a 'health' certificate is ludicrous. A tape measure around the middle is by far the most effective tool in determining one's health status. France is, as I write on August 7th 2021, seeing its 4th week of anti-vaccine certificate protests.

Coercive abuse against the Irish: On December 16th 2020, Ireland announced that people with vaccine certificates were to face fewer restrictions in life. Vaccine certificates were already being considered for air travel in the EU, and also to allow for greater attendance at mass gatherings. Whilst Irish Monster-of-Health, Stephen Donnelly said "nothing is being ruled in or out" and that they were waiting to see if the vaccine prevents the spread of infection and thus can actually impact on reducing transmissibility. Mr Donnelly said, "If it turns out that actually, it's a marginal impact on transmissibility then we might have to think about it differently" (226). A marginal impact? Marginal is scientific for poor. Bear in mind, on this day in June 2021, there were 31 people in intensive care, and Health-Monster Stephen Donnelly is discussing a mandatory vaccine to attend a café (226). Somehow this does not seem proportionate to many of us who lived through the AIDs pandemic and the threat of a nuclear apocalypse. We are currently standing against the introduction of a domestic vaccine certificate in Ireland. Our post-corona era sees Ticketmaster developing a framework for event organisers to require and verify negative tests and/or vaccine status for ticket-holders (227). That may be fair if the vaccine immunised to prevent the spread of infection. The drug cartel that runs the Irish government has ripped the heart out of Ireland. We, the free people, should walk straight into any pub and let the complicit watch us get dragged out and arrested by the new 'COVID compliance officers' (228). Alternatively, join my 'Raging Grannies Pots-&-Pans Protest' group on Telegram.

Coercive abuse against Brazilians: Brazil's Supreme Court ruled COVID-19 vaccinations can be made mandatory, even though around one-fifth of Brazilians said they will refuse the COVID-19 vaccine. The court also ruled that Brazilians may not be vaccinated against their will. Rather than hold people down against their will and plunge a needle in their arm, the court statement said the ruling paved the way for state and municipal governments to approve laws imposing fines or restrictive measures for vaccine refusers. Brazil's President Jair Bolsonaro repeatedly said he will not take any COVID-19 vaccine and opposes mandatory vaccination. Bolsonaro also expressed concern about the potential side effects of the vaccine [229]. Brazil's deputy Monster-of-Health Elcio Franco said that the country has no intention to, as every other country has done as a matter of course, draw up legislation to exempt COVID-19 vaccines manufacturers from liability. Franco said that vaccine manufacturers and the Brazilian government should have a non-binding memorandum on possible future purchases of vaccines against COVID-19, saying that the prices and target populations will be factors in deciding any purchase [230]. In essence, the Brazilian government has said it will mandate COVID-19 vaccines but will not compensate those injured or dying following vaccination.

Coercive abuse against Australians: This one had every human rights activist up in arms. On May 1st 2021, the Australian government Monster-of-Health, Greg Hunt, announced the strengthening of border controls, which included the introduction of AUD$66,600 fine or five years in imprisonment, or both, for rule-breakers. The Australian government had already banned all direct flights from India, leaving 9,000 Australians stranded in India, with 600 of these classified as vulnerable. These rules equate to fines for Australian citizens to simply return home from a 'COVID-ravished' place, even though there is a quarantine in place and testing available [231]. This abhorrent policy is reminiscent of Australia's White Australia policy that only ended in 1973, as it did not include people returning from 'COVID-ravished' UK or 'COVID-ravished' US. As we are seeing, COVID has seen the end of the era of Australians being "young and free".

Coercive abuse against Israelis; the 'freedom pass' and 'freedom bracelet': Israel is the place to watch as to how all our governments will follow suit and introduce the same coercive control measures. Mandatory vaccine certificates will soon be required everywhere to attend social gatherings or sporting events. On February 18th 2021, Israel announced that Israelis would require a 'green pass' to allow Israelis' entry into gyms, hotels and other public venues. The green pass is being issued to those that have proof that they have been vaccinated against, or have recovered from, COVID-19 [232]. On March 3rd 2021, Israel launched a tracking bracelet that monitors the wearer's movements and notifies authorities if the wearer violates mandatory quarantine. The system also alerts authorities when someone attempts to remove the bracelet or travels too far from home quarantine. The indoctrinated could be seen brandishing their 'freedom bracelet' and beaming through their masks like they had just won a prize [233]. This freedom is not the freedom I understand. On February 20th 2021, the daily propaganda reported that Israel's Ministry of Health said the COVID-19 rate of infection had dropped by 96% among those who had received both doses of the Pfizer vaccine. The Ministry of Health also reported that the vaccine was 99.2% effective in protecting against serious illness, 95.8% effective in reducing morbidity and 98.9% effective in decreasing hospitalisations [234]. Please note that this is not the prevention of infection. The daily propaganda fails to highlight that the data for these studies was collected 14 days after the second dose, therefore the vaccine was shown to be effective for 14 days. Additionally, the daily propaganda does not report that people in Israel who have recovered from COVID-19 are not eligible for a COVID-19 vaccine and are eligible for a 'green pass'. The same 'vaccine advertisement' also acknowledges that Israel plans to vaccinate children under 16 [235]. Israel is now vaccinating children for a disease that they are not at risk of, show no symptoms of and are not drivers of.

Israel's Ministry of Health reports that 92% of Israel's COVID-19 fatalities had preexisting chronic diseases. The daily propaganda also reported that deaths in Israelis over 80 had plummeted which suggested that the COVID-19 vaccines are working. This is not entirely correct in its interpretation, as trends in both overall cases and deaths can only reveal so much about the possible impact of vaccines, as these trends may similarly reflect the impact of lockdown or the effect of simple infection control measures such as washing one's hands. Controlled studies are needed to properly quantify the true effect of COVID-19 vaccinations. Instead, the Israeli government sets to rely on individual-level data that tracks who has and has not had the vaccine to untangle to what extent vaccines are driving down cases and deaths [236]. The daily propaganda also fails to report that on January 21st 2021, 12,400 Israeli's tested positive for coronavirus after receiving the Pfizer-BioNTech COVID-19 vaccine [237]. These Israelis got the 'green pass' to pass on their infection. As of June 2021, Israel is back in lockdown due to surging infection rates and is 'boosting' its population; doublespeak for 'boosting Pfizer shareholders' bank balances'.

Mandating vaccines in the workplace: US companies risk a backlash if they introduce mandatory COVID-19 vaccines as a precondition to be able to return to work. Corporate advisers warn that employers' desire to mandate vaccination will clash with deep concerns among many employees. In December 2020, a straw poll announced at a Yale School of Management summit of the chief executive officers (CEOs) of America's largest companies found that 71% of the 150 chief executives said they believed in vaccine mandates. The Society for Human Resource Management reported that 61% of its members planned to "encourage" employees to get the vaccine, and 38% see vaccination as, "very necessary" for the long-term sustainability of the organisation. Employees don't feel the same way, however. A CNBC/SurveyMonkey poll of more than 9,000 US workers found that 41% said they opposed mandatory workplace vaccines, and 25% strongly rejected the idea.

David Nabarro, a special envoy to the World Health Organisation's Director-General on COVID-19 told the *Financial Times*, "I'd be counselling against everybody assuming a mandatory vaccine at work is appropriate". Nabarro said companies had "a very important role" to play in encouraging widespread vaccination but should do so through transparent discussions with workers. CEO of the world's largest public relations firm, Richard Edelman, said that mandatory vaccines were "a venus fly trap for business". Edelman said that companies should be trying to inform and persuade employees about the benefits of vaccinations as opposed to risking the backlash of mandating vaccines. The law firm Gibson Dunn issued guidance to its clients that recommended employers should attempt to stay on the sidelines of the "vaccine wars" but were likely to find themselves at the coal face, "caught between public health imperatives, liability fears, and a restive workforce" (238).

"Vaccine war"; I couldn't have put it better myself. A Harvard Law School post looking at the relevant statutory provision to examine whether an EUA can accommodate vaccine mandates says there is a legal argument that the Secretary of Health and Human Services has the discretion to allow businesses to require vaccines and impose consequences for refusal (239). It appears that businesses can mandate employees and customers get vaccinated with experimental biological agents under EUA. As I write in August 2021, CNN is firing its unvaccinated workforce. At this time also, the FDA gave full authorisation to the Pfizer vaccine on August 23rd 2021. Bear in mind that the FDA also approved birth defect causing thalidomide, heart attack causing Vioxx, deadly addictive OxyContin, ephedrine sulphate injections for pigs aimed for the human consumption, autism causing sodium valproate etc.

Mandating COVID-19 vaccines for Irish healthcare workers: In Ireland, healthcare workers (HCWs) who refuse vaccination are being threatened with removal. The Health Service Executive (HSE) chief executive Paul Reid says Health and Safety Act allows for the removal of staff from frontline positions. The HSE chief has suggested that HCWs who refuse to take the vaccine may be removed from their posts. Mr guilt tripper Reid said it was "inexcusable" for any HCWs who work with patients not to take the vaccine. He said everyone had a right to refuse a vaccine if they wished, but the Health and Safety Act allowed for workers to be removed if they were regarded as a threat to other people [(240)]. The CEO of the HSE knows that HCWs have the highest lack of confidence in vaccines. According to the WHO, vaccination rates among European HCWs are generally less than 30% [(241, 242)]. The vast majority of HCWs refuse to take the recommended vaccines for European HCWs which include, influenza, MMR, hepatitis B, pertussis and varicella (chickenpox) vaccines [(243)]. No one is currently exempt from the threat of mandatory vaccines. HCWs globally are currently being fired left, right and centre.

Mandatory vaccine certificates to travel: The experts say don't do it. On February 5th 2021, the World Wealth Organisation's position (until they changed their position) was that that they were not recommending that national authorities and conveyance operators (transport operators) require proof of COVID-19 vaccination for international travel as a condition for departure or entry. The WHO made this announcement based on what they described as the still critical unknowns regarding the efficacy of vaccination in reducing the transmission of the virus. Additionally, the WHO considered that given that there is limited availability of vaccines, preferential vaccination of travellers may result in inadequate vaccine supplies in priority populations considered at high risk of severe COVID-19 disease. The WHO also recommended that vaccinated people should not be exempt from complying with other travel risk-reduction measures [(244)]. The European Union (EU) are not listening to the 'experts' at the WHO. Instead, the EU 'authorities' rolled out a Digital Green Certificate for the summer of 2021. Gloria Guevara, chief executive of the World Travel and Tourism Council, opposed making COVID-19 vaccinations a requirement for travellers saying such moves would be similar to workplace discrimination. "We should never require the vaccination to get a job or to travel" [(245)].

Travel restrictions violate international law: According to the *American Association for the Advancement of Science* magazine under the International Health Regulations (2005) (IHR), binding on all WHO member states, health measures "shall not be more restrictive of international traffic and not more invasive or intrusive to persons than reasonably available alternatives". Rather than violating IHR obligations, what is supposed to happen is that the necessity of travel bans must be weighed against less restrictive alternatives such as community-based public health measures, including social distancing and contact tracing and are considered proportional. Yet we continue to live under ineffective public health measures and continue to see 'record cases'. We have no right to travel or severe financial limitations set on our right to travel. For my family of six to travel, the compulsory polymerase chain reaction (PCR) tests alone would cost €1800 [(246)]. Financial coercion is bad economics.

More 'green' and 'health' passes than you can shake a stick at: On February 13th 2021, Tony weapons of mass distraction Blair, came out of his cave to push the vaccine passport agenda, telling us they are "inevitable". Blair described the soon to be common cold as a "national security issue" and a "global security issue". Blair's Vaccination Credential Initiative is a coalition of Big Tech and healthcare companies, including Microsoft, the Mayo Clinic, Oracle, Mitre, Cerner, the Carin Alliance and Salesforce. According to the initiative's website, the group is working together to create a "trustworthy, traceable, verifiable, and universally recognised digital record of vaccination status" that would allow people to "safely return to work, school, events, and travel" [(247)]. This is no less that state control.

On December 16th 2020, British cyber technology company VST Enterprises (VSTE) launched a 'fit to fly' V-Health Passport aimed at air travel. The V-Health Passport is a cross-border platform that can be downloaded by the public, airlines and transport carriers and used with multiple forms of COVID-19 testing and vaccination. The V-Health Passport aims to validate a passenger's ID and authenticate their COVID-19 test result and vaccination status. The health passport does not use unsecured bar codes and QR code technology [(248)]. On January 27th 2021, VSTE announced that the V-Health

Passport technology was being produced to avoid the risks facing airports, airlines and passengers from invalid COVID-19 test certificates, vaccination records and the use of health passports using QR and bar code technology which is not General Data Protection Regulation (GDPR) compliant. VSTE say their passport is built on a privacy framework of "self sovereign identity" where the user can choose what information they want to share and is therefore GDPR compliant [249]. Back in November 2020, the International Air Transport Association (IATA) announced that it was in the final stages of developing a mobile phone app called the IATA Travel Pass, which would enable travellers to easily confirm both their identification and COVID-19 vaccine status at airports. The digital travel pass will display a record of an individual's test results, proof of vaccination and link to an electronic copy of the user's passport for identity verification [250]. Travel being dependent on biometric ID and vaccine status was always on the cards.

You don't need a vaccine to travel! People need to know that these passports being introduced by the ruling class won't only be given to vaccinated people. That is propaganda aimed to generate interest in and increase uptake of vaccines. The immune passports, similarly to exemptions from vaccination in Australia, can be provided to people with either vaccine-induced artificial immunity or natural immunity. The issuing of immunity passports can be based on either a laboratory test of immune response (a correlate of protection/specific immune marker) or an immunising event (infection or vaccination). Both methods are equally able to identify individuals less susceptible to acquiring the disease and/ or transmitting the virus [251]. In June 2021, my friend flew from Germany to Romania, 'green' to 'green', no test, no vax, no doc, and has since made this trip again. In June also, mo fhear céile (man together/Irish for husband) went from Ireland to the UK to drink in pubs. He took the ferry; no test, no vax, no doc. The passports are a short-term goal only and a smokescreen. As discussed in Chapter 21, 'Chips, Dots and Bots, on-person vaccine records are coming. A skin scratch test to determine preexisting natural immunity to COVID-19 is also on the cards as discussed in Chapter 17, 'Natural Immunity'.

Mandatory quarantine on arrival: Thanks, New Zealand Prime Minister Jacinda speaks-to-us-like-she's-a-woman Ardern and Australian Prime Minister ScoMo the clown. In January 2021, Ireland, part of the European

Union, decided it identified as New Zealand. Irish public health 'specialist' Professor Anthony Staines on humanity of the Independent Scientific Advocacy Group (ISAG) for COVID-19 in Ireland said that many countries across Europe are concluding that the only way to curb COVID-19 "is to bring this virus sharply under control" introducing tighter measures on isolation and mandatory quarantine. Professor Staines on humanity said that "If this is not done, the consequences will be on all of our heads" (252). Off with your head Professor Staines. Professor Staines is not a specialist in EU affairs, as Ireland was the only country in the EU as of June 2021, to introduce mandatory 'hotel' quarantine.

Re-education centres for COVID dissidents: On January 19th 2020, it was reported that the German government announced it was building a special COVID detention centre in Dresden. The jail is also known as a 'pandemic hotel'. Whilst these detention facilities are currently intended for COVID dissidents, very soon, I am sure with the aim to generate interest in and increase uptake of vaccines, that the impression will be given that those who refuse the experimental biological injection will end up in the gulag (253).

Pure tyranny: Some examples of our ruling class in full swing; In December 2020, a French court ruled that an elderly woman diagnosed with dementia must pay a fine of €166 for incorrectly filling out her 'form for leaving home during lockdown'. The elderly lady put the wrong date on her form (254). In December 2020 also, an Italian man ended up walking 450km after leaving the house to cool off after an argument with his wife and received a €400 fine for breaching the curfew (255). In China, a woman was publicly shamed when a man leaked her personal details online after she tested positive for COVID-19. Publically outing and openly shaming people that are diagnosed with COVID-19 became normalised (256). Tyranny swings both ways; "When the people fear the government, that's tyranny; when the government fears the people, that's freedom". A spurious quote commonly misattributed to Thomas Jefferson (257).

Coercive control using vile media guilt trips: At the end of 2020, Professor of guilt-tripping ICU doctor Hugh Montgomery said COVID-19 rule-breakers "have blood on their hands" (258). That's libel. There is zero proof that anyone's actions to live freely causes harm to another. The award for the vilest piece of fearmongering on the daily propaganda goes to the *LA Times* journalists, Rong-Gong Lin Li and Luke Money, for their jaw-dropping headline "children apologise to their dying elders for spreading COVID-19" [259]. It gets worse. The NHS charity Together made an advertisement showing highly vulnerable Santa ending up as COVID fodder on life support. This disturbing video was withdrawn as it caused post-traumatic stress disorder in children. Together excused this abhorrent display of media scaremongering by saying that they didn't think little children would be paying attention to an advertisement showing Santa getting hospitalised with COVID and the NHS saving the day. The mental health of our children is clearly not at the forefront of their agenda [260].

Coercion of our children through education: Bill Gates is not intent on ruining our existence; he wants to ruin our children's existence. In this video entitled 'The Bill Gates Microsoft Magic Pass', a little girl expressed her fear and anxiety about returning to school. "Mom, I'm scared about going back to school...I don't wanna get sick; I don't wanna get you and dad sick". The video describes an application Gates has designed to make our children feel 'safe'. The app allows you to schedule your COVID-19 test, and as soon as vaccines come online, schedule your vaccination in your "daily task" (WT!). Then "your entrance ticket appears like magic". The school scans the phones on entry whilst the children are muzzled and socially distanced. The child says, "I felt so safe". The only lesson our children need is how to stay safe from their government [261].

Useless testing of our asymptomatic children: On February 13th 2021, the UK government, desperate to keep the pandemonium going, suggested that families of secondary school pupils administer lateral flow tests at home twice weekly to their completely healthy, asymptomatic children [262]. It goes without saying that these lateral flow tests are reliable enough to keep us in lockdown however are not reliable enough to be used for travel.

Mandating COVID-19 vaccines in Irish Schools is on the table: Norma Foley Monster for Education used her time while we were in lockdown to use the Irish Courts to try and exclude home-schooled students from the Leaving Certificate calculated grades process. This is after we parents homeschooled for the best part of a whole year! The court deemed Foley's attempts as unfair and unlawful. A three judge Court of Appeal (COA) concluded it was, *"unreasonable and disproportionate"*, and an unlawful breach of the students' constitutional rights [263]. In a video posted on Twaddle (*Twitter*), Irish journalist Gemma O'Doherty revealed The Teachers' Union of Ireland (TUI) Ireland had scheduled a discussion for their annual meeting in April 2021. Among the topics for the meeting to discuss were mandatory masks for primary and secondary school children and mandatory vaccines. In the video Gemma reads the section on vaccines from the preliminary agenda for the meeting:

> *"It is necessary that society uses all medical tools available to enable a return to face to face classroom teaching...To that end, the uptake of a COVID-19 vaccine should be a requirement for entering and continuing physical attendance in a school. Congress instructs the executive to negotiate with the Department of Education and Skills (DES) that a recognised and required national document be instituted that evidence that a COVID-19 vaccine has been administered other than for those with valid medical exemptions"* [264].

This hasn't happened yet; my lot returned to school on August 30th 2021.

Self-policing: As an Irish republican whose forefathers and foremothers fought for our liberty, self-policing irks me the most. People in Ireland were invited to apply online using a new high-tech system that will track the "rollout of new COVID vaccine"; doublespeak for 'monitoring and tracking those who have complied and taken the shot [265].' In May 2021, a hotline was set up in Donegal to allow people to dob in their neighbours if they were organising an event that was in breach of COVID guidelines. Hilariously, the phone line was inundated with calls from people flooding it with conspiracy theories and crank calls, and the phone line was called a "beacon for lunatics" [266]. Good to see the Irish sense of humour still thriving. I wish the Irish sense of freedom was as astute.

Joints for jabs: This is a new low for the Mardigrassers. On January 11th 2021, earth-loving pot smokers began pushing the pharmaceutical product that will decimate the global shark and horseshoe crab population and pillage and plunder our rivers and lakes for glass. DC Marijuana Justice (DCMJ) which normally fights for equal rights for cannabis and helped legalised cannabis in DC in 2014 released a 'Joints For Jabs' Press Release. The next obvious move after legalising cannabis will be mandating vaccines. Every civil libertarian nowadays wants everybody to be equal and free to identify as a pencil, as long as you don't identify as someone who will not get injected with a foreign substance made in a laboratory by some zany scientist looking to win a Nobel Prize in Physiology and Medicine [267].

Calling us fascists and racists: Name-calling is a tool of coercion which is discussed further in Chapter 4, 'Vaccine Refusal and the Age of Censorship'. A 'reporter' from a local Irish rag, the Connaught trials and tribulations in Galway took words from one of my freedom rally speeches out of context to label me as a fascist and a racist. After a little tête-à-tête, said journalist said to me that someone at the protest had mentioned Sharia Law. At that stage, I understood his agenda. His job is to paint me as a fascist, and my job is to get his attention. In December 2020, it was announced that a group of public figures and various social justice groups launched 'Le Chéile' (Irish for together) to combat the rise of the far-right in Ireland. This movement says that far-right organisations have been present at some Irish anti-lockdown demonstrations. Have they? Freedom rallies have people from all walks of life stand *le chéile* for freedom. Le Chéile's says their primary aim is to "discuss, talk about, raise awareness and educate" about far-right elements. Christy Moore, Damien Dempsey and Vincent Browne support the campaign to denigrate us who want to live freely. The alliance is campaigning under the slogan of #DiversityNotDivision [268]. How about #DiversityInVaccineStatus or #NoDivisionByVaccineStatus?

Antifa are tools of coercive control: Antifa (anti-fascist/anti-racist) label pro-freedom, pro-choice protesters 'fascists and racists'. The Irish off-shoot of Antifa is completely extraneous. An article published in the *Irish Political Studies Journal* remarks that it is unusual for an organisation such as Antifa to exist in Ireland without a coherent far-right. Author Jonathon Arlow, from the School of Law and Government Dublin City University, said Antifa exists in Ireland for three reasons. Firstly, anti-fascism acts to bring the radical left together in a way that rises above the usual ideological divisions to unite a fragmented radical left base. Secondly, Arlow said that in the absence of an effective far-right, anti-fascism acts as prophylaxis. Thirdly, Arlow said that the appeal of anti-fascist activism is due to common ancestry and evolutionary history, which increases the appeal of anti-fascist activism, even in the absence of a far-right threat [269].

Antifa are farcical: By their pro-lockdown and pro-freedom from responsibility counter-protests, Antifa has demonstrated a shameful lack of knowledge of the devastating effects of lockdowns on the very groups of the population they supposedly stand with. Antifa supports black lives matter (BLM). COVID-19 lockdowns don't support BLM. COVID-19 lockdowns disproportionally affect Black and Brown communities. Indigenous and Black Americans have suffered the highest mortality (death) and morbidity (disease) rates, followed by Pacific Islanders, Latinos and Black populations [(270)]. Racial disproportionality in COVID-19 clinical trials exists. Whilst being the demographic overrepresented in the COVID-19 cases and deaths, Black, Asian and minority ethnic (BAME) communities (a UK demographic) are underrepresented in COVID-19 clinical research [(271)].

Antifa supports Free Palestine. COVID-19 lockdowns don't support Palestinian freedom. The UN Office for the Coordination of Humanitarian Affairs (UNOCHA) say Palestinians are suffering from increased hunger, poverty and conflict caused by COVID-19 lockdowns. COVID-19 lockdowns jeopardise the Israel-Gaza ceasefire. Gwyn Lewis, Director of the United Nations Relief and Works Agency for Palestine Refugees in the Near East (UNRWA) Operations in the West Bank, further highlighted the grave socioeconomic conditions facing Palestinians. Lewis said, "With the pandemic, we've seen quite a dramatic impact on the economy. 40% of households on the West Bank kept seeing their income decline by more than half, (and) unemployment increased in the camps by as high as 23%. In Gaza, unemployment has hit 49%, which is very, very dramatic" [(272)]. After Israel's occupation ten year land, air and sea blockade of Gaza, farming in Gaza was already an uncertain way to make a living. COVID-19 lockdowns have made a bad situation worse, with farmers growing increasingly desperate as an already struggling pre-pandemic economy now struggles even more [(273)].

A UN Women's report entitled *COVID-19: Gendered Impacts of the Pandemic in Palestine and Implications for Policy and Programming,* says that Palestinian women are experiencing greater suffering due to COVID-19 lockdown restrictions to other health services. The UN report found that lockdown disproportionally affects women and reinforces patriarchal norms [(274)]. An article published in the *Health and Human Rights Journal* in February 2021 expressed concerns that the global COVID-19 vaccines rollout is creating division between the vaccinated and the unvaccinated. The new subclass of unvaccinated people includes prisoners, Palestinians, and those affected by armed conflict [(275)]. Under Ramallah's coronavirus vaccination plan, Palestinians in the West Bank and Gaza are to receive AstraZeneca, Moderna, the Chinese Sinopharm and the Russian Sputnik V. Palestinians see both Sinopharm and Sputnik V as controversial due to the lack of transparency in their testing procedures and some health experts initially expressing scepticism about their safety and effectiveness. A senior Palestinian Health Ministry Authority official said that Palestinians are vaccine-hesitant about taking the Sputnik V and Sinopharm COVID-19 vaccines [(276)]. Antifa wants Palestinians to be 'free' to shut up obey and take their shot.

Antifa are the true fascists. Antifa doesn't respect a person's right to choose. Antifa supports a woman's right to choose to abort her baby but not that women's right to choose not to vaccinate her baby. Antifa supports a person's right to self-identify, but not a person's right to identify as someone who is pro-natural immunity. Antifa supports boycotting Israeli products to 'Free Palestine' but does not support boycotting drugs to protect the environment. Antifa supports 'Free Palestine' whilst denigrating people who stand to free our countries from the tyranny of emergency COVID laws. If we want to 'Free Palestine', we must first free ourselves then ensure our right to stand for Palestinian freedom is protected. Our right to protest is under threat globally. New security bills mean police can record the public with body cameras and drones, yet the public risk massive fines or imprisonment for filming police. These laws are designed to quash all protests, not only 'anti-lockdown' protests [(136)].

CHAPTER FOUR

VACCINE REFUSAL & THE AGE OF CENSORSHIP

"First they came for the Communists
And I did not speak out
Because I was not a Communist
Then they came for the Socialists
And I did not speak out
Because I was not a Socialist
Then they came for the trade unionists
And I did not speak out
Because I was not a trade unionist
Then they came for the Jews
And I did not speak out
Because I was not a Jew
Then they came for me
And there was no one left
To speak out for me".

Pastor Martin Niemöller (277)

This is the age of censorship. Censorship is a tool used by our coercive controllers. Pro-natural immunity advocates have no voice. I'd like to share here that only now, Barnes & Noble, Kobo, Apple, Tolino and Vivlio blocked distribution of *COVERT-19 What Public Health Won't Tell You*. The front cover didn't pass their compliance test. How naïve I was to think that I could publish my book through the censorship mechanism. If you are reading this, you know I have prevailed. Enough of calling anti-vaxxers stupid! Enough also of calling us vaccine-hesitant! I refuse vaccines because I am pro-natural immunity. Public health uses the daily propaganda to drown our voices and to push the narrative that vaccine hesitancy is a mystery, and the people who don't vaccinate are unable to reason and need educating. One should notice that vaccine refusers are rarely interviewed on the mainstream media. If I were interviewed I would share my opinion of their Gatesist UNICEF campaign calling on parents to vaccinate their children; #VaccinesWork. I have got a few catchy hashtags;

- #COVID-19VaccinesWorkFor7days
- #COVID-19VaccinesAreSafeFor2Months
- #COVID-19VaccineInducedProthromboticImmune-Thrombocytopenia
- # MyocarditisPericarditisFollowingmRNACovid-19Vaccine

The demographics of vaccine refusal in society: Being concerned about vaccine safety is not something that affects people with low IQs, quite the opposite in fact. Demographically speaking, the uneducated and poor vaccinate their children. Parents who do not vaccinate their children at all are statistically the richest and the smartest. There is a stark difference between undervaccinated and unvaccinated. Undervaccinated children tend to be black, born to young single mothers without a college degree, live in poverty and come from the inner city. Completely unvaccinated children tend to be white, born to married mothers with college degrees, and come from a household on an annual income exceeding US$75,000, whose parents expressed concerns regarding the safety of vaccines. The parents of unvaccinated children make their own decision about vaccination for their children, stating their doctors have little influence (278).

The demographics of vaccine refusal in Europe: The 'philanthropic' *Wellcome Global Monitor* website monitors how people around the world think and feel about science and primary health issues. According to Wellcome, in general, the richer a country is, the less its citizens agree that vaccines are safe. 72% of United States (US) and Canadian citizens believe vaccines are safe. 73% of citizens in the northern European arc, including Ireland, the United Kingdom (UK), through the Nordic countries, believe vaccines are safe. Confidence in vaccines is lower in Germany, France, Austria, Switzerland and the Benelux countries, where 59% on average believe vaccines are safe. Only 50% of Eastern Europeans believe vaccines are safe (279).

The demographics of vaccine refusal in Australia: In Australia, the most vaccine-hesitant group in society (other than healthcare workers) are the richest and the smartest. In North Shore Sydney and Byron Bay, Australia's richest suburbs, only 70.5% of five year old children are fully vaccinated. These suburbs also happen to be the most educated areas in Australia, where 48.9% of the population hold a Bachelor degree or higher (280).

The demographics of vaccine refusal in Ireland, the UK and California: The story continues that the richest and the most educated are the least likely to vaccinate their children at all. Parents in the wealthiest parts of Ireland are also the most likely to refuse vaccines for their children. The measles-mumps-rubella (MMR) vaccine uptake among infants in richer southeast Dublin, Dún Laoghaire, south county Dublin and east Wicklow was 87% in 2019, compared with 95% in the poorer Mayo, Galway and Roscommon [(281)]. Berkshire, near Windsor in the UK, has lower MMR vaccination rates than its poorer neighbours [(282)]. According to *Forbes*, Berkshire is one of the wealthiest counties [(283)]. Speaking of Windsor, I wonder, do the Saxe-Coburg-Gothas, or Windsors, vaccinate their prodigies? Statistically speaking, it is highly unlikely. The daily propaganda, of course, reported that the Duke and Duchess of Cambridge received their 'vaccine'. A study looking at the sociodemographic predictors of vaccination exemptions based on personal beliefs in 6,200 California schools published in the *American Journal of Public Health* found that vaccine exemptions were twice as common among those children attending private institutions [(284)]. It is highly unlikely that Zuckerberg's newborn daughters received a hepatitis B vaccine within the first 24 hours of life as Australian babies are compelled to.

Healthcare workers are the most vaccine-hesitant group in society: Healthcare workers (HCWs) are considered to be the most trusted source of vaccine-related information for patients, yet demographically speaking, HCWs have the highest lack of confidence in vaccines. According to the World Wealth Organisation, vaccination rates amongst HCWs are also low throughout Europe, with vaccination coverage among HCWs generally less than 30% [(241, 242)]. This is no conspiracy. 70% of European HCWs refuse recommended vaccines for themselves. According to the WHO, vaccine hesitancy is one of the top ten threats to global health [(285)]. Thus vaccine-hesitant HCWs are one of the ten top threats to global health. This ludicrous name-calling is a purposeful tactic employed by Heidi Larson and her behavioural psychologist peanut gallery to be inflammatory and divisive. Heidi's surveillance and censorship machine, known as the Vaccine Confidence Project, is discussed later in this chapter.

An Irish Health Protection Surveillance Centre (HPSC) report 2017-2018 looked at HCW vaccine uptake in public hospitals and found that influenza vaccine uptake for HCW was 44.8%, up from 34.0% [(286)]. Public Health

England (PHE) fair better at seasonal influenza vaccine uptake ranging from 64.2%-80.8%, yet still only 27.5% of all PHE trusts achieve the desired vaccine uptake rates of 75% or more [(287)]. The 2017 to 2018 influenza season in England saw 68.7% of all frontline HCWs reported as having received the seasonal influenza vaccine [(288)]. An audit of Australian doctors revealed only 28% received influenza immunisation in 2007, down from 44% in any prior year [(289)]. Importantly even with Australia's mandatory vaccinations for HCWs, vaccination uptake rates are still below 50% [(290)]. HCWs need to know they have the power as health authorities cannot logistically fire half the workforce.

Vaccine refusal in general practitioners: In France, 16% to 43% of 1,712 randomly selected general practitioners (GPs) "sometimes or never" recommend at least one specific vaccine to their target patients. It was found that GPs were more likely to recommend a vaccine if they felt comfortable explaining their benefits and risks to patients or trusted official sources of information. GPs recommended vaccines more infrequently if they considered adverse effects likely or lacked confidence in the vaccine's effectiveness [(291)]. A total of 3% of French GPs were 'highly hesitant' or 'opposed' to vaccination, 11% 'moderately hesitant', and 6% were 'not' or only 'slightly' vaccine-hesitant. Both 'highly hesitant', 'opposed to vaccination' and 'moderately hesitant' were themselves less frequently vaccinated [(292)]. An American study found 11% of the 1,251 physicians successfully surveyed did not recommend to parents that children receive all recommended vaccines according to the Centres for Disease Control and Prevention (CDC) schedule [(293)]. Despite current recommendations, a cross-sectional study of Pakistanis GPs published in 2018 showed a very low proportion of doctors in Pakistan were vaccinated against influenza [(294)].

Vaccination practices among general practitioners and their children: In September 2012, 93% of the surveyed GPs agreed with the current official vaccination recommendations and would apply them to their own children. However, the observation that 5% of non-paediatricians would not use Haemophilus influenzae type b (Hib) vaccine if they had a child born in 2004 was said to be "unexpected and concerning". In contrast, both groups gave additional vaccines than those recommended to their own children. Among physicians in Switzerland interested in immunisation, a significant proportion of non-paediatricians decline or delay the immunisation of their own children with the recommended MMR-or DTP-based combination vaccines, with GPs displaying concern due to "immune overload". Members of the Academy of Paediatrics were randomly surveyed with the aim to identify vaccination patterns of both GPs and subspecialists with regard to their own children. Survey questions included how GPs with children vaccinated them in the past and how respondents would vaccinate a child in 2009. Up until 2009, general paediatricians and paediatric specialists largely adhered to the Advisory Committee on Immunisation Practices (ACIP) recommendations. When asked about vaccinating a child in the future, a significant proportion of respondents noted they would deviate from CDC guidelines. 21% of specialists compared to 9% general paediatricians reported a greater willingness to diverge from CDC recommendations due to vaccine safety and other concerns (295). How have these poor paediatrician's belief systems gone so awry?

Global COVID-19 vaccine refusal: A global survey of more than 13,400 people in 19 countries on potential acceptance of a COVID-19 vaccine published in *Nature Medicine* in October 2020, found that Polish citizens had the greatest vaccine hesitancy reporting the highest proportion of negative responses at 27.3%. Sweden, Germany, and Spain were more sceptical than the US and South Korea (296). A more recent University of Warsaw study in May 2021 however, indicated that 40% of the Polish population had refused the COVID-19 vaccine (297). A European survey on willingness to be vaccinated against COVID-19 was published in June 2020. In total, 73.9% of the 7664 participants from Denmark, France, Germany, Italy, Portugal, the Netherlands, and the UK stated that they would be willing to get vaccinated against COVID-19. 18.9% of respondents stated that they were not sure, and 7.2% stated that they would refuse a COVID-19 vaccine. The willingness to be vaccinated for COVID-19 ranged from 62% in France to approximately 80% in Denmark and the UK. Germany and France contained the largest proportions of the population opposed to a COVID-19 vaccination. France also has the largest group of people unsure about receiving the COVID-19 vaccine at 28% (298). The French are the most vaccine-hesitant in Europe. Ironically France also has the strictest mandatory vaccine laws in Europe, proving that mandating vaccines decreases people's confidence in vaccines. In January 2021, a survey by pollster Ifop for the newspaper Le Journal du Dimanche found that 59% of French people do "not have the intention to get a vaccination when it becomes possible". This was up from 46% found in an earlier Ipsos poll from late October 2020. Regarding confidence in vaccines, France ranked last out of 15 countries trailing behind the UK (79%), Germany (69%), and Italy (65%) (299). A Eurofound survey published in May 2021 found that, in general, over 25% of European adults would refuse the COVID-19 vaccine (300). That is 25% of us that are not being represented and need to make our voices heard. It would not surprise me at all if vaccine uptake is overstated and vaccine refusal is understated. The Thought Police know that truth is more contagious than COVID.

COVID-19 vaccine refusal in healthcare workers in Europe: HCWs are also the most COVID-19 vaccine-hesitant group in society. Billions of COVID-19 vaccines are being rolled out globally amid a high degree of vaccine scepticism. The possibility of mandatory COVID-19 vaccines for HCWs raises serious ethical issues and prompts ethical debate; doublespeak for 'promotes censoring' (301). A survey of COVID-19 vaccine hesitancy in Maltese family GPs and their trainees found that vaccine hesitancy is greater in the young, with 33% of senior doctors compared to 66% of junior doctors saying they would refuse the COVID-19 vaccine (302). A video with German Doctor Dr Heiko Schöning introduces Netherlands Dr Elke De Klerk. De Klerk says 87,000 nurses in the Netherlands will refuse the COVID-19 vaccine because they don't want to be, as they say in the Netherlands, a COVID-19 vaccine "rabbit" (303). In 2017 there were 171,140 nurses employed in the care sector in the Netherlands, meaning that greater than half of all Netherlands nurses will refuse a COVID-19 vaccine.

On January 7th 2021, *The Irish Times* reported on a poll conducted by BioNTech that was released in Germany in December 2020, which found that 50% of surveyed nurses and 25% of doctors would refuse the COVID-19 vaccine. The paper reported doctors and nurses as being "vaccine shy" rather than 'anti-vaxxers posing the greatest threat to humanity and global security' (304). A French poll of 2000 HCWs in December 2020 found that 76 % of senior care home staff said they would refuse the COVID-19 vaccine. According to Austria's public broadcaster, half of Austrian care facilities staff in the region of Vorarlberg refused the COVID-19 vaccine (279). The Italian Federation of Medical Professional Associations said about 100 doctors had refused the COVID-19 vaccine. Italian doctors concerned about taking an unlicensed experimental vaccine under Emergency Use Authorisation (EUA) were accused of "promoting anti-vaccination propaganda" [305]. How have these poor European HCW's belief systems gone so awry?

COVID-19 vaccine refusal in healthcare workers in the US: The Kaiser Family Foundation in the US released a survey in December 2020 that found that 29% of US HCWs would 'probably refuse' or 'definitely refuse' a COVID-19 vaccine (304). Following similar lines, in February 2021, a survey in *Medscape* reported that 33% of US HCWs are distrustful about COVID-19 vaccines [306]. The Kaiser Family Foundation released a later survey in March 2021 with a more radical outcome showing that 48% of HCWs had refused the COVID-19 vaccine [307]. In December 2020, an anonymous survey of employees across the Yale Medicine and Yale New Haven Health system conducted at the time the Pfizer-BioNTech vaccine received FDA approval found that 17% of HCWs would refuse the COVID-19 vaccine in the first wave of the rollout [308]. At the beginning of January 2021, *Forbes* reported on the large numbers of American HCWs, emergency service workers and frontline workers who had refused the COVID-19 vaccine. Governor Mike DeWine said that 60% of nursing home staff in Ohio had refused the COVID-19 vaccine. In December 2020, the chief of critical care at Houston's United Memorial Medical Centre, Dr Joseph Varon, reported more than 50% of the nurses in his unit intended to refuse the COVID-19 vaccine [309].

By January 31st 2021, *The Wall Street Journal* was already reporting that efforts to distribute COVID-19 vaccines had plateaued as HCWs were refusing the COVID-19 vaccine. In New York, Governor Andrew Cuomo said that state officials were expecting that 30% of HCWs would refuse the COVID-19 vaccine. A massive 66% of HCWs in a Florida hospital refused the COVID-19 vaccine, leaving so many unused doses that the hospital donated the vaccines to the general proletariat [310]. More than 50% of hospital workers at St Elizabeth Community Hospital in Tehama County refused the COVID-19 vaccine. Dr Nikhila Juvvadi, the chief clinical officer at Chicago's Loretto Hospital, reported that 40% of the hospital staff refused the COVID-19 vaccine [309]. How have these poor American HCW's belief systems gone so awry? This is no conundrum.

COVID-19 vaccine refusal in healthcare workers in the rest of the world: A study looking at the acceptability of COVID-19 vaccination in HCWs from the Democratic Republic of the Congo found that 72.3% of Congolese

HCWs would refuse the COVID-19 vaccine [311]. A survey conducted in April 2020 among Israeli HCWs found that only 61% of nurses and 78% of doctors say they would be willing to get vaccinated, with safety being the biggest concern [312]. Even in the ruling class' precious Israeli model, 22% of Israeli doctors and 39% of Israeli nurses refused the COVID-19 vaccine.

US Military COVID-19 vaccine refusal: The US military is reflecting other frontline professions in having high levels of COVID-19 vaccine refusal. Pentagon officials said that 33% of all military troops have refused the COVID-19 vaccine. Anthony Fauci accused these military servicemen and women of being "part of the problem" [313]. Perhaps they will be healthier in the long run and be part of the national security solution. Nearly 40% of US Marines refused the COVID-19 vaccine. This has prompted some Democrats to urge President Biden-his-time-until-Kamala-takes-over to mandate the COVID-19 vaccines for the military [314]. How have these poor American military service personnel's belief systems gone so awry?

COVID-19 vaccine refusal in non-essential workers: The Firefighters Association president reported in December 2020 that 55% of New York Fire Department firefighters refused the COVID-19 vaccine. In January 2021, *The Los Angeles Times* reported that 50% of frontline workers in Riverside, Calif refused the COVID-19 vaccine and that hospital and public health officials were forced to figure out how best to allocate unused vaccine doses. Between 20% and 40% of LA County's frontline workers refused the COVID-19 vaccine [309]. A probability-based internet panel survey conducted by the CDC in 3,541 adults between September 3rd and October 1st 2020, reported that only 63% of non-essential workers surveyed intended to receive the vaccine [315]. 27% of non-essential workers in the US have refused the COVID-19 vaccine. How have these poor American non-essential worker's belief systems gone so awry?

Supply now outstripping demand: On May 7th 2021, *The Irish Times* reported that the US vaccination rollout was slowing due to diminishing demand and that America was redeploying unused vaccines to regional areas to avoid wastage. Some US states addressed the issue of oversupply of the COVID-19 vaccine by giving out free beer; other states paid people US$100 to take the vaccine [316]. In April 2021, the Associated Press News reported that public health officials and pharmacists were seeing supply outstrip demand for COVID-19 vaccines. Approximately half of Iowa's counties stopped requesting new doses from the state, and the state of Louisiana had not requested shipment of COVID-19 vaccines for the whole month. A pharmacist in Mississippi named Robin Jackson described "practically begging anyone in the community to show up and get shots". The pharmacist said, "Nobody was coming, and I mean no one". Barber County, Kansas, had turned down COVID-19 vaccines from the state in two out of the past four weeks. In early April 2021, Republican Governor Tate Reeves said Mississippi officials had requested that the federal government deliver the COVID-19 vaccine in smaller packages to avoid waste [(317)]. On February 7th 2021, it was reported that the coronavirus vaccination centre in east London has had to close early three days in a row. The temporary facility housed at The John Scott centre in Hackney had been administering vaccines from 10 am until 8 pm every day but had to close at 2 pm due to lack of interest [(318)]. We are not all as eager to inject an experimental unlicensed medical product created at breakneck speed.

The Chinese aren't rushing for their shot either: Chinese health officials aren't making the COVID-19 vaccine mandatory. The reported goal in China was to vaccinate 40% of the population by the end of July 2021, which is what Chinese Health officials say is needed to achieve herd immunity by the end of 2021, in time for the 2022 Beijing Winter Olympics. Perhaps there is some genetic explanation as to why the herd immunity level for the Chinese is 40% and ours is 90%. The reality is that their strict control of the virus (population) paradoxically means that very few people are motivated to get vaccinated. As of March 2021, only about 4% of China's population had received the COVID-19 vaccine [(319)]. Australia's strict control (of the population) measures have also resulted in a very low COVID-19 vaccine uptake. On a positive note, 'successful' suppression of the population successfully increases vaccine hesitancy.

COVID-19 Vaccine Refusal in Sporting Celebrities

Olympic athletes: United States Olympic & Paralympics Committee (USOPC) medical chief Jon Finnoff said take-up of the COVID-19 vaccine in Olympic athletes would not be mandatory. Finnoff said, "I have had athletes raise concerns about are there any long-term ramifications associated with it, if I have the vaccine is there the potential that it will impede my performance?" *Reuters* reported that hesitancy was due to the fear of potentially causing one to fail a doping test however, Finnoff said, "I have not had any athlete raise a concern specifically with me about whether the vaccines can cause a positive (doping) test". The boffins want to paint our world class athletes as unable to reason and reeducate them. The International Olympic Committee (IOC) said COVID-19 vaccines would not be mandated ahead of the Tokyo Games. Finnoff in fact expressed concerns around virus mutations and variants that may escape vaccines (320).

Rugby star Carlin Isles said he feels he has a robust immune system strong enough to fend off any serious illness. Isles said, "I've definitely had my doubts about getting the shot". The near 600 American athletes headed for the Tokyo Olympics in late July had varying opinions about the need to protect themselves against infection. The athletes expressed concerns about the rare but dangerous blood clots linked to Johnson & Johnson (J&J) COVID-19 vaccines. Other concerns expressed were that even mild side effects from a vaccine would disrupt their preparation for the games. Shooting team member Ginny Thrasher scheduled her second dose of the COVID-19 vaccine so that "it would not knock me out for some vital competition days". Swimmer Katie Ledecky said, "The mask-wearing, the distancing, the testing...even if you get the vaccine and you get a positive test, you're still able to spread the virus" (321). Smart woman.

Golf: In April 2021, the PGA Tour announced it was strongly recommending that players get vaccinated for COVID-19 but would not mandate the vaccine to compete in tournaments. The PGA Tour is the organiser of the main professional golf tours played by men in the US. The PGA Tour noted that they would deem players 'inoculated' 14 days after the second dose of the COVID-19 vaccine and those players would no longer be required to test for the coronavirus and that, in accordance with CDC guidelines, these vaccinated players would be able to gather in small groups without a mask (322). How generous of the ruling class.

Rugby: On May 5th 2020, the Australian news reported that National Rugby League (NRL) bosses, as part of rugby league's strict biosecurity measures, asked players to be vaccinated with an influenza vaccine to "not experience a COVID-19 outbreak"; and they say we wear tinfoil hats! More than a dozen NRL players refused to take the influenza vaccine. The players were said to have refused the vaccine as, *"they have had a reaction to the flu shot in the past"*. Gold Coast Titans player Bryce Cartwright refused to take the influenza vaccine and is described as an 'anti-vaxxer'. Gold Coast Titans player Nathan Peats wrote on Insta-gramme-of-soma, *"Another shit story. He wasn't the first in the NRL to say no to it"* [(323)].

Basketball, football and baseball: Professional athletes who care about their bodies are likely to have concerns about COVID-19 vaccine safety. On February 27th 2021, *The Wall Street Journal* reported that a "significant percentage" of the National Basketball Association (NBA), the National Football League (NFL), and Major League Baseball (MLB) players were expressing vaccine hesitancy; doublespeak for 'refused the COVID-19 vaccine'. Leagues are now trying to persuade players by using a doctor to "debunk vaccine myths" [(324)]. This is doublespeak for, *'Cover up 'myths' such as deaths and adverse reactions post COVID-19 vaccine reported to Vaccine Adverse Event Reporting System (VAERS) and EudraVigilance etc.'*

Tennis: On April 1st 2021, BBC News reported that both the ATP Men's Professional Tennis Association and the WTA Women's Tennis Association governing bodies had encouraged players to get the COVID-19 vaccine but insisted they will not mandate the vaccinations. Novak Djokovic and Elina Svitolina expressed COVID-19 vaccine scepticism. Djokovic said that he was "opposed to vaccination" and defied COVID-19 rules by embarking on a controversial exhibition tour in Serbia and Croatia that was attended by fans. Djokovic claimed his comments about vaccinations had been taken out of context and said, *"My issue here with vaccines is if someone is forcing me to put something in my body. That I don't want"*. World number eight, Aryna Sabalenka said she did not "trust" the COVID-19 vaccine as they made it so quickly and that she didn't want either her or her family to take it. Ukrainian player Elina Svitolina is going to, "wait a little while longer to see how it goes". Top ten player Andrey Rublev said, *"If you ask me if I can choose and I can have an option, I will not do it"* [(325)]. Novak Djokovic practically spells out "no vax covid joke".

Motorsport: In July 2020, F1 driver Lewis Hamilton reposted a video on Insta-gramme-of-soma expressing anti-vaccination sentiment. Hamilton reposted a video by actor and former Vine star Andrew Bachelor showing Bill Gates discussing the progress of a COVID-19 vaccine with a caption across it reading, "I remember when I told my first lie". Hamilton has 18.3 million Insta-gramme-of-soma followers. The video was met by widespread criticism among fans claiming they would no longer be fans [(326)]. So fickle! A total of six Formula 1 drivers and three team principals previously tested positive for COVID-19, including Sergio Perez, Lance Stroll, Lewis Hamilton, Charles Leclerc, Lando Norris and Pierre Gasly. Authorities in the Middle East country of Bahrain offered a COVID-19 vaccine to all F1 personnel involved in the Bahrain Grand Prix. Sebastian Vettel refused the COVID-19 vaccine offered to him in Bahrain, saying, "I'll get vaccinated when it's my turn". Additionally, three team principals refused the COVID-19 vaccine, including Alfa Romeo team principal Frederic Vasseur, Williams acting team principal Simon Roberts and Mercedes team principal Toto Wolff [(327)]. Wolff, who contracted COVID-19 during the off-season, said he prefers to wait until he is called for the COVID-19 vaccination by the NHS [(328)]. When you donate your vaccine to someone more vulnerable you are a hero, but when you refuse it, you are the greatest threat to humanity and global security

Reasons for Vaccine Refusal:

> *"Believe half of what you see and none of what you hear. Pay attention to your gut feeling; if it doesn't feel good, walk away".* Grandma

Vaccine refusers don't believe the hype. Vaccine refusers don't think pharmaceutical companies are knights in shining armour. Vaccine refusers know that public health, the media and science has sold out to the pharmaceutical industry and that the pharmaceutical industry is a criminal consortium. Vaccine refusers know their unvaccinated children are healthier and save the taxpayer money. Vaccine refusers don't buy that they are a danger to society. Vaccine refusers know that they don't carry and spread antibiotic-resistant disease. Vaccine refusers don't worship at the altar of allopathic medicine. Vaccine refusers know that doctors are the 3rd biggest cause of death. Vaccine refusers have faith in their God-given immune system. Vaccine refusers are more likely educated, wealthy people more able to afford to see a Complementary and Alternative Medicine (CAM) practitioner as their primary healthcare and therefore more aware of the dangers of suppressing the immune system. Vaccine refusers are less likely to be financially coerced into vaccinating their children. Vaccine refusers know that vaccines aren't safe. Vaccine refusers are strongly intuitive and know when to walk away.

Using the influenza vaccine as an example: Some of us lived in a world before influenza vaccines, and some of us remember this world. Vaccine refusers don't fear influenza and know that the influenza vaccine is ineffective. The daily propaganda leads us to believe that the influenza vaccine is 100% effective. This couldn't be further from the truth. The 'experts' at the CDC state the influenza vaccine's effectiveness in reducing influenza risk between 2005 and 2018 ranged between 10-60% among the overall population [(329)]. Eurosurveillance indicates that the 2017/18 influenza vaccine's effectiveness ranged between 25-52% [(330)]. Vaccine refusers know that observational studies substantially overestimate vaccination benefits. For example, a study published in *The European Respiratory Journal* in 2007 noted that the impact of influenza vaccination on mortality risk has been wildly overestimated as adjustment for confounders and differences in mortality between vaccinated and unvaccinated individuals has not been made. When the figures are adjusted, the reduction in all-cause mortality due to influenza vaccination during three influenza seasons decreased from 50, 46 and 42%, to 14, 19 and 1%, respectively [(331)].

A cyclical regression model published in *Archives of Internal Medicine* in 2005, looked at the impact of influenza vaccination on seasonal mortality in elderly Americans. The study concluded that the decline in influenza-related mortality among people aged 65 to 74 years in the decade after the 1968 pandemic was due to the acquisition of naturally acquired immunity to the emerging A (H3N2) virus and not the introduction of the influenza vaccine. The study's authors could not correlate increased influenza vaccine coverage after 1980 with declining mortality rates in any age group. Because fewer than 10% of all winter deaths were attributable to influenza in any season, the study concluded that observational studies substantially overestimate vaccine efficacy [(332)]. An independent Cochrane review looked at vaccines for preventing influenza in healthy adults and concluded that, for every 100 healthy adults vaccinated, 99 receive absolutely no benefit against laboratory-confirmed influenza. The study concluded that 71 healthy adults need to be vaccinated to prevent one case of influenza, and 29 healthy adults need to be vaccinated to prevent one case of influenza-like illness (ILI) [(333)]. A vaccine refuser weighs up the risk versus benefit and decides not to take the risk for a vaccine that is 1.4% effective. A vaccine refuser questions why one would need an influenza vaccine when the same Cochrane Collaboration says that vitamin D is 100% effective at preventing hospitalisations and deaths from influenza, as is covered in Chapter 19, 'COVID Medical & Natural Medicine Prevention & Treatment'.

Vaccines fear exists because they have not conducted the study that will allay our fear: The US Institute of Medicine's (IOM) Immunisation Safety Review (ISR) Committee does not say vaccines are safe! The ISR say, "There is no study that compares an unvaccinated control group with children exposed to the complete immunisation schedule, nor are there any studies that looked at health outcomes other than those classically defined, such as infections, allergy, or diabetes" [334]. The US Department of Health and Human Services (DHHS) says it will not initiate a randomised controlled trial (RCT) of the childhood immunisation schedule that compares safety outcomes in fully vaccinated children with those in unvaccinated children [335]. A vaccine refuser knows that if they conducted this study, it would prove beyond doubt that vaccines are not safe and end the debate. It is perfectly acceptable to say we have overused antibacterials in the home. It is perfectly acceptable to diagnose fever phobia in parents and say we have overused antipyretics to suppress fever. It is perfectly acceptable to say we have overused antibiotics. However, once we say we have overused vaccines, suddenly we are not 'medically qualified' and should not enter the debate. If a doctor or immunologist suggests it, they are not fit to practice and face suspension. A vaccine refuser knows the subject is not 'hotly debated; it's hotly censored. Lack of vaccine safety studies are discussed further in Chapter 12, 'Vaccines aren't Described as Safe and don't Always Work'.

CHAPTER FOUR – PART II

THE AGE OF CENSORSHIP

2020 was the year the ruling class killed natural immunity. We stand at the altar of allopathic medicine, having taken one gramme of soma, self-flagellating, repeating, "there is no thing like artificial immunity; natural medicine is quackery". Public health wants us all dependent on public health. Public health wants to vaccinate every man, woman, person and child on the planet every year. Parents who choose to use natural medicine to treat their children and don't vaccinate are a danger to society and need to be socially cleansed. Considering these parents avoid public health and save the state money, targeting them for being unhealthy is unsubstantiated. Again a tape measure around the middle is the best health test.

Surveillance and censorship; the Vaccine Confidence Project: The Vaccine Confidence Project (VCP) censors vaccine safety concerns. In 2020 both the concepts of natural immunity and natural herd immunity were targeted by this project. Professor Heidi Larson is an anthropologist and co-founder and Director of the VCP. Heidi previously headed UNICEF's Global Immunisation Communication, chaired Gavi's Advocacy Task Force, and served on the WHO SAGE Working Group on vaccine hesitancy. The VCP is described as a WHO Centre of Excellence on addressing Vaccine Hesitancy. The VCP says "emotions around vaccines are volatile" which makes "vigilance and monitoring crucial for effective public outreach". The VCP team consists of anthropologists, epidemiologists, statisticians, political scientists and 'others'. The VCP have a Vaccine Confidence Index, similar to a consumer-confidence index in which they survey and track attitudes on vaccines. In 2016 the project recognised Europe as having the highest lack of confidence in vaccines. Professor Larson wrote a book about why vaccine rumours don't go away [336]. Heidi's right. Newton's third law is; for every action, there is an equal and opposite reaction. The VCP employs the services of global intelligence and security organisations such as the Five Eyes mentioned again shortly under 'war on anti-vaxxers'.

The VCP seeks to, *'Monitor public confidence in vaccination programmes by listening for early signals of public distrust and providing risk analysis and guidance to engage the public and pre-empt programme disruptions'* which again, is mere doublespeak for, 'Scour the internet and censor free speech!' [337]. Heidi says that there is no single strategy that works for all types of 'misinformation', particularly among those who are already sceptical and that dialogue matters [336]. I am still waiting for an invite to that dialogue. The project is in part funded by GlaxoSmithKline (GSK), and this funding by GSK is not always disclosed [337, 338]. The project does not aim to address the lack of confidence in vaccine safety by conducting the safety study that the ISR say has not been conducted. Aside from the Big Tech companies, Heidi's peanut gallery is called 'fact-checkers'. Fact-checkers are not independent medical professionals. Full Fact was founded in 2009 by businessman Michael Samuel, a renowned 'philanthropist'. Michael is a Conservative Party donor, need I say anymore. The Full Fact team seem to be, by in large ex-politicians or political donors, associated with mainstream media or are recipients of British Empire awards [339]. They likely use ghost-writers. Full Fact is a 'charity' that burns books. Michael Samuel is not a philanthropist; he is a modern-day book burner. Burn this, and I shall be invoicing the VCP for establishing the new category called 'vaccine outright refusal' and for answering Heidi's questions surrounding why our belief systems have gone so awry.

Media manipulation and cronyism: Media manipulation is a group of similar methods used by promoters to create an argument that benefits their own interests. Tactics include the use of logical misconceptions, psychological manipulations, blatant deception and rhetorical and propaganda techniques. The extent of which now goes so far as to actively suppress information and points of view by crowding them out or censoring them and persuading large swathes of people to stop listening to certain arguments. Think vaccine-refusal and 'baby killers' and pro-freedom rallies and 'granny killers' [340]. We live under totalitarian rule and Big Sibling is watching. Social media platforms have partnered with the CDC and the World Wealth Organisation to take unprecedented steps to control what users can see and share [341]. The CDC and the WHO told social media to shut down free speech on vaccine safety concerns. Fascistbook announced a multistep plan to crack down on concerns around vaccine safety. You-will-obey-Tube and Insta-gramme-of- soma have also cracked down on 'anti-vax misinformation' [342]. Vox go so far as to say that anti-vaxxers have scared the media away from covering vaccine side effects [343]. *The Guardian* say that the media should attempt to understand how our belief systems have gone 'so awry' [344].

Whilst Zuckerberg cracks down on us expressing our safety concerns or sharing our vaccine injury experience, Zuckerberg forgot to censor himself from expressing caution. In a video on You-will-obey-Tube, posted by Project Veritas, at 12 minutes and 47 seconds, Zuckerberg violates his own policy by sharing his concerns about the vaccine's safety. Zuckerberg says (in reference to the COVID-19 vaccines) *"but I do just want to make sure that I share some caution on this because we just don't know the long-term side effects of basically modifying people's DNA and RNA"* (345). Fascistbook censors posts describing COVID-19 vaccines as genetically modifying.

Cyberwar on anti-vaxxers: Under their Global Health and Security Agenda, we are being taken out comrades! Not only are we being taken out by the social media giants, we are also being taken out by global security and intelligence agencies. They are waging a cyberwar on us! In November 2020, *Reuters* reported that the UK's Government Communications Headquarters (GCHQ) has been told to "take out anti-vaxxers" online and on social media. The report says that the GCHQ has begun an offensive cyber operation to tackle online 'anti-vaccine propaganda' by 'hostile states'. The GCHQ has, 'a relationship with security and intelligence', which is doublespeak for eavesdropping agencies in the US, Australia, Canada and New Zealand in an intelligence alliance known as the 'Five Eyes' (346). Additionally each WHO member state has a security agency that is 'taking out anti-vaxxers'.

The pseudo professor of complementary and alternative medicine: It is unacceptable that anyone with a concern about vaccine safety is openly discriminated against and their voice silenced. We have every right to choose. We choose not to vaccinate to strengthen our immune systems and prevent chronic disease. When I was investigated by *The Sunday Times*, I had no idea that I was to be rebutted by the world's first Professor of Complementary and Alternative Medicine (CAM), Edzard Ernst. Edzard Ernst is a retired academic physician and researcher who is said to specialise in the study of CAM. As someone who is triple degree qualified in CAM and has 22 years of clinical experience prescribing CAM therapies I am outraged to learn that the world's first Professor of CAM is neither qualified in CAM nor has ever practised CAM. The health czars have appointed Edzard Ernst for one reason only; to scour the internet for evidence on CAM therapies and to downplay them. Ernst is the voice of an industry he does not believe in nor has any practical experience in (347).

Edzard Ernst paints natural medicine as quackery, pseudoscience, containing conspiracy theories and as having extreme right-wing bias.

A fine example of Professor Ernst's work is an article discussing over 100 deaths resulting from three forms of CAM; acupuncture, chiropractic and chelation therapy [348]. Professor Ernst begins by saying that CAM consultants believe that CAM is almost totally devoid of risks. That's a complete falsehood and an insult to the CAM profession. As a level 8 degree qualified Australian acupuncturist, acupuncture is regulated by the Australian Health Practitioner Regulation Agency (AHPRA), the same agency that regulates doctors, nurses and allied health professionals. Australian acupuncturists are required by law to submit an infection prevention and control (IPC) plan to the local authority as a requirement to secure a licence to operate. Australian pharmacies employ degree qualified naturopaths trained in pharmacology to advise the public and the pharmacist on drug-nutrient and drug-herb interactions to protect public health. Professor not in Earnest is a pseudo-Professor.

It is estimated that up to 80% of the world's population living in the developing world rely on herbal medicine for their primary healthcare [349]. The European Information Centre for Complementary and Alternative Medicine (EICCAM) estimates that more than 100 million EU citizens regularly use CAM to treat chronic conditions [350]. Whilst rigorous reporting systems for deaths and adverse events following CAM are needed, given that the European population is 741.4 million, the 100 deaths that Professor not in Earnest mentions could be put into perspective by comparing that medical errors in the US alone result in the deaths of between 250,000 and 450,000 people every year [351]. Contrary to the daily propaganda, life is not about risk avoidance, it is about risk reduction. I look at the available evidence and make an informed choice about my and my family's healthcare. If I were a Professor of CAM and wanted to protect public health, I would facilitate the integration of CAM into mainstream healthcare by ensuring that CAM courses are introduced at universities and taught to an internationally recognised Australian level 8 AQF, Irish level 8 NFQ, European Level 8 EQF, UK Level 6 Ofqual through NARIC etc. degree. This is the pharmaceutical industry's biggest fear. Actually, the pharmaceutical industry's greatest fear is of homeopaths! It would be funny if it wasn't true.

Cleansing society of the unvaxxed (we can't make any money out of them): As I mentioned in my introduction, I have been targeted on a number of occasions in an attempt to single me out and shut me up. Good luck with that. I stand for my descendants. A perspective published in *The New England Journal of Medicine* entitled 'In the Name of Public Health-Nazi Racial Hygiene' discussed Nazi racial hygiene or eugenics in the name of public health. The Nazi policy wasn't only racial hygiene; it was also defective people hygiene. Before 1933, eugenics proposals didn't have widespread support. That changed in 1933 when Hitler wrote in *Mein Kampf* that "the national state...must see to it that only the healthy beget children using modern medical means". Early 20th-century eugenics proponents argued that modern medicine interfered with Darwinian natural selection, which left more defective people in the population, requiring escalating costs [(352)]. No one is suggesting that this is happening in 2021. What people are asking is could we allow this to happen again? Today, daily propaganda portrays unvaccinated people as having inferior immune systems and being the greatest threat to global health and security. That is an inflammatory accusation with no scientific basis. We know a covert eugenics programme was undertaken, with do-not-resuscitate (DNR) orders in place that discriminated against people with disabilities [(353)]. DNR orders are further discussed in Chapter 9, 'Inflated Deaths'.

Social exclusion: The model used to exclude advocates of natural immunity is known as the 'spiral of silence' theory, which had its origins in mass communication. The spiral of silence theory states that a social group or society as a whole might isolate or exclude members due to the members' opinions. This theory stipulates that individuals have a fear of isolation. The spiral of silence stops people from expressing their opinions on controversial public issues as they believe they may be unpopular and lead to social exclusion. The spiral of silence theory results in populations tending to support majority views, resulting in a homogenisation of public opinion [(354)]. This model makes me, a vaccine refuser and CAM consultant, a social pariah.

Discrimination, quarantine and segregation: To discriminate against someone because of their age, gender, religion or sexual orientation is not acceptable however, mentioning that you don't vaccinate provides free rein to discriminate; that, and being ginger. They allow open discrimination against redheads because they know we are the least likely to do what we are told. I believe we should accept our diversity and look to cross over into the mindset of those with opposing views. Not everyone holds the view that vaccines prevent infectious disease and save lives. Vaccine-hesitant communities hail from around the globe and include, Christian scientists, the Somali-American community in Minnesota, the Amish in Ohio, Russian-language immigrants in Washington, Eastern Europeans in Washington State and Orthodox Jewish communities [(355)]. I stand for all these groups. Under-vaccinated groups (UVGs) in Europe include Orthodox Protestant communities, Anthroposophists and Roma and Irish Travellers [(356)]. I stand for all these groups. Other communities that are more likely not to vaccinate their children include, as mentioned, educated professionals living in areas with higher socioeconomic levels in Sydney and Melbourne's rich suburbs, the Hollywood A-lister areas of Byron Bay, and the Northern Rivers in Australia [(280, 357-359)]. Because these people do not want to vaccinate their children to protect their health, these communities in Australia are marginalised, their children are excluded from pre-schools and parents are openly attacked daily in the media. I stand for these families. During a measles outbreak in April 2019, ultra-orthodox Jews in New York state had bus drivers refusing to pick them up and they were having "measles" shouted at them [(360)]. The measles outbreak provided a justification for anti-Semitic sentiment. All these communities are experiencing discrimination, quarantine and segregation for refusing vaccines.

Name-calling, intimidation and bullying: Before COVID (BC) calls were being made by the Royal College of Physicians Ireland for mandatory vaccines for HCWs working in certain settings [(361)]. Anyone who does not comply experiences name-calling, intimidation, bullying, discrimination and ultimately segregation. Names used include "threat to all patients", "danger to society", "blood on their hands", "unable to reason", "neglectful", "vaccine dodgers", "deplorables" etc. In 2019, the WHO have name-called vaccine refusers by describing them as one of, "the ten greatest threats to Global Health" [(285)]. We are up there with the world's most feared war criminals, folks.

Propaganda about Australian child benefit being withheld from anti-vaxxer parents: It is always inaccurately reported in Europe that Australia's 'No Jab No Play' and 'No Jab No Pay' policies prevents unimmunised children from attending schools and their parents from receiving child benefit. Wickedpedia also describes 'No Jab No Play' as an Australian policy initiative that withholds three state payments [362]. Wickedpedia is anti-natural medicine propaganda. The truth is Australia's 'No Jab No Play' policy is for childcare or kindergarten only, not schools. In Australia, child benefit is firstly means-tested and secondly is called Family Tax Benefit (FTB), which is paid in two parts. The 'No Jab No Play' policy affects FTB Part A only. Families with children who are not immunised and do not have an approved exemption have a reduction applied to their FTB Part A [363]. FTB part A is already only paid to families with taxable income of AUD$80,000 or less, making this financial coercion tactic a completely ineffective strategy for the rich least likely to vaccinate [364]. FTB Part A pays a maximum of AUD$182.84 per fortnight for children up to the age of 12 and AUD$237.86 per fortnight for children up to the age of 19 [365]. FTB part B is still paid for unvaccinated children. The rate is FTB Part B pays a maximum of AUD$155.54 per fortnight for children under 5 and AUD$108.64 per fortnight for children aged 5-18 [366]. As the richest are not affected by financial disincentives, this makes the current Australian mandatory vaccination policy inequitable [280, 367]. This policy is having devastating effects on many families who cannot send their children to kindergarten because they want to protect their child's health.

This abhorrent policy is backed by the majority of indoctrinated Australians that have no understanding about vaccines and who blame their children's illnesses on bad genes and bad luck. When their children get mumps and measles in their 20s, these parents will irrationally blame the unvaccinated children that have lifelong protection through natural exposure. The daily propaganda does not tell you also that the official medical exemption in Australia includes, among other things, proof of natural immunity for hepatitis B, measles-mumps-rubella and chickenpox [368]. Thus natural immunity provides proof of an exemption for vaccination in Australia.

Blatant propaganda about Italy and France: The media still reports that Italy has mandatory vaccine laws, however these were met with massive backlash and were overturned, which is never reported [369]. French parents do not go to jail for not vaccinating their children as the daily propaganda will have you believe [370].

A vaccine refuser says no way, never, OVER MY DEAD BODY: My family and I have robust immune systems, and vaccinations go against my professional integrity. My children have had all childhood illnesses and have lifelong immunity. When they reach adulthood, vaccinated children can still catch and spread measles and mumps again at 20 years of age. What a load of poppycock that unvaccinated children are a risk to the vulnerable. Quite the opposite is true. By having lifelong immunity, my children protect the vulnerable in our society. When they had their childhood disease, I isolated them. I did not sit in an emergency department or a doctor's waiting room. They did not spread it to one other child besides those in the home. We have robust immune systems because we have been exposed to, not shielded from, infectious diseases. As a mother with three degrees in CAM, there is not a childhood disease I have not seen nor cannot treat. Whilst I was backpacking heavily pregnant through Southeast Asia during the 2005 H1N5 bird flu, my children got the bird flu. It was a high hallucinogenic fever (classic belladonna in homeopathy); however, I managed it with my first aid kit and a tepid shower. Whilst studying and working as an acupuncturist in Chinese hospitals in 2003, the original SARS outbreak happened. While the other students fled in fear, I knew I was surrounded by the best acupuncturists and Chinese herbalists globally and couldn't have felt safer. I have an arsenal of herbal medicine, homeopathic remedies, nutritional supplements, acupuncture and dietary therapy. I will not fear self-limiting childhood diseases or coronavirus. I fear life-threatening, life-limiting, autoimmune and inflammatory diseases that require lifelong medication. I fear life-threatening drug-drug interactions.

CHAPTER FIVE

DAMAGING LOCKDOWNS

"The people have the power.
All we have to do is awaken the power in the people". John Lennon [371]

Lockdowns are the crux of coercive control. There are two key approaches that public health *could* have adopted to reduce the transmission of coronavirus disease 2019 (COVID-19) as known respectively as 'the nanny state' or 'nightwatchman' approaches. These concepts are derived from what is known in public health as 'the Nuffield intervention ladder', a concept set up by the Nuffield Council on Bioethics in 2006 to examine the ethical issues surrounding public health; doublespeak for, 'examine how public health can ethically justify stripping us of our free will'. I thought we had moved on from gender stereotyping and these terms would have been renamed to the gender-inclusive 'night watchperson' and 'grandparent state'. This 'intervention ladder' is described as a useful way of thinking about the different ways that public health policies can affect people's choices. At the top the intervention ladder sits 'eliminate choice'; at the bottom sits 'do nothing'. The nanny state dictates the state has a duty to look after everyone's health (whether we like it or not) and means guiding or restricting people's choices. The nightwatchman provides only the service of a nightwatchman and requires people to apply common sense and look after themselves. We are all acutely aware that the nanny state puts public health at odds with our freedom [372].

The Nuffield Council on Bioethics' intervention ladder structurally embodies the assumption that personal autonomy (the right to make our own choices) is maximised by non-intervention [373]. Any public health intervention is seen as coming at a cost to personal autonomy. COVID-19 lockdowns have obliterated personal autonomy. The daily propaganda actively engages in the wilful omission of deaths due to lockdown restrictions to push public health policy towards eliminating free choice. Attacks on our freedom to choose remove not only individual choice but also individual responsibility. Public health's effort to silence dissent about lockdowns or concerns regarding vaccine safety will backfire and destroy the public's confidence in public health 'experts' and 'authorities'. Cue the scripted public health counterargument narrative; 'those who want to limit state intervention are the first to complain when the state doesn't intervene'. Try me.

'Lock*down*' is doublespeak for 'lock*up*'. Lockdowns perpetuate fear. Whilst the whole of *COVERT-19 What Public Health Won't Tell You* contains themes surrounding evidence against lockdowns, here I aim to compare and contrast countries that adopted a nanny state approach and went into full lockdown with countries or states that adopted a nightwatchman approach and did not lockdown. A study published in the *Proceedings of the National Academy of Sciences of the United States of America* in April 2021 examined the effects of shelter-in-place (SIP) orders [stay at home orders in the United Kingdom (UK) and Ireland] during the first wave of the COVID-19 pandemic in the United States (US). Study authors did not find detectable effects of these policies on either disease spread or deaths. The team of researchers from the University of Chicago, Harris School of Public Policy found that the states that imposed SIP orders, mandatory business closures and other restrictions didn't see a significant difference in the number of coronavirus infections or deaths during the virus' first US surge in the spring of 2020. Mobile phone data was used to determine that SIP orders had very little impact on people's mobility. Researchers concluded that, regardless of state-imposed restrictions, changes in habits encouraged by public health officials, such as washing hands with soap and water and not lockdowns, had the most significant effect [(374)].

The mandate of the scientists: The Greater Barrington Declaration (GBD) was authored by Dr Martin Kulldorff, Professor of Medicine at Harvard University, Dr Sunetra Gupta, Professor at Oxford University and Dr Jay Bhattacharya, Professor at Stanford University Medical School. The GBD acknowledges the damaging physical and mental health impacts of the COVID-19 lockdown policies. The GBD calls for lifting of all restrictions in healthy people and recommends "focused protection", that is, protecting the vulnerable while letting the disease run its course in the healthy population. On February 20th 2021, the signature count was; concerned citizens 749,895, medical and public health scientists13,618, and medical practitioners 41,244 [(375)]. The retaliatory John Snow Memorandum supporting tighter restrictions to mandate masks, mandate social distancing, mandate travel restrictions, mandate quarantine, mandate vaccines and mandate vaccine passports had 6,000 signatures by comparison at the same time [376]. The science has spoken.

Dr Scott Atlas, former Stanford University Medical Professor and former White House Coronavirus Task Force member, supports using objective science to encourage what the authors of the GBD advocate; to reopen society while protecting the vulnerable. Dr Atlas said:

> *"For people who care about the data...the lockdowns ...were extraordinarily harmful... There is no question that 40% of people didn't get chemotherapy, up to 78% of cancers didn't get diagnosed...All because of fear...and we have a massive public health price to pay as we go forward".* Dr Atlas continued to say. *"We have done the experiment...and can compare what happened...the facts of having an open state which was Florida versus these other states ....when you look at excess mortality rate...it turns out Florida beats 70% of the states...Florida to California...California did 50% worse because of its severe lockdowns. The lockdowns were harmful. They were the opposite of what should have been done...The lockdowns killed people, destroyed lives, destroyed families...our country was willing to sacrifice its children out of fear"* [377].

The GBD authors are discussed further in Chapter 24, 'Speaking Truth to Power'.

Evidence from Europe

Sweden: Sweden relied on voluntary measures focused on social distancing, good hygiene and targeted rules but kept schools, restaurants and shops largely open. Preliminary data from European Union (EU) statistics agency Eurostat compiled by *Reuters* showed Sweden had 7.7% more deaths in 2020 than its average for the preceding four years. Countries that opted for several periods of strict lockdowns, such as Spain and Belgium, had excess mortality of 18.1% and 16.2% respectively [378]. Yet the daily propaganda pushed the narrative that Sweden's outcomes were apocalyptic when compared with Spain and Belgium. Table 1 shows the number of deaths in Sweden between 2016-2020 according to Statista 2021 [379].

Table 1: The number of deaths in Sweden 2016-2020 (Statista 2021)

Year	Number of deaths
2020	97,941
2019	88,766
2018	92,185
2017	91,972
2016	90,982

These figures show 90, 976 (average over 4 years) + 6965 (excess deaths)

Exec. Dir. WHO Health Emergencies Programme says Sweden is the new normal: On a Sveriges Television programme entitled 'WHO on Sweden's strategy: Can be a future model', Executive Director of the WHO Health Emergencies Programme Dr Michael I-am-a-real-boy Ryan discusses the concept of herd immunity. Ryan said, *"with regard to this concept of immunity"*...he goes on to scaremonger;

> *"even in areas of fairly intense transmission, the proportion of people who have seroconverted or have antibodies in their blood is actually quite low, the vast majority of people remain susceptible* (at which stage his nose grows)...*I think if we are to reach a new normal, I think in many ways, Sweden represents a future model, of if we wish to get back to a society in which we don't have lockdowns, then society may need to adapt for a medium or potentially longer period of time in which our physical and social relationships with each other will have to be modulated by the presence of the virus...I think maybe in Sweden, they're looking at how that's done in real-time. I think there are maybe lessons to be learned from what happens in Sweden, Sweden has not avoided controlling COVID-19...what it's done differently...is really has done, is trusted its own communities..."* (380).

Sweden is the new normal. Sweden trusts its own communities. That sounds like the old normal.

Evidence from the United States: Seven states in the US did not introduce stay at home orders back in March and April 2020, although you won't hear about them on CNN because the data coming from these states is damning against lockdowns. These states include Arkansas, Iowa,

Nebraska, North Dakota, South Dakota, Utah and Wyoming. All 43 other states issued stay at home orders [(381)]. An estimation of excess deaths associated with the COVID-19 pandemic in the US, March to May 2020 was published in *JAMA Internal Medicine* on July 1st 2020 (382). Glancing over the figures below one can easily confirm that the states that did not lockdown had the lowest excess all-cause deaths per 100,000. Table 2 compares reported deaths coded as COVID-19 in the US states that locked down compared to US states that did not lockdown [(382)].

Table 2: Reported deaths coded as COVID-19 compared with excess deaths coded as Pneumonia/Influenza/COVID-19 or all causes from March 1st 2020 to May 30th 2020

US State	Estimated excess all-cause deaths per 100 000, median (95% prediction interval)
No Lockdown	
Arkansas	2.2 (-10.1 to 13.5)
Iowa	4.4 (-2.4 to 11.5)
Nebraska	6.4 (-2.1 to 15)
North Dakota	-71.9 (-87.4 to -55.9)
South Dakota	-7.7 (-21.3 to 4.7)
Utah	4.2 (-2 to 9.8)
Wyoming	-58.4 (-76.2 to -43.5)
Early Lifting Lockdown	
Texas	12.4 (10.4 to 14.5)
Florida	16.4 (13.4 to 19.3)
Lockdown	
California	17.2 (15.5 to 19)
New York City	299.1 (295.3 to 302.7)
New York State	111.4 (107.4 to 114.9)
Massachusetts	107.6 (103 to 112.2)
New Jersey	182.3 (178.1 to 186.2)

Texas and Florida: On November 18th 2020, ABC News reported that Texas, Florida and South Dakota governors all refused to go back into lockdown [383]. On March 21st 2021, a Fox News report said that in the over two weeks after Texas Governor Greg Abbott lifted coronavirus mandates, made masks optional and allowed businesses to operate at full capacity, Texas was still reporting decreases in cases and hospitalisations. The lifting of lockdown, of course, coincided with the COVID-19 vaccine rollout. Governor Abbott championed his state's success in a tweet on March 19th 2020, "Today Texas recorded the lowest seven day COVID positivity rate since that data began being calculated at 5.43%" . Abbott also said that "More Texans getting vaccines will keep down the positivity rate", adding that receiving the vaccine was, "always voluntary" [384]. On March 27th 2021, Florida's Fox 29 News reported that the Florida Health Department announced coronavirus deaths had decreased dramatically in one day from 159 to 26, representing the lowest figure since 21 deaths on November 8th 2020 [385]. In March 2021, Mississippi, Alabama and West Virginia also moved to end state-wide pandemic restrictions; more data will ensue [386].

An observational analysis of 27 countries shows lockdowns did not save lives: An article entitled 'Impact of lockdown on COVID-19 prevalence and mortality during 2020 pandemic: observational analysis of 27 countries' published in the *European Journal of Medical Research* in November 2020 concluded that findings indicated that whilst 15 days after the lockdown, daily cases of COVID-19 showed a declining trend, there was no significant decline in prevalence and mortality at all. The lockdowns were completely ineffective [387]. The evidence of lockdowns to prevent deaths from COVID-19 is irrelevant. Shut up! Obey! Stay at home! Develop coviphobia, covibesity and alcohol-related harm to 'save lives'.

CHAPTER SIX

MEANINGLESS PCR TESTS

"In a democracy, you believe it or not;
in a dictatorship, you believe it or else".

Evan Esar [388]

The polymerase chain reaction (PCR) test is the crux of the pandemonium, and the primary tool used by our coercive controllers, so it must be refuted at first instance. Without PCR tests, the house of cards falls. I understand that many fellow non-COVID faithful say that false positives with the PCR tests are very high. My take on this is that whilst this is true, most cases still go undetected. This is very important as this means that the infection fatality rate (IFR) for coronavirus disease 2019 (COVID-19) is vastly lower than reported, and coronavirus is not as deadly as people are being led to believe. Public health uses the case fatality rate (CFR) to drive their fear campaign. CFR only estimates this proportion of deaths in confirmed cases. IFR, on the other hand, takes into account the 80% of people with COVID-19 that are completely asymptomatic. IFR is a much more accurate measurement of fatality [389]. Using IFR would result in a much more proportionate public health response and negate the need for an Emergency Use Authorisation (EUA) vaccine. In April 2020, a seroprevalence study in Santa Clara County, United States (US) concluded that there were 50-85 times as many cases as previously reported. Rather than being a cause for alarm, this means that COVID-19 is 50-85 times less deadly [390]. CFR is frankly as much use as a chocolate teapot and should not be used to inform public health policy. Mass testing for COVID-19 is woefully inaccurate and should not be used to inform public health policy. That is of course if Rockefeller public health policy wasn't to 'vaccinate the world'. CFR and IFR are discussed further in Chapter 9, 'Inflated Deaths'.

The tarnished gold standard: Real-time reverse transcription-polymerase chain reaction (RT-PCR), PCR for short, is the current gold standard for diagnosing COVID-19 and is the most commonly used method worldwide [391]. The accuracy of the real-time RT-PCR test is most commonly reported using 'sensitivity' and 'specificity'. Sensitivity refers to the test's ability to correctly identify those patients with the disease, and specificity refers to the test's ability to correctly identify those patients that do not have the disease. Whilst RT-PCR tests have been widely implemented previously, they have never before been used like this. Under normal circumstances, positive control material for RT-PCR tests from positive patient samples, alternatively viral culture is used to devise the test. Viral culture should be the gold standard, however the age of technology and Klaus' Fourth Industrial Revolution heralded the end of the era of cell culture for virus detection in clinical microbiology. In the early stage of this outbreak, as positive control material from positive patient samples or viral culture was unavailable laboratories instead used synthetic controls either from synthetic DNA fragments or plasmids (double-stranded DNA molecule, distinct from cell's DNA). Whilst synthetic controls are said to have their advantages, depending on the design, great caution must be taken when handling synthetic controls, as trace amounts of this material can cause contamination. Contamination using synthetic controls when testing for severe acute respiratory syndrome coronavirus 2 (SARS-CoV-2) using RT-PCR has been reported [(392)].

There is no standard against which all other tests are compared and calibrated: As viral culture is the gold standard or reference test against which any diagnostic index test for viruses must be measured and calibrated, and as no such standard for SARS-CoV-2 exists, extreme care must be taken interpreting PCR test results [(393)]. A rapid systematic review on the effectiveness of diagnostic tests to detect the presence of SARS-CoV-2 virus and SARS CoV-2 antibodies to inform COVID-19 diagnosis, published in *BMJ Evidence-Based Medicine*, estimated sensitivity (true positive) of 87.8% for an initial real-time RT-PCR test. The study authors said however that, when estimating the diagnostic accuracy of the PCR test, one should bear in mind the absence of a definitive reference standard to diagnose or rule out COVID-19 infection. The study authors concluded that more evidence is needed regarding PCR test accuracy when testing outside of a hospital setting and in mild or asymptomatic cases [(394)].

The PCR test was also issued under EUA: The indiscriminate use of PCR tests is meaningless. Any medical test result is only as good as the context in which it is taken. On May 11th, 2021, 'Labcorp's (Laboratory Corporation of America Holdings) COVID-19 RT-PCR test EUA Summary' stated that LabCorp's COVID-19 PCR test had not been FDA cleared or approved and had been authorised by the Food and Drug Administration (FDA) under an

Emergency Use Authorisation (EUA). The FDA said that positive PCR results are indicative of the presence of SARS-CoV-2 RNA only and that clinical correlation with patient history and other diagnostic information is necessary to determine if the patient is infected. Additionally, the FDA stated that positive results do not rule out bacterial infection or co-infection with other viruses hence SARS-CoV-2 may not be the definite cause of the patient's disease (395). The FDA said that due to the rates of false negatives and false positives, real-time RT-PCR results should never be the only factor in determining or excluding COVID-19. A systematic review and meta-analysis of the accuracy of diagnostic tests for COVID-19 published in the *American Journal of Infection Control* in January 2021, described studies for COVID-19 diagnostic tests as being of moderate methodological quality and recommended a combination of different diagnostic tests to achieve adequate sensitivity and specificity, and to improve accuracy (396).

A positive test does not mean you are infectious: RT-PCR detects whether or not viral RNA is present in samples from a patient (397). Oxford University's Centre for Evidence-Based Medicine (CEBM) says that the RT-PCR test is capable of detecting minute quantities of RNA; however, as the FDA also stated, whether the minute quantities of RNA detected means that the virus is infectious remains unclear (393). The CEBM refers to a *Lancet* study entitled 'SARS-CoV-2 Shedding and Infectivity', which states the viral RNA can be detected long after the disappearance of infectious virus (398). Centres for Disease Control and Prevention (CDC) guidance says that recovered patients can have SARS-CoV-2 RNA detected in their upper respiratory tract samples for up to 12 weeks after the onset of symptoms (399). Up to 12 weeks of false positives and misinformation peddled by the daily propaganda.

The pre-test probability in asymptomatic people: Mass testing of asymptomatic people is not normal practice. Never before in the history of previous epidemics has it been the practice to test asymptomatic people and treat one positive PCR-based test result as confirmation that the person is infected, irrespective of presenting signs, symptoms and past exposure. This practice changed with COVID-19, when all of a sudden, one single positive result was diagnostic of infection with SAR-CoV-2. Under normal circumstances and outside EUA, a positive PCR test would not only be interpreted by taking into account previous medical history, exposure and presenting signs and symptoms, but also check positive results using an ancillary test such as a stool test to confirm viral shedding and that the person is able to spread infection [400]. This is called interpreting the test result in the context of the pre-test probability of disease. The pre-test probability assessment for COVID-19 includes presenting symptoms, past medical history of COVID-19, the presence of antibodies, any potential exposure to COVID-19, and the likelihood of another diagnosis.

A *Lancet Respiratory Medicine* study assessed the hidden issues and costs of false positive COVID-19 test results. This study noted that the pre-test probability underpins the integrity of the testing strategy and that the growing inclusion of testing asymptomatic people negatively affects this key parameter. Simply put, it is not proper science to test symptomatic people. The paper went on to discuss the history of COVID-19 PCR testing in the UK. In March and April 2020, most people tested in the UK were severely ill hospital admissions with a high probability of being infected. After April, this pattern shifted when the number of COVID-19 related hospital admissions decreased from more than 3,000 per day at the peak of the first wave to just over 100 admissions a day in August 2020. Between April 1st and August 1st 2020, the number of daily COVID-19 tests increased from 11,896 to 190,220. This increase resulted in the pre-test probability steadily decreasing as the proportion of asymptomatic cases screened increased. Additionally, this scenario occurred in the midst of new measures to curtail viral transmission, including lockdown, social distancing, hand hygiene and masking, which reduced viral transmission in the population. At the time of publication, September 29th 2020, the authors stated that only one-third of swab tests were being conducted in people with clinical needs or healthcare workers (HCWs) and that the majority of the COVID-19 tests were being conducted in the wider community [401].

PCR tests accuracy: In addition to PCR tests being misused and misinterpreted, false negative and false positive results also occur with real-time RT-PCR [402, 403]. The false positive rate (FPR) and false negative rate (FNR) is difficult to ascertain. False negative RT-PCR results are common when the test is taken within seven days of infection. One study found the FNR to be 9.3% [402]. Researchers at John Hopkins University estimated that those tested for SARS-CoV-2 within four days post-infection were 67% more likely to produce a false negative. If that person was displaying symptoms of the virus, the FNR ranged between 38% on day 1 to 20% on day 8, then increased again to 21% on day 9 and 66% on day 21 [404]. False positives are much more likely. A *JAMA* study published in October 2020 looked at solutions to reducing bias in post-licensure COVID-19 vaccine evaluations. Study authors described RT-PCR test sensitivity as a concern for diagnosing severe COVID-19. They stated sensitivity (true positive rate) ranged between 33% and 80% due to factors including decreased viral shedding due to delayed presentation, inadequate swabbing, or sampling site inaccuracies [405].

Test accuracy depends on how many people have COVID-19: A Brazilian systematic review and meta-analysis on PCR test accuracy in COVID-19 diagnosis found that the accuracy changes according to the prevalence of the disease. The meta-analysis obtained values of sensitivity (true positive rate) (86%) and specificity (true negative rate) (96%). The study however simulated three situations where the prevalence of disease differed;

- With a prevalence of 50%, the post-test probability was 96%.
- With a prevalence of 20%, the post-test probability was 84%.
- With a prevalence of 5%, the post-test probability was 55% [406].

The cycle threshold and false positives: If you test positive for coronavirus, you are likely a 'weak positive', which is also called a 'false positive'. This is due to what is known as the cycle threshold (Ct). Ct values represent the number of cycles of amplification elapsed before the test system signals detection of the target. The Ct correlates with viral load. A lower Ct value indicates a higher viral load in the sample. A higher Ct value indicates a lower viral load in the sample. An article published in *Clinical Medicine* discussed the impact of false positive COVID-19 results in healthcare settings. For the purpose of this study, the authors, affiliated with Public Health Wales Microbiology, defined a Ct 29 as a 'strong positive result', Ct 30-35 as a 'positive result', and >Ct35 as a 'weak positive result'. A weak positive (false positive) result is 'presumed' to be positive. A result is considered as a false positive with a Ct value >35. The study authors reiterated that clinicians need to familiarise themselves with Ct values and how to interpret them, particularly when screening asymptomatic individuals [407]. The tests currently being used on humanity are dialled up to 'Rockefeller public health is pulling history's most audacious scam to coerce us into taking an experimental vaccine'.

At a Ct >35 the rate of false positives is 97%: In September 2020, a letter to the editor in Oxford University's *Clinical Infectious Diseases*, authored by doctors from the Institut Hospitals-Universitaire-Méditerranée Infection, discussed a correlation between quantitative PCR-positives samples and positive cell cultures, which indicated live virus shedding in patients. The study authors referred to more than 100 recent studies that have led to the consensus that the cut-off Ct value and duration of eviction is approximately Ct >30 and at least ten days. The letter to the editor referenced an article published in *Clinical Infectious Diseases*, which reported a Ct >25 meant that patients could not be contagious as the virus as it is not detectable in culture above this Ct value. The authors concluded that at Ct = 35, the value used to determine a positive PCR result, <3% of cultures are positive [(408)]. Significantly this would allow patients with a low viral load to be safely discharged from the hospital (but not allow us to rejoin society) [(409)]. If at a Ct = 35 and <3% of cultures are positive, the probability that the result is a false positive is 97%.

WHO updated guidance on diagnostic testing for SARS-CoV-2: The PCR tests used for COVID-19 are classified as *in vitro* diagnostic medical devices (IVDs). Nucleic acid testing (NAT) technologies use PCR to detect SARS-CoV-2. The NAT is an IVD. All medical tests should be taken in the context of a patient's presenting symptoms, medical history and the Ct value. In January 2021, the World Health Organisation (WHO) updated its guidance on diagnostic testing for SARS-CoV-2 using real-time RT-PCR. In these guidelines, the WHO stated that the Ct required to detect the virus is inversely proportional to the patient's viral load. The WHO requested that those interpreting the results followed the instructions for use (IFU). These IFU require careful interpretation of a weak positive (false positive) result. Updated guidelines now include new recommendations that IVD users must refer to the IFU to determine if a manual adjustment of the PCR positivity threshold is recommended by the IVD manufacturer. The updated guidelines also included new recommendations that when test results do not correspond with the clinical presentation, a new specimen must be taken and retested using the same or different NAT technology [(410)]. These recommendations are not being enforced. Public health does not follow the WHO's advice.

HPSC updated guidance on managing 'weak positive (high Ct value)' PCR results: On April 14th 2021, Ireland's Health Protection Surveillance Centre

(HPSC) updated its guidance on managing 'weak positive (high Ct value)' PCR results. The new guidance said that when testing people for SARS-CoV-2, the interpretation of results is dependent on the availability of Ct values/viral load. The HPSC state that a precise definition of what constitutes a high or very high Ct value is difficult because a Ct value is not comparable to the quantitative output from a calibrated assay, i.e. there is no standard. The Ct value for a given sample will be different in different laboratories depending on the test platform. In general terms, for the HPSC report a Ct value of 30 or greater is considered a high Ct value [(411)]. What Ct values Irish tests are being conducted at is anyone's guess. The aim is to generate interest in and increase uptake of vaccines.

Ct thresholds are rarely reported: When asking people to read the instruction and interpret the results accordingly, the World Wealth Organisation failed to acknowledge that US laboratories rarely report the viral load associated with each positive PCR test, therefore the Ct is never included in the results sent to physicians. In a New York state laboratory, 50% of positives had a Ct value >35. In Massachusetts, 85-90% of positives in July 2020 had a Ct value >30 [(412)]. It is evident that many positive PCR test results run at these high Cts are not actual cases. These false positives have resulted in our freedoms being obliterated, our economy plunged into the worst recession since World War II, and humanity being placed in a global vaccine experiment. I was sure the World Wealth Organisation would finally enforce their guidelines once we had shut up, obeyed and taken our 'effective booster'. What in fact is going to happen is that we will have a completely new test.

The gold standard is now the old standard: The era of the revered RT-PCR test as the the tool of choice by our coercive controllers is coming to an end. A Laboratory Alert posted on the CDC's 'Division of Laboratory Systems (DLS)' webpage states that after December 31st 2021, the CDC will withdraw the request to the FDA for EUA of the CDC 2019-Novel Coronavirus (2019-nCoV) Real-Time RT-PCR Diagnostic Panel which was first introduced back February 2020 to detect SARS-CoV-2. The CDC is now recommending that clinical laboratories and testing sites that have been using the CDC 2019-nCoV RT-PCR assay select and begin their transition to the many FDA-authorised alternatives. The CDC is encouraging laboratories to consider adopting a multifold method that can detect and differentiate

SARS-CoV-2 and influenza viruses [(413)]. After all, our drug lords need to generate interest in and increase uptake of two-in-one vaccines now.

Portuguese court ruled mandatory quarantine unlawful as PCR test unreliable: On November 11th 2020, a Portuguese appeal court rejected the arguments put forward by the *Regional Health Authority* in the Azores that four people could be forced to quarantine after one of the individuals received a positive RT-PCR test for SARS-CoV-2. The other three had been deemed to have undergone a high risk of exposure, thus needed to quarantine.

Citing Jaafar et al. (2020) and Surkova et al. (2020), the court described the reliability of the PCR test as, *"more than debatable"* ("mais do que discutível"). The court ruled that the test was not able to determine infection beyond a reasonable doubt; therefore mandatory quarantine could not be enforced [(414)]. The court concluded:

> *"If someone is tested by PCR as positive when a threshold of 35 cycles or higher is used [as is the rule in most laboratories in Europe, the United Kingdom (UK) and the US], the probability that said person is infected is less than 3%, and the probability that said the result is a false positive is 97%".*

The court's summary of the case to rule against the Regional Health Authority's appeal reads as follows:

> *"Given how much scientific doubt exists, as voiced by experts, about the reliability of the PCR tests, given the lack of information concerning the tests' analytical parameters, and in the absence of a physician's diagnosis supporting the existence of infection or risk, there is no way this court would ever be able to determine whether C was indeed a carrier of the SARS-CoV-2 virus, or whether A, B and D had been at a high risk of exposure to it"* [(415)].

Cue fact-wreckers; 'fact' false-positive equals 97%: Verdict is False.

The infamous goat, papaya and COVID-cola: A *Reuters* video shows a Tanzanian goat and a papaya testing positive for COVID-19. At least the goat is an animate object. Tanzanian President John Magufuli said that people are being told they have COVID-19 when they don't [(416)]. Tanzania had chosen not to adopt the COVID-19 vaccines. Tanzania's President John Magufuli declared that the COVID-19 vaccines are dangerous and unnecessary. Magufuli, a devout Catholic, said God would protect his nation from the disease. Tanzania's Health Minister Dorothy Gwajima taught citizens to blend an immune tonic containing ginger, onions, lemon and pepper [417]. The daily propaganda may teach the world to scoff at herbal medicine we can make in our kitchen, however according to the *Reuters* COVID-19 tracker, as of May 18th 2021, only 509 infections and 21 COVID-19 deaths had been reported in Tanzania since the pandemic began and the country had not been in lockdown since March 2021 [418]. Tanzania's Magufuli died mysteriously in March 2021 [419]. Member of the National Council of Austria, Michael Schnedlitz, was videoed confirming a positive test in cola using a rapid test in the Austrian parliament [420].

Testing positive for COVID-19 after vaccination: After the COVID-19 vaccine became available in the UK, HCWs noticed that positive COVID-19 PCR and rapid antigen tests were occurring in vaccinated individuals. A *Forbes* article explained that mRNA-based vaccines would not result in positive COVID-19 test "since the proteins produced following vaccination are not expressed in the respiratory (nasal tract), which is sampled for COVID-19 PCR or antigen testing". Additionally, the article conveniently concluded that when a vaccinated person tests positive, this 'likely' indicates that they were infected with SARS-CoV-2 just prior to or after being vaccinated [421]. This 'likely' explanation is dubious given that 12,400 people in Israel tested positive post-COVID-19 vaccine, and the UK government Scientific Pandemic Influenza Group on Modelling, Operational sub-group (SPI-M-O) acknowledged in April 2021, that 60-70% of the deaths and hospitalisations in the UK's 3rd wave were occurring in people who have had both doses of the COVID- 19 vaccine [237, 422]. Now the narrative is the 'pandemic of the unvaccinated'. The boffins have managed to finagle statistics to call the vaccinated unvaccinated. According to the CDC (thus the world), you are not fully vaccinated if it has been less than two weeks since your 1st dose of a 2-dose vaccine, or it has been less than two weeks since your second shot of a two-dose vaccine or, alternatively, it has been less than two weeks since your single dose of a single-dose vaccine. In between all these times, you are classed as unvaccinated, Have no doubt that everyone hospitalised with COVID-19 has had their shot. As will be discussed in Chapter 11,'Trial Protocols and Study Design Flaws' the trials only followed participants for seven days after their second dose and concluded that the vaccine works in these 'unvaccinated' by their own definition people!

Pandemic of the unvaccinated: Truth or scare? On October 16th 2021, Ireland's Health Protection Surveillance Centre (HPSC) document entitled 'Vaccination Status of COVID-19 Deaths in Ireland between 1st April 2021 and 16th October 2021' said that in this time there were a total of 402 deaths in people with laboratory-confirmed COVID-19 infection. 224/402 (55.7%) deaths were in people who had received at least one dose of COVID-19 vaccine and 174/402 (43.3%) of the deaths were in people who had died after 14 days or more after receiving both doses of a 2-dose vaccine or 1 dose of a 1-dose vaccine. Queerly, this document also states that 178/402 (44.3%) of deaths were in people not vaccinated (i.e. within 14 days after receiving both doses of a 2-dose vaccine or 1 dose of a 1-dose vaccine), or not registered as vaccinated on Ireland's national COVID-19 immunisation system. Adding these numbers individually, 178, 224 and 174 makes 574, so makes no sense at all given that there were 402 deaths. There is obviously crossover due to classifying vaccinated persons as unvaccinated. Regardless, it hardly indicates a pandemic of the unvaccinated, quite the opposite.

Cross-contamination: *Panorama* went undercover to expose cross-contamination of samples occurring in laboratories. In January and February 2021, *Panorama* investigative reporter Jacqui Wakefield worked 18 shifts undercover at the Milton Keynes laboratory. Wakefield joined one of four teams of technicians preparing and processing PCR test samples. The Milton Keynes laboratory analysed thousands of test-and-trace samples from members of the general public every day. Secretly filmed footage revealed a failing service with shoddy practices and staff complaining they were under pressure to meet targets, despite the laboratory often running well below capacity. The programme discovered that social distancing was poorly maintained and that three outbreaks of COVID-19 had occurred among staff. Test samples sometimes arrived poorly packaged and labelled, with equipment frequently malfunctioning and leading to contamination of results. The programme also discovered that tests, including some intended to find new variants of coronavirus, have been wrongly discarded or lost.

Expert Chris Denning, Director of the University of Nottingham Biodiscovery Institute, described a scene from the undercover footage where a technician wipes up a sample with a tissue as "crazy" and said,

"There is almost zero question that this would lead to contamination". Standard practice is for contaminated plates to be retested [(423)].

What Kary Mullis had to say about the PCR test he invented: Kary B Mullis invented the PCR test, a technique vital in DNA research and technology. Kary, who shared the Nobel Prize in Chemistry in 1993 with Michael Smith, died suddenly of pneumonia on August 7th 2019, aged 74 years. There is no doubt that Kary would have spoken out about the misinterpretation of his PCR test in the current crisis. In a conference about HIV, when questioned about the possible misuse of PCR to estimate all these supposed free viral RNA that may or may not be there, Kary replies:

> *"I don't think you can misuse PCR. The results...the interpretation of it...if you can say...if they can find this virus in you at all and with PCR if you do it well you can find almost anything in anybody...If you can amplify one single molecule up to something that you can really measure, which is what PCR can do...then there are just very few molecules that you don't have at least one single one of in your body, so that can be thought of as a misuse...to claim that it's meaningful...The measurement for it (HIV) is not exact at all...With HIV, the results are inferred in a sense. PCR is separate from that; it's just a process to make a whole lot of something out of something. It doesn't tell that your sick or the thing you ended up with was gonna hurt you"* [(424)].

The acquired immunodeficiency syndrome (AID) pandemic was also fuelled by a PCR test for human immunodeficiency virus (HIV). HIV had not been proven to cause AIDs. In a video entitled *'Kary Mullis didn't find single proof that HIV causes AIDS'* on You-will-obey-Tube, Kary discusses meeting AIDS discoverer and fellow Nobel Laureate Luc Montagnier. Kary says:

> *"I went over to Montagnier, and I said Dr Montagnier, can you help me?"* (Mullis was talking about his work at the Speciality Laboratories in Santa Monica). *"I was a consultant there...we were working on that, and at some point, we needed to re(new) our grant from the NIH (National Institute of Health), and I had to write it and so...The first line* (of a paper Mullis was writing) *was 'HIV is the probable causes of AIDS' (acquired immune deficiency syndrome), and I wrote it, and I said well I need a paper, some kind of scientific paper to reference that statement"*.
>
> *"By the time I had met Luc Montagnier, I had met a lot of AIDS researchers...I always went up to them afterwards, and I said, where can*

I find a scientific reference that I can use ...remember I said I had a sentence there that HIV is the probable cause of AIDS...and I needed to have to back that up by something before I could write it and submit it...I can't find it...There's got to be someone that knows this...so I asked all these people...none of them had it... none of them...and I was getting really freaked, they don't know nobody knows this whole thing is a big sham...it's ridiculous".

"Finally Montagnier came to a...seminar... down in San Diego... lots of federal money... wine and cheese. I went over to Luc Montagnier afterwards, I said Dr Montagnier... I can't find a reference that goes with the statement that says HIV is the probable cause of AIDS. I'm sure you can help me... He said, Why don't you quote this new work about ...a virus that can kill monkeys... some kind of monkey...a little ape...a model system for studying AIDS... some kind of retrovirus... It killed (chimpanzees) in about a week... it was nothing like AIDS there... it doesn't kill you in a week... I read that paper, and I didn't see any connection... I wouldn't wanna use that as a reference...I don't remember exactly what he said, but then he walked away... Before (he walked away)...he told me about that paper he said why don't you use the NIH... the CDC report, and I said I looked at that and that was not a scientific paper, then he said what about...this, this paper that had just come about a month before... a lot of fanfare associated... but it was total crap... yeah if you get two million dollars you can figure out how to kill a primate with a retrovirus so what, it doesn't have anything to do with AIDS...it didn't look like AIDS, it didn't smell like AIDS, just because it was a retrovirus... I didn't get anything more out of him... And the people standing around who were his colleagues looked at him as if he should come up with a better answer than that, but he didn't. I really thought he would have an answer... I really did... Montagnier will know why he thinks HIV causes AIDS...but he didn't" (have an answer) [(425)].

Kary on Fauci: In another video, Kary lets us know his feeling about Master Mason Fauci.

"What is it about humanity that wants to go to all the details? Guys like Fauci get over there and start talking, I mean, he doesn't know anything about anything, and I'd say that to his face. Nothing! The man thinks you can take a blood sample and stick it in an electron microscope, and if it's got a virus in there, you will know it. He doesn't understand

electron microscopy... he doesn't understand medicine. He should not be in the position he is in. Most of those guys up there on top are just total administrative people and don't know anything about what's going on at the bottom. Most guys have got an agenda, which is not what we would like them to have, being that we pay for them to take care of our health in some way. They've got a personal kind of agenda...they make up their own rules as they go, they change them when they want to. Tony Fauci does not mind going on television in front of the people who pay his salary and lie directly into the camera".

"You can't expect the sheep to really respect the best and the brightest; they don't know the difference...The vast majority of humans do not possess the ability to judge who is and who isn't a really good scientist...That is the main problem with science this century. Because science is being judged by people. (Science) Funding is being done by people who don't understand it...Who do we trust? Fauci? Fauci doesn't know enough. If Fauci wants to get on television with somebody who knows a little bit about this stuff and debate them, he can easily do it because he's been asked. I've had a lot of people...the President of the University of South Carolina (ask Fauci to) come down there and debate me on the stage in front of the student body because I wanted somebody who was from the other side to come down here and balance my...".

The interviewer replies, *"But he didn't wanna do it"* [(426)].

Conflict of interest: A cataclysmic conflict of interest exists in Ireland. In February 2021, the EU's Health Security Committee agreed on a common list of antigen tests that can be included in COVID-19 test result certificates. Whilst these rapid antigen tests are allowed to be recognised in the 27 countries of the bloc, Ireland's National Public Health Emergency Team (NPHET) do not allow rapid antigen tests to be used. Cillian De Gaston is a member of NPHET and the Director of the National Virus Reference Laboratory (NVRL). NPHET is Ireland's public health police power [(427)]. The NVRL and Cillian De Gascun financially benefit from PCR testing. Ireland's Health Service Executive (HSE) said the executive's carried out 2.4 million COVID-19 tests and spent a total of €280.48 million on Ireland's 'test and trace' in 2020. Clonmel, Tipperary-based Enfer processed the COVID-19 tests from its Kildare laboratories on behalf of the NVRL.

Businessman Louis Ronan who controls Enfer was paid €122.4 million in 2020 to process COVID-19 tests [428].

A person with free will may express concern that the Irish government defers to 'NPHET guidelines'; that NPHET defers to WHO guidelines; and that the WHO defers to the World Health Assembly. As previously mentioned, the World Health Assembly is the world's highest health policy-setting body that makes all the decisions for the WHO's 194 Member States regarding the Global Health and Security Agenda (GHSA). The Irish government, and indeed all governments take orders from above. NPHET 'guidelines' are WHO 'guidelines', which are the World Health Assembly, thus the decisions regarding our countries health are not made by our elected representatives.

Back in December 2020, UK Minister of Innovation at the Department of Health and Social Care, James Bethell, in response to an MP's concerns about blanket PCR testing put to him by one of the constituents, admitted that COVID-19 mass testing is inaccurate and gives a false sense of security [429]. PCR tests are being misused, misinterpreted and are wholly inaccurate, yet public health continues to push this false narrative to generate interest in and increase uptake of vaccines. Refuse to get tested and the pandemonium ends, so to the reason for Rockefeller's public health 'emergency'.

CHAPTER SEVEN

DOES SARS-COV-2 EXIST?

"No one is more hated than he who speaks the truth". Plato [430]

In order to answer the question does the virus exist, the question that needs to be asked is, does severe acute respiratory syndrome coronavirus 2 (SARS-CoV-2) cause coronavirus disease 2019 (COVID-19)? In order to answer that question, certain criteria have to be met. Controversy exists as to whether the SARS-CoV-2 virus has met these criteria.

In the beginning, there was no viral culture: As previously mentioned in Chapter 6, 'Meaningless PCR tests', polymerase chain reaction (PCR) is classified as an *in vitro* diagnostic (IVD) COVID-19 test. In viral culture, viruses are injected into laboratory cell lines to see if they cause cell damage and death, thus releasing a whole set of new viruses that can go on to infect other cells. As previously mentioned also, Klaus' Fourth Industrial Revolution and the Age of Technology heralded the end of the era of cell culture for virus detection in clinical microbiology. The boffins now use computers. The Centres for Disease Control and Prevention (CDC) Division of Viral Diseases made recommendations for IVD use. On January 1st 2020 the CDC reported on page 42 of these recommendations that no quantified virus isolates of the 2019-novel coronavirus (nCoV) were available for CDC use at the time the test was developed [431]. As no positive control material from positive patient samples or viral culture was available to be used to devise the test, laboratories had to use synthetic controls either from synthetic DNA fragments or plasmids. As aforementioned also, handling synthetic controls can lead to trace amounts that can result in cross-contamination [392]. Oxford University was surprised that SARS-CoV-2 had not been isolated. In August 2020, Oxford University's Centre for Evidence-Based Medicine (CEBM) published an *Open Evidence Review* of oral-faecal transmission of COVID-19. Study authors stated that few studies had attempted or reported culturing live SARS-CoV-2 virus from human samples. This surprised the study authors, as viral culture is regarded as the gold standard or reference test against which any diagnostic index test for viruses must be measured and calibrated to understand the predictive properties of that test [393].

Computers, not SARS-CoV-2 viral culture, were used to develop PCR tests: The development of the PCR test did not use viral culture and instead relied on computational science. The term *in silico* refers to biological experiments performed by computer or via computer simulation that utilises databases and computational power. *In silico* relates to *in vivo* and *in vitro*. *In silico* primer design is utilised in PCR detection of novel SARS-CoV-2 [(432)]. When the first quantitative reverse transcription PCR (RT-qPCR) methods were being developed in January 2020, limited numbers of SARS-CoV-2 genomes were available for initial *in silico* specificity (true negatives) evaluation [(433)]. On January 17th 2020, the World Wealth Organisation (WHO) published the very first primers and probes for RT-qPCR. Computer scientists used known SARS-CoV and related bat coronaviruses genomic data to create a non-redundant alignment (an alignment not characterised by repetition). Upon release of the first SARS-CoV-2 genome sequence, the first diagnostic RT-qPCR test was developed using this sequence and an alignment with other known SARS-CoV sequences. The original PCR tests for SARS-CoV-2 were also reactive to the original SARS-CoV and bat SARS-like-CoV. On January 23rd 2020, a third monoplex RT-qPCR was added. This is currently the test used by many laboratories worldwide [(434)].

Isolation and genomic sequencing: SARS-CoV-2 has been isolated, but only in a handful of cases and never in 'pure culture'. The global initiative on sharing all influenza data (GISAID) was established to provide open access to genomic data of influenza viruses and coronaviruses. The WHOs Global Influenza Surveillance and Response System (GISRS) laboratories submit genetic sequences data to GISAID and Genbank or similar databases in a timely manner consistent with the Standard Material Transfer Agreement [(435)]. In February 2020, SARS-CoV-2 was isolated from the oropharyngeal swab specimen of the first laboratory-confirmed patient with COVID-19 infection in Korea. Phylogenetic analyses of whole-genome sequences using sequences downloaded from the National Centre for Biotechnology Information (NCBI) and GISAID showed that it clustered with other SARS-CoV-2 reported from Wuhan. Vero cell cultures were used to isolate SARS-CoV-2. Vero cells are African green monkey (*Chlorocebus aethiops*) kidney cells [(436)]. In March 2020, a complete genome sequence was obtained for a SARS-CoV-2 strain isolated from an oropharyngeal swab specimen of a patient with COVID-19, who had returned to Nepal from Wuhan, China [(437)]. In March 2020, SARS-CoV-2 was isolated from confirmed by PCR COVID-19 cases in Northern Italy, and full-length genome sequencing occurred. The swab contents again were seeded on Vero E6 and the sequences were submitted to GISAID [438].

Koch's postulates: Microbiology is a component of public health, and my master's dissertation was entitled 'Systematic Review and Meta-Analysis of Plant-Derived Antimicrobials in WHO Priority Pathogens', so I have some understanding of microbiology. The rules that scientists use to determine if an infectious microorganism causes a specific disease are called "Koch's postulates". Koch's postulates are the criteria required to identify the causative factor of an infectious disease. The major groups of microorganisms are bacteria, archaea, fungi (including yeast and moulds), algae, protozoa and viruses. The question remains; have the scientific rules required to prove SARS-CoV-2 according to Koch's postulate been satisfied?

Koch's Postulates state;

1. The microorganism must be found in abundance in all organisms suffering from the disease but should not be found in healthy disease-free organisms.
2. The microorganism must be isolated from a diseased organism and grown in pure culture.
3. The microorganism (from the pure culture) should cause the disease when inoculated into a healthy organism.
4. The microorganism must be re-isolated from the inoculated, diseased experimental host and identified as being identical to the original specific causative agent.

Applying Koch's Postulates to prove if SARS-CoV-2 causes COVID-19 requires isolating the virus from a diseased organism; growing of the viral agent in pure culture; and observing the onset of disease when the virus is reintroduced into a healthy organism. This is the approach that has, up until the new normal, been used for over a century to identify viruses in diseased organisms and isolate viruses from their natural reservoirs that harbour them [439]. There is no doubt whatsoever that Koch's postulates have not been satisfied for SARS-CoV-2. The 2nd criteria require that SARS-CoV-2 be isolated in pure culture. This hasn't been satisfied. The 3rd criteria require that SARS-CoV-2 should cause the disease when inoculated into a healthy person. This hasn't been satisfied. The 4th criteria require that SARS-CoV-2 be re-isolated from that inoculated person. As the 3rd criteria are not established, the 4th criteria cannot be satisfied as a matter of course.

How the scientists avoid being scientists: *WebMD*, an apparently credible medical information website, states SARS-CoV-2 has been found and grown from several individuals who have been suffering from coronavirus disease, thereby fulfilling the first two of Koch's postulates. However, *WebMD* goes on to excuse that as it would be 'unethical' to expose people to SARS-CoV-2, and that public health scientists used 'epidemiology' to prove that only people exposed to the virus got infected. Scientists say they have shown that SARS-CoV-2 is associated with people with COVID-19, and SARS-CoV-2 has been isolated (in Vero cells) from these patients. The epidemiology is said to show that COVID-19 occurs in people who are exposed to SARS-CoV-2 "more often than people who have not been clearly exposed" to SARS-CoV-2. 'More often' is not proper science. Finally, *WebMD* explains the virus has been grown (in Vero cells) from the people who were subsequently exposed. In addition, scientists are able to use animals to demonstrate these last two rules by exposing the animal to SARS-CoV-2 and see if it causes COVID-19 [(440)]. Scientists have not however done this step, as will be explained shortly.

Why SARS-CoV-2 has not been proven to cause COVID-19: SARS-CoV-2 has not been proven to cause COVID-19 for two reasons. Firstly SARS-CoV-2 has not been isolated in pure culture; thus, the 2nd criteria have not been met, and secondly, SARS-CoV-2 hasn't been shown to cause COVID-19 in a healthy person; thus, the 3rd criteria have not been met. In all fairness, virologists may have provided themselves with a valid excuse not to isolate the virus in a 'pure culture', however there is no excuse not to inoculate a healthy person and then re-isolate the virus from that inoculated person in order to prove the existence of the virus.

Firstly SARS-CoV-2 has not been isolated in a pure culture: At the time Koch's postulates were proposed, knowledge regarding viruses was in its infancy. The procedure of 'growth in pure culture' in virology differs substantially from 'growth in pure culture' required for bacteriology. Historically viruses were isolated by inoculating laboratory animals or eggs with small quantities of tissues or fluids obtained from biological specimens. Modern-day propagation of viruses requires host cells which inevitably results in a mixed population of viruses. Additionally, multiple steps are necessary for a virus to replicate in cell culture. Each of these steps has the potential to impose strong selective pressure, meaning that individual organisms have an increased chance of survival over others. With SARS-CoV-2 'pure culture' virus isolation requires propagating viruses using for example, mammalian cell (animal cells) culture *in vitro* preparations. Modern-day *in vitro* culture techniques to isolate viruses are the inoculation of susceptible, generally immortalised cells with biological material containing the desired agent (SARS-CoV-2). The starting and final virus populations are not the same as there is always some degree of genetic mutation resulting from 'adaptation' to the cultured cells. Therefore the selective pressure placed on the prorogation of viruses in this manner and the degree of genetic mutation that occurs creates several limitations for viruses generated using this method. These limitations have the potential to reduce the biological relevance of *in vivo* studies performed with cell culture-derived viruses [(439)].

Cell cultures are used to isolate SARS-CoV-2: Culture of SARS-CoV-2 takes place in certified Physical Containment Level 3 (PC3) laboratories. Culture of SARS-CoV-2 requires either non-human cell lines: Vero and Vero E6 cells, human cell lines or engineered cell lines.

Non-human cell lines/Vero cells: Vero CCL-81 or Vero E6 cell lines contain an abundance of ACE2 receptors, which are commonly used. Vero CCL-81 and Vero E6 cell lines are derived from the kidney of an African green monkey (*Cercopithecus aethiops*). The African green monkey is also called the grivet monkey [(441)]. Other monkey cells used to isolate SARS-CoV-2 are LLC-MK2 rhesus monkeys (*Macaca mulatta*) kidney cells [(442)].

Human cell lines: Human continuous cell lines that support the growth of SARS-CoV-2 include Calu3 (pulmonary cell line) and Caco2 (intestinal cell line). Modest growth is also seen in Huh7 (hepatic cell line), 293T (renal cell line) and U251 (neuronal cell line). I have not come across any studies isolating SARS-CoV-2 that use human cell lines.

Engineered cell lines: Cell lines can be genetically engineered to express proteins that assist in the entry of SARS-CoV-2, potentially producing higher viral loads in cells that did not support the growth of SARS-CoV-2. Vero E6 cells have been engineered to be superior to human lung tissue and Calu-3 cells for SARS-CoV-2 culture. Other engineered human cell lines include HEK 293 cell line (human kidney cells), HT1080 cell line (human fibrosarcoma cells), BHK-1 cell line (baby hamster kidney cells) and HeLa (housewife Henrietta Lacks' cells) [(441)].

Whilst SARS-CoV-2 is isolatable using Vero E6 cell line, Huh7 or human airway epithelial cell line (BEAS-2B), the engineered cell line, Vero E6 is highly susceptible to SARS-CoV-2 infection and Vero E6 are the predominant cell lines used to isolate SARS-CoV-2 in humans [(443)].

Secondly, SARS-CoV-2 hasn't been shown to cause COVID-19 in a healthy person: As SARS-CoV-2 hasn't been shown to cause COVID-19 in a healthy person the 3rd criteria have not been met. The technique of satisfying the 3rd criteria (and therefore 4th criteria) of Koch's postulate should, under normal circumstances, rely on studying groups of people who have become ill and then comparing them with people who have not become ill. Investigators can reasonably make the assumption the disease would occur if a healthy person was exposed to the virus. The researchers would then look to see if newly unintentionally exposed people come down with the disease and then attempt to isolate and grow the virus from them.

It is a complete double standard to say that it is unethical to expose people to the SARS-CoV-2 virus to satisfy Koch's postulates and prove that SARS-CoV-2 causes COVID-19. The same scientists have no ethical dilemma deliberately infecting a healthy person with SARS-CoV-2 in human challenge trials designed to improve the speed at which vaccines are developed. In February 2021, the UK government announced it would run a COVID-19 human challenge study, following approval from the country's clinical trials ethics body, the National Health Service (NHS) Research Ethics Service (RES) [(444)]. The WHO is actively encouraging human challenge trials. '1 day Sooner' advocates for people who want to participate in high-impact medical trials, including COVID-19 challenge trials where they will be deliberately infected with SARS-CoV-2 [(445)].

To 'satisfy' Koch Postulates scientists used two monkeys back in 2003: As previously mentioned, scientists are able to use animals to demonstrate the last two of Koch's postulates. I cannot see that the following study has been conducted for the current SARS-CoV-2. The study I am about to describe was conducted back in 2003 for the original severe acute respiratory syndrome (SARS-CoV). Back in 2003, in an attempt to prove that SARS-CoV caused SARS disease, scientists inoculated two rhesus macaques with Vero cell-cultured SARS coronavirus (SCV) isolated from a person who had died of SARS, then monitored their clinical signs, antibody response and virus excretion. Both macaques became lethargic and developed a skin rash and one suffered from respiratory distress. The macaques excreted virus from the nose and throat, confirmed by reverse transcription-polymerase chain reaction (RT-PCR) and virus isolation. The isolated virus was identical to that inoculated, as shown by electron microscopy and RT-PCR analysis. Vero cells were used to demonstrate seroconversion to SARS-CoV. The virus was isolated from the faeces of one of these animals (446). Two monkeys back in 2003! You zany scientists! Scientists are now too complacent to reconstruct this study for the current SARS-CoV-2, and it remains 'unethical' to prove the virus exists in humans.

Caution against using electron microscopy to identify coronaviruses: In 2020, the American Society of Nephrology (ANS) issued caution when identifying coronaviruses by electron microscopy. The ANS said care should be taken to prevent mistaking cell organelles for viral particles. The study authors, Farkash et al. noted that electron microscopic images, whilst appearing to look like a coronavirus, did not demonstrate coronaviruses. Instead, the structure referred to were clathrin-coated vesicles (CCVs), normal subcellular organelles involved in intracellular transport (447).

Public Health Ireland failed to produce evidence of isolation of SARS-CoV-2: Irish journalist and activist Gemma O'Doherty produced a letter from the Health Service Executive (HSE) dated December 23rd 2020. *Reuters* fact-wreckers need to stop spreading misinformation. *Reuters* report it as a letter from the United Kingdom's (UK's) Department of Health and Social Care (DHSC). The letter O'Doherty refers to is a response to a Freedom of Information Request (FOI) from Ireland's HSE. In the video, O'Doherty concludes, *"the virus...does not exist"* (448). O'Doherty made a request for:

> *"A full, accurate and complete list of records held by HSE or under the authority of the HSE which describes the isolation of the* SARS-CoV-2 *virus, taken directly from symptomatic patients with COVID- 19 where the same was not combined or mixed with any other source of genetic materials such...as monkey kidney cells or cancer cells thereby eliminating contamination as a possible alternative source of sampling"*.

The response Gemma received said;

"Following consultations with my colleagues both from the scientific and medical areas of the HPSC (Health Protection Surveillance Centre), I can confirm that we would hold no records. In relation to your request, these are the reasonable steps I have taken to ascertain the whereabouts of the existence of such records, and unfortunately, I must inform you that having undertaken these searches, we were unable to locate the records in question. I am satisfied that all reasonable steps have been taken to locate the record that you have requested and must refuse, therefore, your request".

According to O'Doherty, the phrase, *"the record concerned does not exist"* is highlighted in yellow. The letter dated December 23rd 2020, is from Sinead Roche Moore, FOI decision-maker. Sinead's other title is Business Manager at HPSC [(449)].

Public Health England failed to produce evidence of isolation of SARS-CoV-2: As of October 12th 2020, PHE had failed to produce evidence that SARS-CoV-2 had been isolated. A lady called Mrs Sear made a FOI request to PHE to provide proof that the virus has been isolated and purified to enable the PCR tests to be correctly used to identify the virus SARS-CoV-2 and not just pick up any coronavirus. PHE's response was;

"PHE can confirm that it holds the information you have specified. However, the information is exempt under section 21 of the FOI Act because it is reasonably accessible by other means, and the terms of the exemption mean that we do not have to consider whether or not it would be in the public interest for you to have the information [(450)].

Not in the public interest? SARS-CoV-2 has not been isolated in pure culture as is required to satisfy Koch's postulates. Whilst using engineered monkey kidney cells to isolate SARS-CoV-2 may be satisfactory from a virologist's perspective, it can be disputed that using human lung epithelial cells to study the effect of a human respiratory virus would be more clinically relevant. Scientists have deemed that satisfying the 3rd and 4th Koch's postulate using humans is unethical, so this has not been met for SARS-CoV-2. In addition, no evidence exists that the 3rd and 4th Koch's postulate has been satisfied using monkeys for the current SARS-CoV-2. As Koch's postulates have not been satisfied for SARS-CoV-2, it has not been proven that SARS-CoV-2 causes COVID-19.

CHAPTER EIGHT

MEANINGLESS CASES

"Those who cannot remember the past are condemned to repeat it".
George Santayana (451)

Inflated cases are a tool for exerting control and power. The new era of public health is supposed to depend on good science (452). I am not suggesting that estimating mortality in a global pandemic due to a novel virus is an exact science. Rationally speaking however, the data informing current public health policy should reflect accurate infection rates and actual mortality rates in order to determine the actual infection fatality rate. The public is being provided with neither. The recording of both COVID-19 cases and COVID-19 deaths is highly misleading and, in fact, overinflated. Why? Fear is the foundation of government control. Again, fear is the main ingredient in the public health seven-step recipe for generating interest in, and increasing demand for, influenza (or any other) vaccination as discussed in Chapter 3, 'Coercive Control' (177).

Casedemic: Anyone may think listening to the daily propaganda that COVID-19 disease has a 100% fatality rate. The media have nonsensically reported cases which is a meaningless measure. To view the statistics on the incidence of COVID-19 cases in the past seven days in Europe, go to *Statistica*. I visited this site on May 23rd, 2021. Whilst it showed that Ireland has the lowest case rates in Europe, Irish businesses still suffered, and other health conditions were still being sidelined (453). In September 2021, Ireland had both the highest vaccination and case rates in Europe. Go figure. COVID-19 is a disease that is so deadly that most people have to be tested to know they have it. Undocumented cases of COVID-19 occur in asymptomatic cases. A study conducted for the Chinese social media and technology company Tencent published in *Science* on May 1st 2020, used a mathematical model of infectious disease transmission to estimate that nearly 80% of confirmed COVID-19 cases originated from undocumented cases in people who experienced mild, limited or no symptoms at all (454).

Everyone remembers, in the beginning, it was two weeks to 'flatten the curve'. Flatten the curve is a public health strategy aimed to slow down the spread of the SARS-CoV-2 to prevent overwhelming the hospitals. Then, thanks to New Zealand Prime Minister Jacinda speaks-to-us-like-she's-a-woman Ardern doing such as 'great job' (on us), New Zealand moved without consensus to suppressing the virus cases using a zero COVID strategy. To drive this change in policy, the pharmaceutical owned daily propaganda created COVID-19 pandemonium by fabricating a 'casedemic'. In September 2020, calls were made in Ireland for the "meaningless" daily COVID-19 updates to be changed for weekly figures as they were causing people to suffer from severe anxiety [(455)]. These calls went unheeded.

Meaningless graphs and shoddy modelling: The behavioural psychologist's advice was to barrage us with meaningless graphs showing exponential growth. We have been observed to mistakenly perceive the coronavirus to grow linearly, thereby underestimating its potential for exponential growth, and thus less likely to adhere to COVID-19 social distancing laws. The ruling class thus ordered the daily propaganda to use repeated displays of exponential graphs to correct our "perceptual error" and increase our compliance. Mathematical models that do not account for us all being different are also used to manipulate COVID-19 statistics. At the beginning of the pandemonium, Professor Martin COVID-69er Ferguson's notorious modelling assumed that society was culturally homogenous (that we are all of the same and equally susceptible), resulting in Ferguson's overinflated figures, which in part, led to the global shutdowns [(456)].

Ireland cooks the books on cases: A video of a Dáil debate at the Irish Oireachtas (National Parliament) shows Aontú party Peadar Tóibín questioning Ireland's ex-Taoiseach Leo Varadkar on how Ireland's methods for counting cases differed from other countries. Leo-the-Liar says that when compared to other countries, Ireland is "doing their own thing". The video shows Varadkar seemingly pleased with himself that Ireland counts cases that aren't cases [(457)].

> *"One thing we always did in Ireland was to count cases in care homes from day one; other countries didn't do that. We counted suspected cases even when there wasn't a laboratory test confirming that the patient had COVID...and we didn't discount people who had underlying conditions like other countries did. If someone had stage four cancer, was in a nursing home and was suspected of having COVID but didn't test positive for COVID, we counted that!".*

Inflated strain on hospital intensive care units: I am not suggesting that healthcare workers have not worked hard to save lives during the emergence of this novel coronavirus, and acknowledge that there has been a strain on the hospitals at certain periods. In Ireland, these were during April 2020 and January 2021 (post-vaccine rollout). I believe this strain has been overstated, however. Every year since 2000, we have been bombarded with reports of our hospitals being on the brink. In 2017, before COVID (BC), *Health Manager* journal described Irish intensive care units (ICU) as being very busy, with 91% bed occupancy in adult ICUs and 94% bed occupancy in paediatric ICUs in 2017. The recommended occupancy levels are 70-80% [(458)]. In 2020, Health Service Executive (HSE) CEO Paul Reid said the number of fully staffed ICU beds across the hospital system pre-March 2020 was 225, with temporary surge capacity during the pandemic bringing this figure up to 354. During the pandemic, the HSE put 55 permanent and fully-staffed beds in place, increasing capacity by 25% pre-March and bringing the current permanent capacity number to 280. Additionally, the Winter Plan funding was to add an extra 17 beds, increasing the number to 297 in total.

On September 30th 2020, there were 41 of the current 280 fully staffed ICU beds available in Ireland [(459)]. On January 15th 2021, during Ireland's 3rd lockdown, Ireland recorded the highest COVID-19 transmission rate in the world, driving absolute panic, fear and hysteria throughout the susceptible population. There were 287 patients in Irish ICUs on this day, with 169 of these having tested positive for COVID-19. The HSE's Director of Acute Services, Liam Woods, acknowledged that with a surge capacity limit of up to 350, the health system had the capacity to accommodate 63 further patients in ICU before exceeding surge capacity [(460)]. The Irish government provides up-to-date figures on ICU data and acute hospital and testing data. On January 15th 2021, confirmed cases in ICU were 173 out of 321/350 surge capacity [(461)]. At this time we Irish were being held responsible for killing our grandparents in nursing homes we didn't visit during Christmas 2020.

Inflated hospitalisations: We have all seen a busy hospital and a full hospital car park. We've all seen a heaving Accident & Emergency (A&E). Every year, we have all read the headlines of the hundreds waiting on trolleys in hospitals; 'Thousands of people were left lying on trolleys', 'number of patients on trolleys reaches record highs'. We have all seen endless footage on the news of the 'trolley crisis', Far from being an arrestable offence, peoples videos of the trolley crisis made the news. My generation was raised to believe half of what we see and none of what we hear; apparently our eyes are deceiving us altogether.

The announcement of the COVID-19 vaccine being approved was met with the daily propaganda bombarding us with repeated images of ambulances parked outside hospitals. I worked in an A&E. Ambulances parking outside a hospital is very ordinary. Watching the daily propaganda, one soon recognised the people specific personal protective equipment (PPE) stock images of the 'overwhelmed COVID-19 ward'. Curious truth seekers could easily see with their own two eyes if their hospital was busy. Our local hospital was conducting major road works in the car park during our 'crisis'.

Nightingale debacle: Despite repeated 'surging' COVID-19 cases, the Nightingale hospitals, the seven hospitals built to cope with the perceived pressures on the National Health Service (NHS) in England from the first COVID-19 wave lay empty and remained on standby, as medics warn of staff shortages. Indeed, most Nightingale facilities were yet to start treating COVID-19 patients, despite the number of people in hospitals during the April 2020 peak [(462)]. The Nightingale debacle is a prime example of crony capitalism at its finest. In May 2020, *The BMJ* reported that the COVID-19 Nightingale hospitals were to shut down after seeing very few patients [(463)]. Fifty-four patients were admitted to the Nightingale Hospital London between April 7th and May 7th 2021 [(464)]. On January 20th 2021, it was revealed that the Nightingale hospitals cost British taxpayers half a billion pounds [(93)]. The Nightingale hospitals existed for one purpose only, and that was to drive project fear.

Gloucestershire and Croydon: A video posted on Fascistbook by freedom protester Debbie Hicks entitled 'All Quiet on the Medical Front' shows Gloucestershire Hospital main entrance, A&E, the Injury Unit etc., empty. In the video, the hospital looks completely deserted [(465)]. The hospital's official response was;

> *"Contrary to what you may have seen through secret filming, our hospitals are and remain extremely busy. We are currently caring for more than 200 patients with COVID-19, including many who require*

treatment in our critical care departments and a further 500+ non-COVID patients who need our care and expertise".

Where they were, who was looking after them, and where exactly where these people were entering and leaving the hospital and parking remains anyone's guess. Hicks was arrested on suspicion of a public order offence. Apparently, filming *no one* in an A&E is so intrusive and upsetting to the hospital's policy of 'maintaining patient confidentiality'; doublespeak for, 'maintaining the promotion of fear so as to generate interest in, and increase the uptake of vaccines' (466). The daily propaganda's official narrative at the time of Hick's filming on December 14th 2020, was that the NHS had issued an "urgent plea" as Gloucestershire's two main hospitals and their staff were under considerable pressure, with the number of COVID-19 hospital admissions having risen to 186 (467). Another video posted on Fascistbook shows Croydon Hospital empty (468). In true form, the official spiel by the daily propaganda aiming to generate interest in and increase uptake of vaccines was that Croydon University Hospital was "very, very busy" as coronavirus cases surge (469).

Enter hospital spokesperson to refute claims by delegitimisation and censorship: Hospitals' spokespeople have had to justify why our hospitals are quiet (empty), including visitor's restrictions, fewer outpatient or elective appointments, and according to the time of day. This hardly explains why the car parks, entrances and A&E entrances are empty. Where are the trolleys? Everyone understands patients will be in wards, but we know if this is the case, the hospital will have movement and activity – right? Governments can track this activity from space as they did in China to prove how busy the hospitals were (470). In an aim to censor videos of empty hospitals, one study looked at what authors described as the 'Film Your Hospital Conspiracy Theory'. After analysing Twaddle data, the study authors concluded that hashtags that were using and sharing so-called conspiracy theories could be targeted in an effort to delegitimise content, and that social media platforms should boost efforts to label or remove this content. The authors also suggested that public health authorities could enlist the assistance of influencers to spread an antinarrative message (471).

There are more cases than we are led to believe: Cases do not mean hospitalisations! Actual cases are much higher than the daily propaganda lead us to believe. Public health does not want us to know, as this means that COVID-19 is far less deadly than we are being led to believe. Between March and May 2020, the Centres for Disease Control and Prevention (CDC) stated the true number of COVID-19 cases in the US was anywhere from six to 24 times higher than the confirmed number of cases. The CDC obtained this information from a *JAMA Internal Medicine* seroprevalence antibody study which tested people's blood for antibodies to determine if they had been previously infected and had immunity to the virus (472). Back in April 2020, a seroprevalence study of Santa Clara County, US, discovered that there were 50 to 85 times more cases than previously reported, meaning a far lower CFR, and concluded that seroprevalence studies should be used to determine COVID-19 parameters to inform public health policy (390). Back on November 30th 2020, FDA's Deputy Commissioner for Medical and Scientific Affairs and member of the board of Pfizer, Scott Gottlieb said that up to 30% of Americans may have been infected with coronavirus by the end of 2020 and that some US states will have had a rate of prior infection as high as 50% (473). This is good news as Gottlieb said;

> *"You combine a lot of infection around the country with vaccinating 20% of the population (and) you're getting to levels where this virus is not going to circulate as readily, once you get to those levels of prior immunity"* (473).

Pfizer's Scott Gottlieb certainly did a summersault, going from vaccinating 20% of adults to vaccinating babies over six months (474).

CHAPTER NINE

INFLATED DEATHS

"A statesman is an easy man, he tells his lies by rote. A journalist invents his lies and rams them down your throat. So stay at home and drink your beer and let the neighbours vote".

William Butler Yeats [475]

Inflated deaths are a tool for exerting control and power. Before COVID (BC), we had seasonal influenza, seasonal, being the operative word. Now we have seasonal coronavirus, the uncommon cold, soon to be the common cold. At the height of summer in the northern hemisphere, the daily propaganda did not acknowledge natural ebbs and flows of the current severe acute respiratory syndrome coronavirus 2 (SARS-CoV-2). In 2019 the United States (US) Centres for Disease Control and Prevention (CDC) and the World Health Organisation (WHO) estimated that up to 650,000 deaths annually are associated with respiratory diseases from seasonal influenza [64, 476]. A *Lancet* study on influenza mortality 2019/20 showed that previous estimates of annual influenza deaths were outdated. Vital death records and influenza surveillance data estimates of country-specific influenza-associated respiratory excess mortality rates in 33 countries confirmed that the global influenza-associated respiratory mortality estimates are higher than previously reported [476]. The death rate from seasonal influenza is typically put at around 0.1% in the US [477]. Yet we didn't hit the global panic button for influenza. Watch this space.

Meaningless graphs and shoddy modelling: As for cases, behavioural scientists discovered that using a logarithmic scale to display coronavirus (COVID-19) disease-related deaths gives the public a 'less accurate' understanding of how the pandemic is developing; doublespeak for 'we are less likely to comply'. So, mass media and policymakers were told to communicate to the general public using a graph on a linear scale instead [478].

SARS-CoV-2 mortality: Even after a year, there is no scientific consensus on how fatal SARS-CoV-2 is. There are three measures epidemiologists use to describe the risk of fatal outcomes during and after an infectious disease outbreak. The first measure is the case fatality rate (CFR) which is used by the daily propaganda. CFR estimates this proportion of deaths among identified confirmed cases only. The second measure is the infection fatality rate (IFR), which includes deaths among all cases, including undocumented mild and asymptomatic cases. IFR is a more accurate figure of mortality as it estimates this proportion of deaths among all infected individuals. There are discrepancies also in fatality rate usage by the National Institute of Allergy and Infectious Diseases (NIAID), the CDC and the WHO. Estimation of the IFR in coronavirus disease 2019 (COVID-19) is urgently needed to assess the scale of the coronavirus pandemic. As previously mentioned, many cases go undiagnosed. Policymakers and the public are calling on using the IFR, which is a much more accurate figure but remains an important unknown [479]. While the actual IFR remains unknown, the daily propaganda continues to indoctrinate us that the estimated mortality rate for the coronavirus is ten times higher than for seasonal influenza to coerce us into their global experiment.

IFR in Iceland was found to be 0.3%; 3 times that for influenza: A systematic review and meta-analysis of research data on COVID-19 IFRs were published in the *International Journal* of *Infectious Diseases* in December 2020. Study authors again reiterated that whilst the CFR is extremely valuable for experts, IFR is increasingly being called for as a more accurate estimate of the overall mortality from COVID-19. The authors found that until July 2020, the IFR of COVID-19 across populations was 0.68%; however, they concluded that due to very high heterogeneity in the meta-analysis, it was difficult to know if this represented an entirely unbiased point estimate. Heterogeneity refers to differences in susceptibility of the population that result in variability in the data that poses a risk of bias. Different places and people will experience different IFRs. High heterogeneity includes factors such as age and underlying comorbidities in the population [480].

Iceland is the place for good data on COVID-19 cases and mortality rates. Reykjavik-based deCODE Genetics is a subsidiary of the US biotech company Amgen, with several hospitals, universities and health officials in Iceland. A deCODE Genetics study analysed antibodies and the death rate in COVID-19 in the Icelandic population. The country tested 15% of its population since late February 2020, when its first COVID-19 cases were detected, giving a solid base for comparisons. In a subgroup that tested positive, further testing found that antibodies rose for two months after their infection initially was diagnosed and then plateaued and remained stable for four months. The overall conclusion is that antibodies against the SARS-CoV-2 virus did not decline within four months after diagnosis and that the risk of death from infection was 0.3% (481). As previously mentioned, the death rate from seasonal influenza is typically around 0.1% (477). Icelandic data showed that COVID-19 is three times as deadly as influenza. As previously mentioned also, bear in mind that A *Lancet* study confirmed that the global influenza-associated respiratory mortality estimates are higher than previously reported (476).

The science is settled, the CFR is anywhere from 15% to 0·1%: The *Lancet Journal of Infectious Disease* describes a wide range of the many estimates of the CFR ranging from reports of 15% initially from a small cohort to, as more data emerged, the CFR decreasing to between 4.3% and 11.0% and later to 3.4%, with rates reported outside China in February 2020 even lower at 0.4% (482). On February 28th 2020, an editorial released by NIAID and the CDC published online in the *New England Journal of Medicine* stated, "...the overall clinical consequences of COVID-19 may ultimately be more akin to those of a severe seasonal influenza (which has a case fatality rate of approximately 0.1%)" (479). Yet, here we stand, a year and a half later threatened with mandatory unlicensed 'vaccines' for a disease with the same mortality as influenza. Evidence of the virus' lethality is irrelevant. We have the saviour vaccines! Shut up! Obey! Take your shot!

COVID-19 deaths are not necessarily deaths from COVID-19: Accurate estimates allow us to keep things in perspective. 'Dying from' or 'dying with' COVID-19 are two completely different things and open to different interpretations by medical practitioners having difficulty determining which categories a death falls into. The current reporting system works to overinflate COVID-19 death statistics and mislead and frighten the public. COVID-19 deaths are not all confirmed. An undisclosed amount of reported COVID-19 deaths are 'deaths from any cause within 28 of a positive PCR test', or 'suspected', 'probable' and 'possible' deaths from COVID-19. According to the WHO guidelines, a COVID-19 death is defined for surveillance purposes as a death resulting from a clinically compatible illness in a probable or confirmed COVID-19 case unless there is a clear alternative cause of death that cannot be related to COVID-19 disease (e.g., trauma). There should be no period of complete recovery between illness and death [483]. Additionally, WHO guidelines in April 2020 stated;

> *"COVID-19 should be recorded on the medical certificate of cause of death for ALL decedents (dead person) where the disease, or is assumed to have caused, or contributed to death, i.e. COVID-19 is the underlying cause of death".*

Such an example would be someone who has developed pneumonia as a result of COVID-19 and dies from acute respiratory distress. Alternatively, COVID-19 may be present on the death certificate as a significant condition contributing to death but not the underlying cause. These guidelines are clear that in such cases, these deaths "are not deaths due to COVID-19 and should not be certified as such" [483]. The WHO doesn't listen to the experts at the WHO.

Public Health England (PHE) changed its definition of COVID-19 deaths. The new definition is now death in a person with a laboratory-confirmed positive COVID-19 test within (equal to or less than) 28 days of the first positive specimen date [484]. The BBC reports COVID-19 deaths as, *"deaths from any cause with 28 days of a positive COVID diagnosis".* Public Health Ireland, in general and before Brexit, follows PHE. In Ireland, the 'Guidance in Relation to the Coroners Service and Deaths due to COVID-19 infection' says that confirmed and suspected or possible COVID-19 related deaths are reportable to the relevant District Coroner [485]. The Health Protection Surveillance Centre (HPSC) supplies statistics to the Chief Medical Officer (CMO), Dr Tony cervical botch job Hooligan, who admitted to the reporting of 'suspected' deaths from COVID-19 in people who have not tested positive for COVID-19 [486]. Since April 2020, in fact, a positive COVID-19 test in the US was no longer required to confirm a COVID-19 death [487]. The CDC is the US's health protection agency; doublespeak for 'public health police'. The European Centres for Disease Prevention and Control (ECDC) is the European Union's counterpart. Doctors were told COVID-19 can be a cause of death even if patients are not tested. The National Vital Statistics System (NVSS), part of the CDC, and 'CDC Guidance for Certifying Deaths due to COVID-19' stated that testing for COVID-19 should be conducted, however it is acceptable to report COVID-19 on a death certificate without this confirmation if the circumstances are compelling within a reasonable degree of certainty [488]. Their reasonable is unreasonable. After being criticised for being the only country listing COVID-19 deaths where an autopsy confirmed the virus was the main cause of death, on December 28th 2020, Russia revised their COVID-19 deaths statistics. This revision happened to coincide with the Russian COVID-19 vaccine rollout, in a fortunate upturn of events to generate interest in and increase uptake of the COVID-19 vaccine. Deaths from COVID-19 in Russia increased exponentially [(489)].

Oxford University says one-third of COVID-19 deaths were not COVID-19 deaths: While death certification is regarded as a gold standard for ascertaining the cause of death, again it is important to distinguish between deaths where COVID-19 was a contributory cause and those where COVID-19 was the underlying cause of death. In September 2020, Oxford University's Centre for Evidence-Based Medicine (CEBM) stated that in full, approximately one in thirteen (7.8%) of deaths that had COVID-19 on the death certificate did not have COVID-19 as the underlying cause of death. By September 2020, the CEBM said that this proportion had risen substantially to one-third (29%) [(490)].

Error on death certificates in the old normal: The pandemonium aside, error on deaths certificates is exceedingly common. In March 2020, a retrospective review of the accuracy of cause and manner of death certification in cases in which autopsy was performed at the University of Wisconsin Hospital (UWHC) found that, in 85% of cases, death certificates contained ≥ one error, with 51% containing multiple errors and 33% containing single errors [(491)]. A Vermont study found that 53% of death certificates had errors, with 51% having major errors; and 10% having minor errors [(492)]. One may safely deduce that 51% of COVID-19 deaths have major errors on their death certificate and that not all COVID-19 deaths are deaths from COVID-19.

The IMHE model used by the CDC overshoots figures: In relation to COVID-19 death projections by the Gates financed Institute for Health Metrics and Evaluation (IHME) at the University of Washington, epidemiologist Marc Lipsitch of the Harvard T.H. Chan School of Public Health said, "It's not a model that most of us in the infectious disease epidemiology field think is well suited". Others experts, including some of the model maker's colleagues, are even more critical. Epidemiologist Ruth Etzioni of the Fred Hutchinson Cancer Centre, who has served on a search committee for IHME said,

"That the IHME model keeps changing is evidence of its lack of reliability as a predictive tool. That it is being used for policy decisions and its results interpreted wrongly is a travesty unfolding before our eyes".

The primary cause for concern in relation to the IHME projections of COVID-19 deaths, according to Etzioni, is that, *"the fact that they overshot will be used to suggest that the government response prevented an even greater catastrophe, when in fact the predictions were shaky in the first place".* The IHME initially projected 38,000 to 162,000 US deaths. At the beginning of the pandemic, the White House combined these estimates with others to alert citizens of the potential for 100,000 to 240,000 deaths [(493)]. The whole shebang is pretty shaky.

Financial incentives exist to inflate COVID-19 deaths: Why is it acceptable to report a COVID-19 on a death certificate without confirmation? Money talks. A video from a coronavirus response meeting discussing that US state COVID-19 deaths statistics were overinflated shows US Representative Blaine Luetkemeyer questioning CDC Director Dr Robert Redfield about the "perverse incentive" to record a death as a COVID-19 death. Speaking at 1 minute 8 seconds, Dr Redfield acknowledges that monetary incentives existed in the past with HIV, whereby a patient may die of a heart attack, however a financial incentive for a hospital existed to record this as a HIV death. Dr Redfield also acknowledges a monetary incentive for hospitals to report deaths as from COVID-19 even when the actual cause is not COVID-19 [(494)].

Early in the pandemic, the US Senate passed the Coronavirus Aid, Relief and Economic Security (CARES) Act. The CARES Act is the largest of the three federal stimulus laws enacted in response to the coronavirus and was signed into law on March 27th 2020. During this emergency period, this legislation provides a 20% add-on to the diagnosis-related group rate for patients with COVID-19. This add-on applies to patients treated at rural and urban inpatient prospective payment system hospitals. Medicare pays hospitals the 20% 'add-on' to the regular payment for COVID-19 patients. Wilson H. Taylor Scholar in Health Care and Retirement Policy Joeseph Antos said,

"This is no scandal. The 20% was added by Congress because hospitals have lost revenue from routine care and elective surgeries that they

can't provide during this crisis, and because the cost of providing even routine services to COVID-19 patients has jumped" [495].

It would be no scandal if our current situation wasn't so scandalous.

In Minnesota: Republican state senator Scott Jensen, who is also a medical doctor, said the American Medical Association (AMA) is encouraging doctors to over-count COVID-19 deaths. Jensen revealed that "Medicare is determining that if you have a COVID-19 admission to the hospital, you get US$13,000. If that COVID-19 patient goes on a ventilator, you get US$39,000, three times as much". The document that Dr Jenson refers to is entitled 'Guidance for Certifying Deaths Due to Coronavirus Disease 2019 (COVID -19)'. Jensen told local media he received a directive from the Minnesota Department of Health to list COVID-19 as the cause of death on death certificates even if patients were never tested for it. When asked why officials would want to inflate the death statistics, Jensen said, "Fear is a great way to control people, and I worry about that" [496].

The *Kaiser Family Foundation* website also confirms these financial incentive figures. The Kaiser Family Foundation provides in-depth information on key health policy issues, including Medicaid, Medicare, health reform and global health. To project how much hospitals would get paid by the federal government for treating uninsured patients, the foundation examined payments for admissions for similar conditions to COVID-19. For less severe hospitalisations, the foundation used the average Medicare payment for respiratory infections and inflammations with major comorbidities or complications in 2017, which was US$13,297. They also used the average Medicare payment for a respiratory system diagnosis with ventilator support for greater than 96 hours for more severe hospitalisations, which amounted to US$40,218. These average payments were then increased by 20% to account for the add-on to Medicare inpatient reimbursement for patients with COVID-19 that was included in the CARES Act [497].

Ireland cooks the books on deaths (and cases again): If Irish Tánaiste Leo-the-Liar being caught on tape describing how Ireland cooks the books on cases, here is the Irish government's National Public Health Emergency Team (NPHET) for COVID-19 spokesperson admitting to Michael McNamara, Chair of the Special Committee on the COVID-19 Response, how Ireland also cooks the books on deaths.

McNamara questions; *"Dr Cuddy if somebody who is asymptomatic ...shows no symptoms whatsoever of COVID and they had a heart attack, and they are brought to a hospital and tested, and it is found that they have COVID (what he means is tested positive for SAR-COV-2), and they die soon thereafter, but this is somebody who has demonstrated no symptoms whatsoever, are they recorded as a COVID death or not?...if they tested positive for COVID, but ultimately they came to hospital because they've had a heart attack or a stroke or fallen off a building or something like that?"*

NPHET answers, *"Well, we adhere to the WHO uh case definitions in terms of the recording and reporting of deaths, so in the situation, you've just described where someone has a positive COVID test, then it is a death in a confirmed COVID case, but such a case would be subject to a coroner's report...as part of the ongoing validation of the data in our surveillance system we would take additional...(continued drivel)"*.

McNamara questions, *"Ok but a coroners' report sorry, I'm trying to be very reasonable ...obviously, a coroner's report takes a very long time to make its way through the system so, for now, they are recorded as a COVID death, but it may be that they are taken off that list at a later date is that what you're saying?"*

NPHET answers, *"That's it exactly"*.

McNamara questions: *"If somebody is admitted to a hospital, they're asymptomatic with a broken leg, for example, and require hospitalisation they're tested they're asymptomatic, but test positive, are they included among the statistics of those in hospital with COVID?"*

NPHET answers, *"Yes, they are"*.

McNamara's questions: *"Even though the reason they're admitted may not have been COVID, they may have been admitted with a broken leg or heart attack or something unrelated to COVID, they are included in the stats of people in hospital with COVID at the moment?"*

NPHET answers, *"They're included in the surveillance data, that's right"* (498).

The United Kingdom cooks the books on deaths: The United Kingdom (UK) government is also inflating COVID-19 deaths. In July 2020, an article published by Oxford University's Centre for Evidence-Based Medicine (CEBM) website entitled 'Why no one can ever recover from COVID-19 in England' described a 'statistical flaw' in the way data is gathered by Public Health England (PHE). Using the current PHE definition, no one with COVID-19 in England ever recovers from their illness. A patient who tests positive and is successfully treated and discharged from the hospital will still be counted as a COVID death, even if they have a heart attack or are run over by a bus three months later [(499)]. 'Statistical flaw' is doublespeak for 'massaging statistics'.

Age-stratified case data and underlying medical conditions: In the US, the CDC state that 94% of COVID-19 deaths have occurred in people with underlying multiple chronic coexisting diseases [(500)]. The CDC reported that only 6% of these COVID-19 deaths record COVID-19 as the only cause of death [(501)]. There is an absence of age-stratified case data in the UK and Ireland. According to Ireland's Central Statistics Office (CSO), 92% of deaths occur in people over 65 years of age [(502)]. 63% of COVID-19 deaths in the Republic of Ireland occurred in nursing homes and other long-term care settings [(503)]. Older and/or obese populations are more likely to suffer from multiple, chronic, coexisting diseases known as comorbidities or multimorbidities. Patients with comorbidities such as diabetes, hypertension, or obesity have a higher risk of getting seriously ill and dying from COVID-19, and a higher risk of dying in general. According to Ireland's CSO, over 93% of people who died with COVID-19 had an underlying medical condition.

The median age of COVID-19 deaths in Ireland is 83 and life expectancy in this country is 82, yet the lives of the young and fit have been sold down the river to protect people that have lived full and productive lives. No one would take issue with these policies if they had actually worked, however the policies drove infection into our nursing homes. The virus entered our care homes as underpaid care home staff simply couldn't afford to take time off work to self-isolate when they had symptoms. Staff moved between different nursing homes, and personal protective equipment (PPE) was inadequate [(504)]. Public health blamed nursing home outbreaks on most of the population who went nowhere near them. In true Catholic style the Irish public blamed themselves for enjoying Christmas as the daily propaganda had taught them to.

Drop in COVID-19 mortality: When reporting COVID-19 deaths, public health and the media neglect to reassure us that these are deaths are predominantly in older populations. Policymakers should maintain rationality and focus on age-specific IFRs, not the broad spectrum sledgehammer to crack a walnut approach currently being used. German data reports cases and deaths by age categories. This data shows that the fatality rate from COVID-19 declined in all age groups, with the older age groups driving the overall reduction [(505)]. A percentage point is a difference between two percentages. For example, moving up from 40% to 44% is a four percentage point increase, but is a 10% increase. Horwitz and colleagues looked at death rates among 5,000 hospitalised patients at New York University (NYU) Langone Health from March to August 2020 and found that mortality rates were lower, thought to be due to improved treatments. Early reports showed high mortality from COVID-19. Mortality decreased by 18 percentage points, with chances of dying once hospitalised decreasing from 25% at the beginning of the pandemic to approximately 7%. Death rates declined for all groups. After factoring in age and comorbidities, the research team found that the drop in deaths in patients being diagnosed with COVID-19 later in the pandemic was because patients were younger and suffering from fewer comorbidities [(506)]. Another study conducted in England showed similar declines in death rates among 21,000 hospitalisations between March and June 2020. Mortality decreased by 20 percentage points, including in different ages, racial groups and underlying conditions [(507)].

German government cover-up: As granny said, "there are two people you can never trust; a politician and a statistician". All statistics can be finagled. Germany is the country with the greatest number of Members of the European Parliament (MEPs), therefore has the greatest influence in the European Union (EU) and world affairs. Germany has been widely reported as experiencing a lower CFR than other European countries. This wholly inaccurate reporting by the daily propaganda results in people assuming that Germany is somehow superior. In reality, Germany's lower CFR is in part attributed to higher testing rates, and therefore more confirmed cases, which subsequently lowers the CFR. Germany has a robust testing programme that tests people with and without symptoms. The fact is that in many countries, only high-risk patients and those critically ill are tested, dramatically underestimating case numbers, as cases with either no symptoms or mild illness are not tested [508]. Data comparing excess deaths with COVID-19 deaths in 2020 from 35 countries showed that Germany had an excess death rate of 3%, which was surprisingly low in comparison with other countries such as Italy (19%), the UK (17%) or Spain (23%) [509].

A German-language report challenging the established coronavirus pandemic narrative was leaked from the German interior ministry. The report entitled *Coronakrise 2020 aus Sicht des Schutze's Kritischer Infrastrukturen (Corona Crisis from the Perspective of Critical Infrastructures)* evaluated the previous coping strategy and made recommendations for action [510]. According to the so-called 'Russian propaganda', known as the Strategic Culture Foundation, the leaked report said that the risk of COVID-19 was vastly overestimated, so much so that at no point was the danger posed by the novel virus going to rise above the normal level.

The document stated that worldwide, within a quarter of a year, there were no more than 250,000 deaths from COVID-19, compared to 1.5 million deaths (25,100 in Germany) during the influenza wave 2017/18. The leaked report focused on the "manifold and heavy consequences of the corona measures" and warned that these are "grave" and that more deaths are would be due to state-imposed COVID-19 lockdowns due to the German healthcare system focusing on coronavirus, and postponing life-saving surgery and delaying or reducing treatment for non-COVID patients [511].

My German-speaking friend confirmed this. In May 2020, *The Times* reported that the interior ministry civil servant leaked the report to the right-wing website after being frustrated that his concerns were not being taken seriously by his superiors. He was subsequently fired. The report says;

> *"The (entirely unforced) collateral damage of the corona crisis has by now become gigantic".* It also says, *"The protection measures ordered by the state...have meanwhile lost any purpose but remain largely in force"* and *"we urgently recommend completely lifting them in short order in order to prevent (further) damage to the population..."* [512].

Disability discrimination and do-not-resuscitate orders: Mencap charity for people with a learning disability said that people with disabilities suffered from 'shocking discrimination' during the pandemic. A covert eugenics programme was undertaken during the pandemic with do-not-resuscitate orders (DNR) in place. Mencap found that among the 120 patients with disabilities without COVID-19 who died during this period, 91.7% had a DNR order when admitted [513]. DNR patients were, in general, found to be older and had more comorbidities. The risk of death from COVID-19 was significantly higher in patients with DNR orders [353].

The Antibiotic Apocalypse and the Obesity Pandemic as a Cause of Death

Two concurrent pandemics as an unrecognised cause of death are occurring concomitantly. Prior to COVID-19 pandemonium, the obesity pandemic and the antibiotic apocalypse existed. Both the obesity pandemic and the antibiotic apocalypse were predicted to crash the health system and the global economy. I firmly believe COVID-19 is a cover-up for what we are largely witnessing, which is deaths due to obesity impairing the immune response combined with deaths from drug-resistant secondary bacterial infections that can no longer be 'cured' with antibiotics.

Antibiotic apocalypse: BC, I applied to do a PhD in Biomedicine at a research centre to answer the question are plant-derived antimicrobials (PDAm) suitable for the treatment and control of multidrug-resistant (MDR) pathogens causing healthcare-associated infections. I also have experience in treating antimicrobial-resistant infections using herbal medicine. Antimicrobial resistance (AMR) occurs when microorganisms, including bacteria, fungi, viruses and parasites, adapt to become resistant to their counterpart antimicrobial drugs. Overprescribing antimicrobials is the main driver of AMR [514]. Data regarding bacterial superinfections in COVID-19 pneumonia is still emerging [515]. Superinfections can be resistant to antibiotics. A report by Jim O'Neill entitled *Antimicrobial Resistance: Tackling a crisis for the health and wealth of nations*, found that antimicrobial-resistant infections contributed to 700,000 deaths in 2016 and that this figure is predicted to reach ten million deaths annually by 2050 [516]. The foreword of this report admitted that this figure did not account for the secondary effects of AMR, such as the risks imposed by surgery and subsequent post-operative resistant infection [516].

Additionally, former UK Chief Medical Officer (CMO) Sally Davies highlighted the magnitude of underreporting of AMR deaths and called for AMR to be put on relevant death certificates [(517)]. A Royal Institute of International Affairs review on AMR progress estimated a cumulative cost to the global economy of US$100 trillion by 2050 [(518)]. In 2012 multidrug-resistant (resistant to three or more classes of antimicrobials), extensively drug-resistant (resistant to all but one or two classes) and pan drug-resistant bacteria (resistant to all available classes), particularly in pathogens causing pneumonia, was described in *Clinical Microbiology and Infection*, the official publication of the European Society of Clinical Microbiology and Infectious Diseases. Antimicrobial drug resistance in pathogens causing pneumonia is an emerging public health challenge worldwide [(519)]. In 2017 the WHO published a WHO priority pathogens (WHO PPs) list of antibiotic-resistant (AR) bacteria requiring urgent research and development (R&D) for new antibiotics [(520)]. The WHO PPs are a catalogue of twelve families of bacteria that are categorised into three priority levels. The WHO PP list was developed in collaboration with the Division of Infectious Diseases Tübingen University, whereby a multicriteria decision analysis was used to prioritise these AR bacteria. These criteria included infections with the highest mortality, length of hospital stay required, how frequently resistance is encountered once community spread occurs, the ease of zoonotic (animal to human or human-to-human) transmission, preventability through hygiene practices and/or vaccines, therapeutics, and whether new antibiotics were already in the R&D channel [(521)].

Eurosurveillance, Europe's journal on infectious disease surveillance, reported that the prevalence of antibiotic-resistant Gram-negative bacteria is escalating in many European countries. Furthermore, bacterial isolates characterised as multidrug-resistant extensively drug-resistant or pan drug-resistant are increasingly isolated in hospitalised patients. There are no adequate therapeutic options for these infections [(522)]. A 2017 point prevalence survey of healthcare-associated infections (HCAIs) and antimicrobial use (AMU) in European Acute Care Hospitals identified methicillin-resistant *Staphylococcus aureus* (MRSA), vancomycin-resistant Enterococci (VRE), extended-spectrum β lactamase (ESBLs) and carbapenem-resistant or carbapenemase-producing Enterobacterales (CPE) as the pathogens associated with higher healthcare costs, increased length of hospital stay and higher mortality [(523)]. The Antimicrobial Resistance and

Infection Control (AMRIC) division section of Ireland's Health Protection Surveillance Centre (HPSC) state the pathogens associated with AMR in Ireland are CPE, VRE, *Escherichia coli* (*E. coli*), *Klebsiella pneumoniae* (*K. pneumoniae*), *Pseudomonas aeruginosa* (*P. aeruginosa*) and *Neisseria gonorrhoeae* (*N. gonorrhoeae*) [(524)].

Sir William Osler once described pneumonia as the most widespread and fatal of all acute infectious diseases. Osler also described pneumonia as the "captain of the men of death" and "the old man's friend" [(525)]. Pneumonia associated mortality receives specific attention during global outbreaks, including the Spanish flu 1918-1920 and the current COVID-19 pandemic. However, it is important to recognise that even before SARS-CoV-2, pneumonia was already the most frequent cause of death among all infectious diseases in both adults and infants [(526)]. Secondary bacterial pneumonia is one of the risk factors associated with COVID-19, and recent studies on COVID-19 patients provide evidence that secondary bacterial infections were significantly associated with worse outcomes death despite antimicrobial therapies [(527)]. According to an article published in *The Lancet Global Health* in 2020, infections such as seasonal influenza and COVID-19 impair both innate and adaptive immunity antibacterial defences. Opportunistic infections such as *Streptococcus pneumoniae* (*S. pneumoniae*), *Staphylococcus aureus* (*S. aureus*) etc., take advantage of this compromised immunity, resulting in secondary bacterial pneumonia that leads to severe disease with high morbidity in people with preexisting comorbidities. Drug-resistant secondary bacterial infections, secondary bacterial pneumonia, and antibiotic-resistant healthcare-acquired infections (HAI) during the COVID-19 pandemic are currently an unrecognised public health challenge [(528)]. It is virtually impossible that drug-resistant infections are being accurately reported as the cause of death on the death certificates of many 'COVID-19 deaths'.

Obesity pandemic: In 2010, *Global Burden of Disease* study, published in *The Lancet*, noted that obesity had become a bigger public health challenge than hunger. The World Economic Forum (WEF) says that obesity threatens the global economy. The WEF states that more than 2.1 billion people, 30% of the world's population, are classified as overweight or obese. The obesity pandemic costs about US$2 trillion a year which equates to 2.8% of the world's GDP. The McKinsey Global Institute research says obesity costs our global economy the same as armed violence, war, and terrorism combined [529]. Obesity is the main risk factor in COVID-19 disease and is associated with increased risk of hospitalisation, admission to critical care and fatalities [530]. In 2017 a study looking at the health effects of overweight and obesity in 195 countries over 25 years published in the *New England Journal of Medicine* found that high body mass index (BMI) accounted for four million deaths globally, with nearly 40% of these deaths occurring in people classified as non-obese overweight. More than two-thirds of deaths related to high BMI were due to cardiovascular disease [531].

A systematic review and meta-analysis published in *Environmental Science and Pollution Research International* in 2020 described higher BMI as one of the main risk factors in COVID-19 patients [532]. Individuals with obesity experience significant increases in morbidity and mortality from COVID-19. Many mechanisms explain this impact. An article entitled 'Individuals with obesity and COVID-19: A global perspective on the epidemiology and biological relationships' was published in *Obesity Reviews* in 2020. Study authors conducted a systematic search of the Chinese and English language literature on COVID-19 and used 75 studies to conduct a series of meta-analyses on the relationship of individuals with obesity and the spectrum of risk through to mortality. Individuals with obesity were more at risk for hospitalisation. Risk for intensive care unit (ICU) admission was 113% higher, mortality risk was 74% higher, and deaths were 48% higher when compared to healthy BMI people [533]. A major concern is that vaccines will be less effective for individuals with obesity due to primary vaccine failure. Primary vaccine failure refers to an individual not mounting an immune response (making antibodies) after vaccination. Obesity adversely affects the immune system, and obese populations have been shown to respond poorly to vaccines. Data on the effect of obesity on vaccine immunogenicity is limited, and efficacy suggests that obesity is a factor that increases the likelihood of poor vaccine-induced immune response [534]. Primary vaccine failure is discussed further in Chapter 12, 'Vaccines aren't Described as Safe and don't Always Work'. A more proportionate, targeted approach would have been to shield obese patients and let healthy weight people live as normal.

Excess Mortality and COVID-19 Deaths

Excess mortality statistics can help ascertain the actual toll of COVID-19. However, a major limitation in using excess mortality statistics to monitor a global pandemic is that these statistics are only available for a small number of countries. One study showed there were, in fact, no excess total deaths at all in the US. The author of a John Hopkins newsletter article entitled 'A closer look at US deaths due to COVID-19' Genevieve Briand, Assistant Programme Director of the Applied Economics master's degree programme at Hopkins University, critically analysed the effect of COVID-19 on US deaths using data from the CDC in her webinar titled 'COVID-19 Deaths: A Look at US Data'. Briand focused on total deaths per age group and per cause of death in the US instead of looking directly at COVID-19 deaths. In her webinar, Briand explained that the significance of COVID-19 on US deaths could only be fully understood by comparison with the number of US total deaths. Using CDC data, Briand compiled a graph representing percentages of total deaths by age category from early February to early September 2020 and included the time frame before the outbreak. Briand discovered that the CDC data did not show an increase in the percentage of deaths in the older age group, as we are led to believe. Briand also found the percentages of deaths among all age groups remained relatively the same. Briand concluded that COVID-19 had no effect on the percentage of deaths in older people or on the increase in the total number of deaths [(535, 536)]. This upset the applecart and the study was quickly retracted. Undoubtedly Briand got a sharp rap on the knuckles.

Ireland experienced 3.5 % fewer deaths in 2020: In Ireland, deaths are typically reported within two days by family members or the funeral directors through a forum called *RIP.ie*. On November 2nd 2020, a CSO analysis of historic RIP.ie data against official death data was published by the CSO. The CSO released a statement that the continued analysis showed death notices on the website *RIP.ie* provide close to "real-time" mortality trends in Ireland. The CSO statement said there was a rise in death notices between March and April 2020, in line with the impact of the COVID-19 pandemic. By September 2020, the number of death notices stood at 2,353 and was described as being "broadly in line with previous years' mortality statistics". This contrasted with the pronounced increase in death notices reported in April 2020, when the number of death notices rose from 2,861 in March to 3,502 in April. Based on the analysis of thousands of death notices, the CSO concluded that excess mortality for the period between March and September 2020 was between 876 and 1,192 additional deaths than would have normally been expected [(537)]. At the end of 2020, the CSO updated these figures to show that there was, in fact, a drop in deaths reported in 2020. The CSO's 'Vital Statistics' webpage shows that deaths in Ireland decreased from 7358 in 2019 to 7111 in 2020. This figure represents a fall of 3.5% in Irish deaths [(538)]. Yet we are being coerced into taking part in the global experiment. The sharp rise in deaths seen post-vaccination rollout in Irish nursing homes in January 2021 is discussed in Chapter 13, 'COVID-19 Vaccines are Safe for Two Months'.

135,960 deaths in three years and one-quarter months globally: A study published in *Nature* in October 2020, looking to determine the effect of the first wave of the COVID-19 pandemic on all-cause mortality in 21 industrialised countries, found that from mid-February until the end of May 2020, there were 206,000 (95% credible interval, 178,100 -231,000) excess deaths. The authors of this study were from the School of Public Health at the London Imperial College. Bear in mind that some of these deaths will be due to COVID-19, and some will be due to lockdown [(539)]. As previously mentioned in Chapter 2, 'Money, Power and Control', the CDC states that 44% of all excess deaths are caused by the consequences of lockdown [(152)]. Extrapolating the data published in *Nature* provides a total of 135,960 deaths in three and a half months globally, which equates to approximately 500,000 deaths during the course of the year. Poor countries have inadequate death registration systems, but 500,000 is a far cry from 5,000,000.

Look on the bright side, we 'cured the flu'! The *Contagion Live Infectious Disease Today* website states that COVID-19 may have also impacted influenza-like illness reporting, with preliminary data from the CDC estimating between 24,000-62,000 influenza-related deaths in the US in the 2019/20 influenza season [(540)]. We 'cured' influenza by not testing for it. Following the widespread adoption of COVID-19 community mitigation measures to reduce transmission of SARS-CoV-2, the percentage of respiratory specimens submitted for influenza testing in the US testing positive decreased from >20% to 2.3%. Data from Southern Hemisphere countries also confirmed little to no influenza activity [(541)]. Another study published in *The Morbidity and Mortality Weekly Report* stated the dramatic decrease in influenza cases was because the number of samples submitted for testing for influenza dropped by 61% during 2020 [(542)].

Lessons from history never learned: A *Disaster Medicine Public Health Preparation* article entitled 'Public Health Lessons Learned from Biases in

Coronavirus Mortality Overestimation' published in August 2020, stated that public health lessons learned for future infectious disease pandemics include safeguarding against research biases that either underestimate or overestimate an associated risk of COVID-19 mortality. Another lesson to be learned included reassessing the ethics of fear-based public health campaigns and providing full public disclosure of adverse effects from severe mitigation measures to contain viral transmission [(479)]. Don't hold your breath. Public health exists to drive fear to generate interest in and increase uptake of vaccines.

CHAPTER TEN

MASKING

"You wear a mask for so long, you forget who you were beneath it".
Alan Moore [543]

Masks are another tool for exerting control and power. Masking is divisive and pits non-mask wearers against maskers. Hiding our face is historically, culturally and ethically questionable. While health professionals initially refuted mandatory universal masking, more than 100 countries subsequently issued nationwide mask mandates, and the COVID party faithful took to wearing them like ducks to water [544]. How ironic that around the same time, on March 7th 2021, the Swiss donned face masks to vote in a referendum banning burkas and niqabs that cover the face! [545] The referendum passed. I do scoff at the 'biohazard waste' pollution on my bike ride.

Masks exist to act as a reminder of the pandemonium to increase compliance. Masks exist to obscure your identity, smother your voice and weaken your immune system. Masks perpetuate fear and are a tool of coercion. The newly coined 'coronaphobia' results from public health measures to control us. Social distancing, masking, hand sanitising, and avoiding touching one's face creates a vicious cycle of fear and anxiety. Human beings typically touch their face an average of 23 times an hour. We have literally been reprogrammed to avoid a practice we have practised mindlessly since birth [546]. Face masks strongly confuse how other human beings read human emotion [547]. Common sense says that breathing in stale air can't be good for you and masks are dirty.

Flip-flop Fauci: The experts say whatever their drug lords want them to say. If they say the 'wrong' thing, the expert gets a slap on the wrist and are told to do a U-turn, hence the flip-flops scientists. Flip-flop Fauci, was anti-mask one minute, pro-mask the next. Many will remember the *60 Minutes* interview where flip-flop Fauci says;

> *"Right now, people should not be ... there is no reason to be walking around with a mask. When you're in the middle of an outbreak, wearing a mask might make people feel a little bit better, and it might even block*

a droplet, but it's not providing the perfect protection that people think that it is. And often, there are unintended consequences...people keep fiddling with the mask, and they keep touching their face" [(548)].

The next minute Fauci was sporting not one but two masks of different colours to show how conscientious he is, and the Fauci followers were wearing 'I Love Fauci' masks. More appropriate would be 'Masks are Fausty'.

Flip-Flop CDC: Prior to the pandemonium, the Centres for Disease Control and Prevention (CDC) told us that masks didn't reduce influenza virus transmission. A systematic review and meta-analysis conducted by the CDC was published in the CDC's *Emerging Infectious Diseases* Journal in May 2020. The authors identified randomised controlled trials (RCTs) of each measure for laboratory-confirmed influenza. In their systematic review, the authors identified ten RCTs that reported estimates of the effectiveness of face masks in reducing laboratory-confirmed influenza virus infections from literature published between 1946 and July 27th 2018. The pooled analysis found no significant reduction in influenza transmission with the use of face masks [(549)]. Evidence of mask effectiveness is irrelevant. The purpose of masks is to perpetuate fear to generate interest in and increase uptake of vaccines.

'The science' depends on who you get on the day: Oxford University's Centre for Evidence-Based Medicine (CEBM) completely contradicts the CDC's systematic review and meta-analysis by stating that standard surgical masks are as effective as respirator masks for preventing healthcare worker (HCW) infections during viral respiratory diseases outbreaks such as influenza. The CEBM do acknowledge, however that there are no published head-to-head trials of these interventions in severe acute respiratory syndrome coronavirus 2 (SARS-CoV-2) infection, coronavirus disease 2019 (COVID-19), and no trials in primary or community healthcare settings [(550)].

Flip-flop Lukey Kooky: In this video, educated Irish clown, Professor of Immunology, Trinity College Dublin, Luke O'Neill, was at one time an anti-masker. Professor Lukey Kooky says, *"The virus can penetrate the eyes. There's no evidence that wearing a facemask can protect you at all. Just wash your hands, and if you're not infected, don't wear a facemask"* [(551)]. By

July 2020, Professor Lukey Kooky was full steam ahead, backing mandatory face masks for secondary schools [552]. O'Neill's understanding of the human immune system is wanting. O'Neill should know that children are not the drivers of the coronavirus pandemic. In November 2020, Professor Lukey Kooky spoke to a full classroom of Irish students via Zoom in on taking advantage of the disadvantaged to fill their impressionable minds with propaganda and his plans for their dystopian future. In the video, O'Neill says;

> *"We may wear masks every winter in shops like you see in China, and so I think it's gonna be vaccines plus, keep doin' what yer doin' (lockdowns distancing and masks) certainly for six months. Everybody should get vaccinated. You're not doing it for yourself, you're doing it for the vulnerable people in society. I mean, what we're discussing at the moment, the passport ID...you might have a thing on your iPhone that says I've been vaccinated...you may have a wristband that can't get off, so there may be wristbands that can't come off that's one thing, now that could be, people may say 'not on my wrist', there'll be civil liberty questions there...some civil libertarians will kick us a fuss about dat... hardy har, hardy har...I'll bet you'll take your vaccine to get to your debs probably..hardy har, hardy ha.."* [553].

You zany scientists! People forget that they wear masks in China because of air pollution. I was in China during the original SARS outbreak and didn't see one single mask.

Mask that: Wastewater screening is used to monitor SARS-CoV-2 in wastewater globally. One of the biggest concerns is that SARS-CoV-2 survives, even for a limited time, in sewage treatment plants and drinking water supplies. SARS-CoV-2 has been found to persist in aquatic systems and has been found in drinking water. Chlorine is used as a disinfectant to inactivate SARS-CoV-2 in drinking water, however delicate ecosystems are being damaged by the use of chlorine [554]. Trihalomethanes (THMs) are a by-product of chlorine disinfection and are a risk factor for cancer, with unsafe limits of THMs detected in drinking water [555]. SARS-CoV-2 has been found to persist in hospital wastewater, household wastewater, domestic sewage and survives in tap water for 2-3 days at 20°C and up to 14 days at 4°C [556]. It does not matter that SARS-CoV-2 is in our drinking water, keep wearing your mask. The impossibility of masking the human microbiome is discussed in Chapter 17, 'Natural Immunity'.

Masks carry antimicrobial-resistant genes and respiratory viruses: I understand there have been many studies proving that 'masks are safe and effective', however there are many to the contrary. Before science, we had common sense. To anyone with an ounce of common sense, masks are bacteria-ridden. It is becoming common knowledge that where bacteria congregate, antibiotic-resistant bacteria may be present. Multidrug-resistant bacteria are found on everyday items, including mobile phones and computer keyboards of student healthcare workers (HCWs) [557, 558]. It can be safely postulated that multidrug-resistant bacteria are on the new everyday item; the facemask. An article published in the *BMJ Open Respiratory Research* found that face mask samples revealed antimicrobial-resistant (AMR) genes in exhaled aerosols from patients with chronic obstructive pulmonary disease and also healthy volunteers. AMR genes give bacteria the ability to evade antibiotics and become resistant. This study raised the possibility that masks may be transmitting AMR bacteria within the hospital setting [559]. Since the beginning of the COVID-19 outbreak however, there has been no further study on the potential of masks to spread AMR genes, thereby potentially spreading healthcare-acquired antibiotic-resistant bacterial infections. Instead, 'the science is settled', 'masks work'. Masks act as a vector (carry) for respiratory viruses. Two pilot studies in laboratory and clinical settings published in *BioMed Central Infectious Diseases* in 2019 were carried out to determine the contamination by respiratory viruses on the outer surface of medical masks used by hospital HCWs. Study authors found evidence that respiratory pathogens on the outer surface of the medical masks may result in self-contamination [560].

Breathing in plastic: As an environmentalist, I've been speaking out about this from the off. Most masks are made of non-renewable petroleum-based plastic. A performance study during COVID-19 pandemonium published in the *Journal of Hazardous Materials* found that wearing masks increased the risk of microplastic inhalation. Surgical, fashion and activated carbon masks were found to pose a higher fibre-like microplastic inhalation risk. Reusing masks increased the risk of granular microplastic particles and fibre-like microplastic inhalation. N95 masks were found to pose less fibre-like microplastic inhalation risk [561]. N95 masks are respirators masks. An article published in the *Journal of Medical and Biological Engineering* concluded that respirators interfere with many physiological and psychological aspects of task performance [562].

Rebreathing of carbon dioxide: A paper published in *Results in Physics* looking at masks used for COVID-19 protection discussed the potential side effects and solutions. Rebreathing of carbon dioxide (CO2) is a key concern regarding facemask use. Rebreathing CO2 occurs when expired air, rich in CO2, lingers longer than normal in the breathing space of the respirator. The paper provided a literature review on the use of facemasks with the aim to determine which facemasks could be used to avoid re-inhaling rejected CO2. Hypercapnia (excess CO2 in the bloodstream due to deficient inhaled oxygen) is recognised as being related to symptoms including fatigue, discomfort, muscular weakness, headaches and drowsiness. The paper concluded that the rebreathing of CO2 due to mask use has not been taken into consideration. No studies have been conducted to determine and recommend which mask is effective in reducing the spread of coronavirus while simultaneously avoiding CO2 inhalation of the mask wearer [(563)].

Surgical mask induced deoxygenation: A Stanford University surgical mask study published in *Medical Hypotheses* in January 2021 concluded that the existing scientific evidence does not show masks are safe or effective as a preventive measure for COVID-19 and are detrimental. The data suggested that both medical and non-medical facemasks are ineffective in blocking the human-to-human transmission of viral SARS-CoV-2 or COVID-19 disease. Wearing surgical masks has been demonstrated to have adverse physiological and psychological effects, including hypoxia, hypercapnia, shortness of breath, fatigue, headaches, cognitive impairment, activation of the stress response, immunosuppression, and depression and anxiety. Long-term consequences of mask-wearing may cause health deterioration and exacerbate the development and progression of chronic disease. The author advised against the use of masks. The study upset the applecart and was quickly retracted [(564)].

In 2008 a preliminary report published in *Neurocirugía* on surgical mask induced deoxygenation during major surgery evaluated whether the surgeons' oxygen saturation of haemoglobin was affected by the surgical mask or not during major operations. Preoperative and postoperative pulse oximeter readings revealed a decrease in the oxygen saturation of arterial pulsations (SpO2) and a slight increase in pulse rates postoperatively in all surgeon groups [(565)]. I know the zany TicTok docs have refuted this 'conspiracy theory' by placing a pulse oximeter on them while looking cool in their trendy masks and white coats. The point is however, to place a pulse oximeter on while wearing a surgical mask under the duress of a busy emergency room or operative theatre.

Masking during COVID-19 decreases competence, autonomy and relatedness: A commentary entitled 'Physiological and Psychological Impact of Face Mask Usage during the COVID-19 pandemic', published in the *International Journal of Environmental Research and Public Health* in 2020, discussed the physiological effects of wearing masks for prolonged periods. The author noted that mask-wearing does not appear to cause any harmful physiological effects in healthy populations, and the benefits of face masks in protecting against COVID-19 disease seem to outweigh the documented side effects such as headaches. Theoretical evidence, however, suggests that there may be consequential psychological impacts of mask-wearing on the basic psychological needs of competence (the need to produce desired outcomes and to experience mastery), autonomy (the need to feel ownership of one's behaviour) and relatedness (the need to feel connected to others). The study also acknowledged concerns surrounding mask-wearing in those engaging in exercise training and in individuals with preexisting chronic diseases [(566)]. Up to 86% of older Americans have a preexisting chronic disease, and one in two Americans will soon have a preexisting chronic disease [(567)]. The evidence that masks may have detrimental health effects in people with preexisting chronic disease is irrelevant; 'masks work' (to drive fear).

RCTs show cloth masks increase the transmission of viruses: A cluster randomised trial of cloth masks compared with medical masks in HCWs published in the *BMJ Open* in 2015 explained that this study was the first RCT of cloth masks. The study authors cautioned against the use of cloth masks and concluded that this is an important finding to inform occupational health and safety. Moisture retention, reuse of cloth masks and poor filtration may result in an increased risk of infection. The authors concluded that further research is needed to inform the widespread use of cloth masks globally. However, as a precautionary measure, study authors noted that cloth masks should not be recommended for HCWs, particularly in high-risk situations, and guidelines need to be updated [(568)]. A systematic review and meta-analysis on the effectiveness of personal protective measures to reduce pandemic influenza transmission published in *Epidemics* in 2017, found that during the 2009 swine influenza (H1N1) pandemic, encouraging the public to wash their hands reduced the incidence of infection significantly, whereas wearing facemasks did not [569]. The evidence from previous pandemics is irrelevant; 'masks work' (to drive fear).

COVID-19 mask studies say masks are irrational and ineffective: A *Lancet Respiratory Medicine* article published in 2020 said there is no solid evidence that facemasks protect the public against infection with respiratory viruses, including COVID-19 and said there is no rational reason for the use of face masks during the COVID-19 pandemic [570]. A study entitled 'Effectiveness of Adding a Mask Recommendation to Other Public Health Measures to Prevent SARS-CoV-2 Infection in Danish Mask Wearers', was published in the *Annals of Internal Medicine* in March 2021. The Danish RCT was the first in the world to test for the efficacy of face masks to prevent wearers from contracting the coronavirus. The study authors were from Copenhagen University Hospital. The authors concluded there was no statistically significant difference in COVID-19 cases between mask wearers and non mask wearers [571]. The evidence that masks are ineffective is irrelevant; the masquerading continues.

The standard spiel: The European Union (EU) describes masks as 'community masks' or 'hygienic masks'. As masks became part of EU citizens daily lives, the EU introduced new European Committee for Standardisation (CEN) guidelines for community masks in relation to quality and compliance. The CEN Workshop Agreement (CWA) guidelines say this standard is identified as CWA 17553 or CEN/CWA 17533 [572]. The standard is not a guarantee that the mask can protect against SARS-CoV-2. In Ireland, the National Standards Authority of Ireland (NSAI) worked with the Department of Health, the Health Service Executive (HSE) and the Competition and Consumer Protection Commission to fast track a new standard for coverings known as SWiFT 19. The standard should be printed on the packaging for products that meet the criteria and tells consumers that a mask has been tested and deemed suitable for use in adhering to public health advice during the pandemic [573]. Again the standard does not guarantee that the mask can protect against SARS-CoV-2.

If you're going to mask, mask: The two major classes of facemask are medical/surgical masks which are loose-fitting, disposable masks that filter out droplets, and tight-fitting N95 or P2 'respirator' masks. In general, surgical masks are designed to protect the environment from the wearer, whereas respirators are designed to protect the wearer from their environment. A respirator mask contains a particulate matter (PM) 2.5 activated carbon (also known as activated charcoal) filter, which blocks up to 95% of airborne particles [574]. N95 masks are designed to remove more than 95% of all particles that are at least 0.3 microns (μm) in diameter. Measurements of the particle filtration efficiency of N95 masks show that they are capable of filtering ≈99.8% of particles with a diameter of ≈0.1 μm. SARS-CoV-2 is an enveloped virus ≈0.1 μm in diameter [575]. On the other hand, surgical masks may let a significant fraction of airborne viruses penetrate through their filters, providing very low protection against aerosolised virus particles [576].

Everyone is equal, but some are more equal than others: During the inauguration party at the White House, President Biden-his-time-until-Kamala-takes-over wore no mask. The White House's new press secretary was asked why President Biden wore no mask at the Lincoln Memorial on the night of his inauguration, as Biden had signed an executive order hours earlier mandating face coverings on all federal property. Jen Psaki replied that he was, *"celebrating an evening of a historic day"* and that there are *"bigger issues to worry about at this moment in time"* [577].

Corruption in procurement: Corruption risks in procurement are even more pronounced during times of emergency, and robust government procurement practices are required. An article published in The *Journal of Pharmaceutical Policy and Practice* in September 2020 called for an urgent need for transparency and accountability in the procurement of medicine and medical supplies during the COVID-19 pandemic times. During disaster response, huge amounts of additional funding are directed to rapidly resolve critical and complex problems, often through acquiring limited resources under large amounts of pressure. An estimated US$16 trillion has already been spent by governments globally on their responses to COVID-19 [578]. In November 2020, a doctor-led nonprofit legal organisation called the Good Law Project and Every Doctor took legal action against the UK government for awarding personal protective equipment (PPE) contracts to companies without the normal procurement procedures surrounding advertising and a competitive tender process. The Good Law Project said that in the two weeks of inviting tenders for PPE back in March 2020, the government received offers from 16,000 suppliers, many experienced in providing PPE for HCWs. The three largest beneficiaries awarded contracts were a jewellery company called Saiger, a pest control company called Postfix, and an opaque 'family office' called Ayanda owned through a tax haven [(579)].

Masking is a tool of tyranny: If we question the efficacy of masks and refuse to comply, An Garda Síochána (the Irish Police) have been given additional powers under Health Act 1947 [Section 31A-Temporary Restrictions (COVID-19) Regulations], including arrest without warrant. Face mask breaches are punishable by a fine of up to €2500, or up to six months imprisonment, or a combination of both [(580)]. In 2021 Germany mandated the use of FFP1 masks or the more protective FFP2 filtering mask, with France saying it was considering the same mandate [(581)]. FFP1 masks are €1 each; proving that government officials are so far removed from the reality of how the lockdown of the economy has pushed people into extreme poverty and further divided the socioeconomic gap. Food or mask? Heating or mask?

Overturning mandatory mask mandates: On November 9th 2020, mandatory masking of Italian school children was imposed. By January 26th 2021, the Italian Council of State issued a resolution prohibiting children between six and 11 years of age from using masks in schools. This U-turn came after the parents of a child sued the Bolzano regional government in Italy. The judge noted that "the minor cannot be forced to wear a mask during the duration of the classes due to the risk of respiratory fatigue" and that no oximeter was installed to monitor the first sign of respiratory distress in very young students [(582)]. On December 30th 2020, Estonian news reported that 45 complaints had been submitted to the court in an attempt to overturn the government's mandatory mask order requiring people to wear masks in public and other complaints related to the coronavirus restrictions [(583)].

On December 23rd 2020, Austria's Constitutional Court ruled that compulsory mask-wearing and splitting classes and teaching them in alternate shifts was illegal. The court made this decision after two children and their parents brought the case before the court, saying the measures violated the principles of equality before the law, the right to private life and the right to education. The Constitutional Court ruled that the measures in question were illegal and explained this decision by saying that the "ministry has not made clear why it considered these measures necessary" [584]. On November 9th 2020, it was reported that the German city of Düsseldorf lifted a mandatory mask mandate order after a citizen successfully sued against the blanket rule. The Düsseldorf authorities had ordered masks in public across the city unless a social distancing measure of five metres could be maintained. Parks and cemeteries had been excluded from this rule [585]. How magnanimous that we don't have to wear a mask to 'save the dead'.

CHAPTER ELEVEN

TRIAL PROTOCOLS & STUDY DESIGN FLAWS

"There are three kinds of lies: lies, damned lies, and statistics".
Benjamin Disraeli [586]

This chapter summarises the COVID-19 vaccine trial protocols. The data is in tabulated form and includes the inclusion and exclusion criteria, intervention, placebo, endpoints, immunogenicity endpoints, and safety and efficacy to allow data to be compared and contrasted. Secondly, study design flaws and discussed. Both the breakneck speed at which the trials were conducted, and flaws in the study design, negatively impacted the gathering of proper safety and efficacy data. The trials did not prove if the vaccines prevented transmission of severe acute respiratory syndrome coronavirus 2 (SARS-CoV-2) or proved nothing about the safety and efficacy of the COVID-19 vaccine candidates in the populations of most interest, that is, the people most susceptible to coronavirus disease 2019 (COVID-19). Tables 3-6 display adapted data from the 'Clinical Study Protocols' issued by the vaccine manufacturers for;

- Moderna mRNA-1273 vaccine-(Spikevax) [587]
- Pfizer-BioNTech mRNA BNT162b2 vaccine (Comirnaty) [588]
- Oxford-AstraZeneca AZD1222 vaccine (Vaxzevria/ Covishield in India) [589]
- Janssen Ad26.COV2.S vaccine (no trade name) [590]

Design flaws in the COVID-19 therapeutic trials: In relation to COVID-19 therapeutic trials, many design flaws have been acknowledged. A study from researchers at Johns Hopkins Bloomberg School of Public Health published in *BMJ Open* in June 2021 analysed 201 clinical trials for COVID-19 therapeutics (not vaccines) that had been registered under *ClinicalTrials.gov* and in the international clinical trials registry maintained by the World Health Organisation (WHO) by March 26th 2021. Researchers found that most of these trials demonstrated design flaws. 33% of trials lacked defined clinical endpoints such as hospital discharge or survival, nearly 50% of trials enrolled fewer than 100 patients, and 27% enrolled fewer than 50 patients. 25% did not have a randomised design, and just under 50% were open-label; therefore, these studies...*(continued on p.162)*

Table 3: Moderna COVID-19 vaccine candidate; inclusion/exclusion criteria, intervention, placebo, endpoints, safety and efficiency

Inclusion	Healthy adults > 18 or adults with preexisting medical conditions who are in stable condition. At least 25% of enrolled participants, but not more than 40%, will be either ≥ 65 years of age or < 65 years of age and "at-risk". Female participants of nonchildbearing potential (Moderna TX. Protocol mRNA-1273, amendment 3. 2020 p.43).
Exclusion	Individuals under 18 years. Women who are pregnant or breastfeeding. Known history of SARS-CoV-2 infection. A baseline (Day 1) evaluation for SARS-CoV-2 infection and ongoing surveillance for COVID-19 throughout the study. All participants had no immunologic or virologic evidence of prior COVID-19 (negative nasopharyngeal (NP) swab test at Day 1 and/or binding antibody (bAb) against SARS-CoV-2 at Day 1 before first dose (Moderna TX. Protocol mRNA-1273, amendment 3. 2020 p.88). Known or suspected allergy or history of anaphylaxis, urticaria, or other significant adverse reaction to the vaccine or its excipients. bAbs are not neutralising antibodies (nAbs). Immunosuppressive or immunodeficient state (Moderna TX. Protocol mRNA-1273, amendment 3. 2020 p.44).
Inter-vention	Two doses of COVID-19 vaccine candidate the first on Day 1 and the second on Day 29 (Pfizer. PF-07302048 (Moderna TX. Protocol mRNA-1273, amendment 3. 2020 p.8).
Placebo	0.9% sodium chloride (normal saline) injection, which meets the criteria of the United States Pharmacopeia (USP) (Moderna TX. Protocol mRNA-1273, amendment 3. 2020 p.12).
Endpoints	Vaccine efficacy (VE) of mRNA-1273 to prevent, mild, moderate or severe COVID-19 including serologically confirmed SARS-CoV-2 infection regardless of symptomatology or severity (Moderna TX. Protocol mRNA-1273, amendment 3. 2020 p.16).
Immuno-genicity Endpoints	SARS-CoV-2 -specific neutralising antibody (nAb) on Day 1, Day 29, Day 57, Day 209, Day 394, and Day 759 (Moderna TX. Protocol mRNA-1273, amendment 3. 2020 p.36).
Safety	Solicited adverse reactions (ARs) will be assessed for 7 days after each dose and unsolicited ARs will be assessed for 28 days after each dose (Moderna TX. Protocol mRNA-1273, amendment 3. 2020 p.41).
Efficacy	In the primary analysis of vaccine effectiveness (VE) of COVID-19, cases will be counted starting 14 days after the second dose (Moderna TX. Protocol mRNA-1273, amendment 3. 2020 p.14).

Table 4: Pfizer COVID-19 vaccine candidate; inclusion/exclusion criteria, intervention. placebo, endpoints, safety and efficiency

Inclusion	Male /female participants 18-55 years and 65-85 years, inclusive (Phase 1 only), or ≥16 years (Phase II/III), at randomisation. Healthy participants with preexisting stable disease, defined as disease not requiring significant change in therapy or hospitalisation during the 6 weeks before enrolment, can be included. Female contraception included (Pfizer. PF-07302048 (BNT162 RNA-based COVID-19 vaccines) protocol C4591001. 2020. p.41).
Exclusion	History of severe adverse reaction with a vaccine and/or severe allergic reaction (e.g., anaphylaxis) to any component of study intervention (s). Phases 1 and 2 only: Known infection with virus HIV, HCV or HBV. <u>Previous clinical or microbiological diagnosis of COVID-19. Asymptomatic COVID-19 cases may thus have been included.</u> Women who are pregnant or breastfeeding (Pfizer. PF-07302048 (BNT162 RNA-based COVID-19 vaccines) protocol C4591001. 2020. p.41).
Inter-vention	Two doses of COVID-19 vaccine candidate given 21 days apart (Pfizer. PF-07302048 (BNT162 RNA-based COVID-19 vaccines) protocol C4591001. 2020. p.29).
Placebo	Normal saline (0.9% sodium chloride solution for injection) (Pfizer. PF-07302048 (BNT162 RNA-based COVID-19 vaccines) protocol C4591001. 2020. p.41).
Endpoints	To describe the safety and tolerability profiles of prophylactic BNT162 vaccines in healthy adults after 1 or 2 doses. COVID-19 incidence (up to 7 days after receipt of last dose) of past SARS-CoV-2 infection. The number of severe COVID-19 cases (Pfizer. PF-07302048 (BNT162 RNA-based COVID-19 vaccines) protocol C4591001. 2020. p.41).
Immuno-genicity Endpoints	*SARS-CoV-2* neutralisation assay (Pfizer. PF-07302048 (BNT162 RNA-based COVID-19 vaccines) protocol C4591001. 2020. p.57).
Safety	Adverse events (AEs) from Dose 1 to 1 month after the last dose. Serious AEs (SAEs) from Dose 1 to 6 months after the last dose (Pfizer. PF-07302048 (BNT162 RNA-based COVID-19 vaccines) protocol C4591001. 2020. p.10).
Efficacy	Efficacy of RNA vaccine candidates against COVID-19 in healthy individuals complying with the key protocol criteria at least 7 days after second dose (Pfizer. PF-07302048 (BNT162 RNA-based COVID-19 vaccines) protocol C4591001. 2020. p.11).

Table 5: Oxford-AstraZeneca COVID-19 vaccine candidate; inclusion/exclusion criteria, intervention, placebo, endpoints, safety and efficiency

Inclusion	Male /female adults ≥ 18 years who are not immunosuppressed, but are at increased risk of SARS-CoV-2 infection. Adults with medically stable chronic diseases (AstraZeneca. Clinical study protocol-amendment 2 AZD1222-D8110C00001. 2020. p. 35). 1,500 participants 18-55 years, 750 participants 56-69 years and 750 participants ≥ 70 years (AstraZeneca. Clinical study protocol-amendment 2 AZD1222- D8110C00001. 2020. p.15).
Exclusion	Pregnant / breastfeeding women. Individuals < 18 years. Participants who have been previously diagnosed with laboratory-confirmed SARS-CoV-2 only. Participants with previous asymptomatic or undiagnosed infection are not excluded. Participant's baseline serostatus will be determined but not used as basis for exclusion as vaccine will be distributed to millions who will not be tested prior to vaccination (AstraZeneca. Clinical study protocol-amendment 2 AZD1222- D8110C00001. 2020. p.35-36).
Inter-vention	Two doses of COVID-19 vaccine candidate on days 1 and 29 (AstraZeneca. Clinical study protocol-amendment 2 AZD1222- D8110C00001. 2020. p.15).
Placebo	0.9% sodium chloride for injection (AstraZeneca. Clinical study protocol-amendment 2 AZD1222- D8110C00001. 2020. p. 42). Or Meningococcal conjugate vaccine (the conjugate MenACWY vaccine) as control (Pedro M Folegatti et al., *Lancet*, 2020 p.1).
Endpoints	COVID-19 case if their first case of SARS-CoV-2 RT-PCR-positive symptomatic illness occurs ≥ 15 days post second dose. Otherwise, a participant is not defined as a COVID-19 case (AstraZeneca. Clinical study protocol-amendment 2 AZD1222- D8110C00001. 2020. p.13).
Immuno-genicity Endpoints	Anti-SARS-CoV-2 neutralising antibody levels in serum following 2 IM doses of AZD1222 or placebo (AstraZeneca. Clinical study protocol-amendment 2 AZD1222- D8110C00001. 2020. p. 63).
Safety	AEs will be recorded for 28 days post each dose of study intervention. Solicited AEs will be recorded only for participants in the substudy for 7 days post each dose (AstraZeneca. Clinical study protocol-amendment 2 AZD1222-D8110C00001. 2020. p.55).
Efficacy	Participants who present with at least one COVID-19 qualifying symptoms. With exception of fever, shortness of breath, or difficulty breathing, symptom must be present for 2 or more days within 7 days following each dose (AstraZeneca. Clinical study protocol-amendment 2 AZD1222- D8110C00001. 2020. p.49).

Table 6: Janssen COVID-19 vaccine candidate; inclusion/exclusion criteria, intervention. placebo, endpoints, safety and efficiency

Inclusion	Male /female adults ≥ 18 to <60 years of age. Participants must be good or stable health. Participants may have underlying illnesses (not associated with increased risk of progression to severe COVID-19a,13 as specified in Exclusion Criteria 15), as long as their symptoms and signs are stable and well-controlled. Not of childbearing potential (Janssen Vaccines and Prevention. VAC31518 (JNJ-78436735) clinical protocol VAC31518COV3001 amendment 1. 2020. P.69).
Exclusion	Participant has a known or suspected allergy or history of anaphylaxis or other serious adverse reactions to vaccines or their excipients. Participant has abnormal function of the immune system, autoimmune disease and immunodeficiency. The study did not exclude people with a history of SARS-CoV-2 infection (Janssen Vaccines and Prevention. VAC31518 (JNJ-78436735) clinical protocol VAC31518COV3001 amendment 1. 2020. p.70).
Inter-vention	Two doses of COVID-19 vaccine candidate (Janssen Vaccines and Prevention.VAC31518 (JNJ-78436735) clinical protocol VAC31518COV3001 amendment 1. 2020. p.47).
Placebo	0.9% sodium chloride solution (Janssen Vaccines and Prevention. VAC31518 (JNJ-78436735) clinical protocol VAC31518COV3001 amendment 1. 2020. p.22).
Endpoints	Symptomatic COVID-19 cases after vaccination from at least 14 days post-vaccination (Janssen Vaccines and Prevention. VAC31518 (JNJ-78436735) clinical protocol VAC31518COV3001 amendment 1. 2020. p.4).
Immuno-genicity Endpoints nAb	Neutralising antibody responses against SARS-CoV-2 (Janssen Vaccines and Prevention. VAC31518 (JNJ-78436735) clinical protocol VAC31518COV3001 amendment 1. 2020. p.178).
Safety	To evaluate safety in terms of serious adverse events (SAEs; during the entire study), medically-attended adverse events (MAAEs; until 6 months post-vaccination) (Janssen Vaccines and Prevention. VAC31518 (JNJ-78436735) clinical protocol VAC31518COV3001 amendment 1. 2020. p.16).
Efficacy	Symptomatic COVID-19 cases after vaccination from at least 14 days post-vaccination (Janssen Vaccines and Prevention. VAC31518 (JNJ-78436735) clinical protocol VAC31518COV3001 amendment 1. 2020. p.4).

(con't from p. 157) ...were, *"likely to yield only preliminary evidence of a given treatment's safety and effectiveness against COVID-19"*. Study authors also acknowledged the benefits of global registries for urgent clinical trial research as a platform for coordination and cooperation in research [591].

Design Flaws with the COVID-19 Vaccine Trials

Trials too fast to gain adequate safety and efficacy data: COVID-19 vaccines have been issued for use under Emergency Use Authorisation (EUA) [592]. This means that time required to assess safety and efficacy for each phase of clinical research from phase I to phase IV was massively reduced. The shortened timelines under Operation Warp Speed (OWS) and EUA are discussed further in Chapter 13, 'COVID-19 Vaccines are Safe for Two Months'.

The COVID-19 trials enrolled immune people! COVID-19 vaccine trials did not exclude people with a history of SARS-CoV-2. Some trials in fact actively sought people with a history of infection with SARS-CoV-2. A study published in *Vaccine* noted that changes in immunoassays are expected during the vaccine development process in order to understand the immune response to vaccines [593]. It isn't proper science to enrol participants in a vaccine trial to prevent a disease without proper screening for preexisting immunity to that disease. As 80% of people who have SARS-CoV-2 are completely asymptomatic, vaccine manufacturers likely trialled their COVID-19 vaccine candidates in people with preexisting natural immunity to COVID-19 [75].

The Moderna mRNA-1273 trial excluded people with an active COVID-19 infection and people with a known history of SARS-CoV-2 infection. Some participants, however, were described as seropositive at baseline, having antibody (bAb) levels against SARS-CoV-2 (Moderna TX. Protocol mRNA-1273, amendment 3. 2020 p.61) [587]. Baseline antibodies (bAb) titers reliably predict neutralising antibodies (nAb), therefore participants with antibodies at baseline may have had preexisting immunity to SARS-CoV-2 [594].

The Pfizer-BioNTech mRNA BNT162b2 trial excluded people with a previous clinically diagnosed (on signs and symptoms alone where a PCR test result wasn't available) and microbiologically diagnosed

COVID-19 (Pfizer. PF-07302048 (BNT162 RNA-based COVID-19 vaccines) protocol C4591001. 2020. p.41). As 80% of people experience asymptomatic COVID-19 participants in this trial may have had preexisting immunity [588].

The Oxford-AstraZeneca AZD1222 trial did not exclude participants with previous asymptomatic or undiagnosed infection (AstraZeneca. Clinical study protocol-amendment 2 AZD1222-D8110C00001. 2020. p.35). Oxford-AstraZeneca openly enrolled participants with preexisting immunity [589].

The Janssen Ad26.COV2.S trial study did not exclude participants with a history of SARS-CoV-2 infection (Janssen Vaccines and Prevention. VAC31518 (JNJ-78436735) clinical protocol VAC31518COV3001 amendment 1. 2020. p.70). Janssen also openly enrolled participants with preexisting immunity [590].

COVID-19 vaccine trials didn't show the vaccine prevents transmission of SARS-CoV-2: On December 29th 2020, WHO Chief Boffin Dr Soumya Swaminathan said coronavirus vaccine trials didn't tell us if they stopped transmission. Dr Swaminathan said;

"I don't believe we have the evidence on any of the vaccines to be confident that it's going to prevent people from actually getting the infection and therefore being able to pass it on".

Swaminathan said that people should still quarantine when travelling to countries with lower coronavirus transmission rates even if they have had the vaccine [595]. Roll on six months later, and Tony Blair wants a new British unvaccinated subclass, and in July 2021, medical apartheid was introduced in France, Greece, Ireland, Portugal etc. [247].

Whilst the daily propaganda purport that COVID-19 vaccines prevent transmission, the daily propaganda is telling porkies. The daily propaganda reported that new data from the Oxford-AstraZeneca COVID-19 vaccine suggests that one dose of the 'jab' could cut transmission of the virus by 67% [596]. The study that the daily propaganda refers to, published in *The Lancet* in November 2020, does not in fact conclude that the vaccine prevents transmission. The study discusses immunogenicity, which is the ability of an antigen to provoke an immune response. The 69% efficacy rate the study refers to is the percentage of people in which antibody levels were maintained 90 days after the second dose with minimal warning. The study also found that the efficacy to prevent COVID-19 disease was higher with a longer prime-boost interval of 12 weeks. The study makes no mention of whether the antibodies are neutralising antibodies that can bind a virus in a manner that blocks infection. This correct interpretation relates to the vaccine's efficacy to reduce or prevent COVID-19 disease only and not to prevent the spread of infection. Humoral immunity, also called antibody-mediated immunity, is a type of adaptive (later) immune response. Whilst humoral immune response was assessed using immunoassay to measure antibodies in the 18-55 years cohort, and volunteers who were seropositive to SARS-CoV-2 were excluded, T cell adaptive immunity was not determined [(597)]. Both preexisting T cells and cross-reactive T cell immunity to COVID-19 should have been assessed [(598)]. The innate (early) and adaptive (later) immune system is discussed further in Chapter 17, 'Natural Immunity'.

The study urgently needed to determine if COVID-19 vaccines can prevent transmission was halted. Researchers looking to conduct a large study on 20 US college campuses that sought to assess whether Moderna's COVID-19 vaccine could prevent person-to-person spread on college campuses by comparing nasopharyngeal swab samples between vaccinated an unvaccinated students said they couldn't get federal funding. Thus the critical question as to whether the new COVID-19 vaccines stop the virus from spreading has not been answered [(599)]. It is irrelevant if COVID-19 vaccines prevent transmission; we have our weapon of mass salvation. When the vaccinated spread COVID-19, public health will use the daily propaganda to generate interest in and increase uptake of COVID-19 vaccines by blaming the 'pandemic of the unvaccinated'.

Placebos were not used in all COVID-19 vaccine trials: A study by a WHO expert panel published in *Vaccine* in 2014 discussed the controversy surrounding the appropriate design of vaccine trials and the use of unvaccinated controls. Randomised, placebo-controlled trials (RCTs) are considered the gold standard in evaluating the safety and efficacy of a new vaccine. In these trials, participants are randomised to receive either the vaccine under investigation or a placebo, an inert substance, often a saline injection. Randomisation and the use of placebo allow researchers to control for confounding effects (events that may be associated but not necessarily causally related) and allows for differences in disease incidence or adverse effects between the vaccinated and unvaccinated control groups determined. The 'science' says that RCTs designs raise ethical concerns when participants in the control arm are deprived of an existing vaccine. The 'science' says testing a new vaccine against a placebo is scientifically and ethically fraught when the hypothesis being tested is whether an experimental vaccine is more efficacious than a vaccine already in use. Therefore, what usually occurs in vaccine trials is that researchers compare the effects of one vaccine to another vaccine currently on the market. The WHO expert panel acknowledges there is insufficient and inconsistent guidance on how to evaluate the use of placebo controls in vaccine trials. Most ethical guidelines for research do not address vaccine trials specifically, and in those that do, the guidance regarding placebo use is limited [(600)].

When a placebo is not a placebo: A placebo is not a placebo when it is not an inert substance. Using another vaccine in the control arm of a trial may be 'vaccine science', but it's flawed science. Another vaccine contains multiple elements known as immune system irritants that have been known to cause allergic reactions. These ingredients include, but are not limited to, adjuvants such as aluminium, preservatives such as mercury-based thimerosal and formaldehyde, food proteins such as egg, yeast and gelatine, and human serum albumin, antibiotics etc. [(601)]. All these ingredients in vaccines can cause adverse events following immunisation (AEFI), making it impossible to accurately compare the placebo to the vaccine. These irritants and allergens are discussed further in Chapter 12, 'Vaccines aren't Described as Safe and don't Always Work'.

Oxford-AstraZeneca did and didn't use a placebo: A data analysis published in *The Lancet* in December 2020 discussed the global trial designs for the Oxford-AstraZeneca COVID-19 vaccine. The UK trial arm used an approved conjugate meningococcal ACWY (MenACWY) meningitis vaccine in the control group rather than saline. The Brazil trial arm used MenACWY as the control for the first dose and saline for the second dose. The South African trial arm used only saline controls [(602)]. However, the clinical study protocols did not report that the Oxford-AstraZeneca vaccine was compared with a meningococcal vaccine in the UK. This lack of transparency is potentially more than an error of omission. The meningitis vaccine also contains similar components ingredients with the potential to cause adverse reactions. These can influence how beneficial or harmful the active intervention appears to be. Without adequate descriptions of placebo or sham controls, it is difficult to interpret results about the benefits and harms of active interventions within placebo-controlled trials [603]. Moderna, Pfizer-BioNTech and Janssen all used 0.9% sodium chloride (normal saline) injection as a placebo control [587, 588, 590].

Vaccines were tested in countries where social distancing and masking was mandated: It is not scientifically plausible to test the efficacy of a vaccine against a virus whilst concurrently suppressing that virus with public health interventions. French doctors spoke out against vaccine trials being conducted in countries practising public health measures. Dr Camille Locht, Research Director at the French National Institute of Health and Medical Research (Inserm) and Dr Jean-Paul Mira, head of the intensive care unit at the Cochin Hospital Paris, suggested doing a study in Africa where the infection is not suppressed. Whilst it harkened back to French colonialism and caused uproar, the doctors were being matter of fact. Whilst African clinical trials by large pharmaceutical companies are ethically suspect, these doctors were genuinely asking how the efficacy of a therapeutic or vaccine can be assessed in a country where the population are suppressing the virus using public health measures. There was no such uproar when AstraZeneca conducted their COVID-19 vaccine trials in the developing countries suppressing the virus, including India, Brazil and South Africa [604]. The pull of lower labour costs motivates pharmaceutical companies to conduct many ethically questionable trials in low-to-middle-income countries (LMICs) [605].

Out-and-out dosing mistake: There was an out-and-out mistake in handling and formulating the Oxford-AstraZeneca COVID-19 vaccine in the UK arm. The UK trial arm participants were accidentally given different doses. A subset of patients in the UK trial arm got a half dose of vaccine first, followed by a full dose as a booster. The news of the global trial error came out after the headline figure for the vaccine's overall efficacy was put at 70%. In the subset of fewer than 3,000 people in the UK who were given the lower dose regime by accident, the efficacy rose to 90%. In most trial volunteers in Brazil and the UK, the overall efficacy of the Oxford-AstraZeneca COVID-19 vaccine was 62% [606].

The COVID-19 vaccine trials have been unblinded: A WHO Expert Working Group made recommendations in a letter to the editor published in *Nature*

Medicine on March 16th 2021. The letter discussed ethical considerations for current and future COVID-19 placebo-controlled vaccine trials and trial unblinding. The WHO Expert Working Group said a severe threat to public health posed by the COVID-19 pandemic warrants the unblinding of COVID-19 vaccine trials [607]. With no 'emergency', there is no excuse for EUA vaccines. With no 'emergency', there is no excuse to unblind the trials and thereby avoid a direct comparison of the health outcomes in the vaccinated to the unvaccinated.

'Healthy Vaccinee Bias'.. (yes, with the double-ee, is the person receiving the vaccine) means many groups are underrepresented in trials. Effectiveness is related to efficacy; however, it refers to how the vaccine works in the real world. Clinical trials participants do not represent the general population thus, results cannot be generalised. Healthy vaccinee bias occurs when the general population is a lot unhealthier, affecting how the vaccine works in a real-world scenario. Because vaccines are administered to entire populations, they need to be tested using volunteers from the whole population. The Food and Drug Administration (FDA), however, allows vaccine manufacturers to exclude or under-represent certain populations from the sampling. Therefore pharmaceutical companies commonly exclude or under-represent those at higher risk and people with preexisting conditions. As a result, there is simply not enough known about how well the COVID-19 vaccines protect the elderly, minorities, and other high-risk groups against serious COVID-19 [608].

Challenges of studies used to determine vaccine effectiveness after rollout: RCTs are used to establish vaccines efficacy prior to licensure, although as discussed, comparing one vaccine to another is not a placebo-controlled RCT. After a vaccine rollout, vaccine effectiveness (VE) in the population is determined using observational study designs including cohort, case-control and observational studies once the vaccine is in use. In our dystopian future, vaccine manufacturers will pay for observational studies to determine the efficacy of their COVID-19 vaccines, with these observational studies being inherently at risk of chance, selection bias and confounding. Selection bias is the selection of healthy people to get a positive result. Confounding is something other than what is being studied that may be causing the results seen in a study, such as someone preventing infection by washing their hands more frequently [609].

Case-control VE studies can provide useful information to guide policy decisions and vaccine development; however, rigorous preparation and design are essential. A study published in *Vaccine* stated that case-control studies do not measure the impact of vaccine introduction on disease at a population level and are subject to bias and confounding. Study authors concluded that this bias may lead to inaccurate results that can misinform policymakers' decisions and provided recommendations of that group of experts regarding best practices for planning, design and enrolment of cases and controls [(610)].

Observational studies report that influenza vaccination reduces winter mortality risk from any cause by 50% among the elderly. This efficacy reported by influenza vaccine manufacturers is highly questionable as observational studies are prone to bias. A systematic review published in *BMC Infectious Diseases* in 2015 discussed the frequency and impact of confounding by indication and healthy vaccinee bias in observational studies used to assess the effectiveness of the influenza vaccine. The review concluded that both confounding by indication and healthy vaccinee bias are likely to operate simultaneously in observational studies on influenza vaccine efficacy studies [(611)]. A study reported in *Archives of Internal Medicine* now *Geriatrics JAMA Internal Medicine* used a cyclical regression model to estimate seasonal influenza-related excess mortality in the elderly from pneumonia and influenza and all-cause deaths for the 33 seasons from 1968 to 2001. In the US, influenza vaccination coverage in the elderly (≥65 years) increased from between 15%-20% pre-1980 to 65% in 2001. The study authors attributed the decline in influenza-related mortality in the decade after the 1968 Hong Kong influenza (H3N2) pandemic to the acquisition of natural immunity to the emerging H3N2 virus. The study authors were unable to correlate increasing vaccination coverage post-1980 with declining mortality rates in any age group. Study authors concluded that observational studies substantially overestimate vaccination benefits [(332)]. Many challenges lie ahead in evaluating the best practices required to achieve robust unbiased results from observational studies for COVID-19 vaccines, challenges that will unlikely be met.

Immunocompromised patients were excluded from COVID-19 vaccine trials: Immunocompromised patients, including those with autoimmune disorders or on immunosuppressive medications, were excluded from the vaccine trials, therefore the efficacy of the vaccine in this population still needs to be determined [612]. 20% of the US population have an auto-immune disease [613].

People with a history of allergic reactions were excluded from COVID-19 vaccine trials: Both Pfizer-BioNTech and Moderna's clinical trials excluded people with a history of the severe allergic reaction known as anaphylaxis. Both Pfizer-BioNTech and Moderna's clinical trials excluded people with a history of allergies to components of the COVID-19 vaccines. Pfizer also excluded those who previously had a severe adverse reaction to any vaccine. People with previous allergic reactions to food or drugs were not excluded but were likely underrepresented when compared to the general population [614]. The UK's medicine regulator, the Medicines and Healthcare Products Regulatory Agency (MHRA) said in December 2020 that people with a history of significant allergic reactions should not receive the Pfizer vaccine [615]. The peak professional body for allergy in Australia and New Zealand, the Australasian Society of Clinical Immunology and Allergy (ASCIA) stated that one in five (20%) Australians were affected by allergies and anaphylaxis in 2013 [616].

BAME communities were underrepresented in COVID-19 clinical trials: As previously mentioned, racial disproportionality in COVID-19 clinical trials exists. Black, Asian and minority ethnic (BAME) communities (a UK demographic) are the demographic overrepresented in the COVID-19 cases and deaths, yet they are underrepresented in COVID-19 clinical research (271). In 2018 13.8% of the UK population was from a BAME background, with London having 40% of its population from BAME communities [617].

Vaccine trials weren't conducted in the elderly with frailty and co-morbidity: Despite the frail, elderly with co-morbidities being most at risk and prioritised in national vaccination programmes, COVID-19 vaccine trials have by and large excluded care home residents and frail, older people. As such, there are no published data on safety and efficacy in this group [618]. It is a disincentive to test a therapeutic or vaccine in a population when that therapeutic or vaccine is far less likely to show a positive result. Vaccine manufacturers have too much to lose by trialling vaccine candidates on vulnerable populations too early in the process.

Clinical Professor of Pathology at the University of Hong Kong and coronavirus expert, John Nicholls said,

"They need to produce a vaccine, and they're not going to try it out on a 55 to 70 year old population because there's definitely less chance of getting an immune reaction and an immune response" (619).

An analysis of 26 global studies by researchers at Dartmouth College in the United States (US) published in the *European Journal of Epidemiology* in August 2020 found that the risk of mortality from COVID-19 rises substantially from 0.4% for individuals aged 55 to 15% for those aged 85 (620). Whilst people over 65 years of age constitute 9% of the global population and account for between 30%-40% of all COVID-19 cases and 80% of COVID-19 deaths, older people haven't been included in COVID-19 vaccine trials to the extent that younger people have. A research letter reviewing all COVID-19 treatment and vaccine trials on *ClinicalTrials.gov* to evaluate their risk for exclusion of older adults (≥65 years) published in *JAMA Network* in September 2020 found that the exclusion of the elderly from COVID-19 vaccine trials missed the target. Findings indicated that older adults (over 65) were likely to be excluded from greater than 50% of COVID-19 clinical therapeutic trials and 100% COVID-19 vaccine trials (621).

An interim analysis of four RCTs in Brazil, South Africa, and the UK on the safety and efficacy of the Oxford-AstraZeneca COVID-19 vaccine by age was published in *The Lancet*. Study authors concluded that, as studies only enrolled healthy volunteers aged 18-55 years, there was a lack of certainty over the effectiveness of the vaccine in those over 55 (602). On January 28th 2021, the German vaccine committee announced that it would no longer recommend the Oxford-AstraZeneca COVID-19 vaccine for those aged over 65, citing a lack of data to recommend use in older age groups (622).

On February 3rd 2021, Switzerland also announced it had banned the Oxford-AstraZeneca COVID-19 vaccine for all its citizens. The Swiss medical regulator Swissmedic claimed the lack of data on the efficacy of the COVID-19 vaccine meant they could not reach a conclusion (623).

On April 14th 2021, Denmark completely withdrew AstraZeneca from its COVID-19 vaccination programme, citing a lack of data (624). US biotech giant Moderna enrolled a grand total of 22 adults over age 55 in their trials (619). It is estimated that a quarter to a half of people over 85 years are frail (625).

Pregnancy

The exclusion of pregnant women from COVID-19 vaccine trials and flip-flop advice on the use of these vaccines in pregnancy is called the "pregnant 'person's' paradox" and is discussed in Chapter 15, 'COVID-19 Vaccines and Pregnancy Safety Concerns'

Other problems encountered during vaccine trials

In February 2021, Pfizer withdrew an application for EUA of its COVID-19 vaccine in India after failing to meet the drug regulator's demand for a local safety and immunogenicity study [626].

CHAPTER TWELVE

VACCINES AREN'T DESCRIBED AS SAFE & DON'T ALWAYS WORK

"The earth has music for those who listen". George Santayana [627]

COVID-19 vaccine safety cannot be considered without discussing vaccine safety as a whole. In Switzerland, vaccines are considered to be 'generally' safe [628]. Generally, in most cases, usually. That's not science that inspires confidence in vaccines, Heidi. Whilst I'm Irish Australian and have a particular affinity for these places, when I discuss public health, I discuss the Global Health Security Agenda (GHSA) whose regulations are underpinned by the United States (US) Food and Drug Administration (FDA) [629]. The GHSA, including recommendations for routine immunisation, is set by the World Economic Forum (WEF) members [630]. When discussing vaccine injury, I think it prudent not to focus on studies that link vaccines to autoimmune, inflammatory and allergic diseases. These are too numerous and are used as a smokescreen for the study that has not been done. I choose to focus on the simple truth, the lack of a single safety study to prove beyond doubt that vaccines are safe, and suggest how this censored debate around vaccine safety can be put to bed. I also focus on the acknowledged and hugely underreported adverse events following immunisation (AEFI) or adverse reactions (ADRs), which I use interchangeably.

A camel is a horse designed by a committee: When it comes to assessing safety, there are a number of committees. The Vaccines and Related Biological Products Advisory Committee (VRBPAC) reviews and evaluates data concerning the safety, effectiveness, and appropriate use of vaccines and related biological products intended for use in the prevention, treatment, or diagnosis of human diseases, and where applicable, other products for which the FDA has regulatory responsibility [631]. The Advisory Committee on Immunisation Practices (ACIP) consists of medical 'experts' and public health 'authorities' who develop recommendations on vaccines and related biological products in the US population. These recommendations provide public health guidance for the safe use of vaccines and related biological products [632].

The National Vaccine Advisory Committee (NVAC) was established to provide advice and make recommendations to the Director of the National Vaccine Programme on standards for implementing the ACIP recommendations [(633)]. The NVAC 'White Paper' reports NVAC's findings and makes recommendations based on a review by the current federal vaccine safety system, the Vaccine Supply Working Group (VSWG) [(634)].

The National Immunisation Advisory Committee (NIAC) is the Irish equivalent. The Immunisation Safety Review (ISR) Committee is a project within the Institute of Medicine (IOM). The IOM is said to be an American nonprofit, non-governmental organisation (NGO) that addresses current and emerging vaccine safety concerns. The ISR is said to provide independent, non-biased advice to policy-makers, practitioners and the public on vaccines. The ISR evaluates the evidence on possible causal associations between immunisations and provides this information to the public [(334)]. The IOM is now called the National Academy of Medicine (NAM) since 2015.

No study exists comparing the health outcomes of unvaccinated and vaccinated: The ISR committee does not say that vaccines are safe.

> *"There is no study that compares an unvaccinated control group with children exposed to the complete immunisation schedule"* (VSD, 2016 p. 7) [(635)].

The ISR further state; In relation to addressing the concern that multiple immunisations (trivalent, quadrivalent, pentavalent, heptavalent vaccines) can adversely affect the developing immune system, the ISR asks the following three questions;

- Do multiple immunisations have adverse short-term effects on the infant immune system that are reflected in increased susceptibility to heterologous (other) infection?
- Does exposure to multiple antigens in vaccines directly and permanently redirect or skew the immune system toward autoimmunity, as reflected in type 1 diabetes (T1D)?
- Does exposure to multiple antigens in vaccines directly and permanently redirect or skew the immune system toward allergy, as reflected in asthma?

What the ISR says about vaccine safety:

> *"There is no study that compares an unvaccinated control group with children exposed to the complete immunisation schedule, nor are there any studies that looked at health outcomes other than those classically defined, such as infections, allergy, or diabetes. Thus the committee recognises with some discomfort that this report addresses only part of the overall set of concerns of some who are most wary about the safety of childhood vaccines".*

The ISR could not address the concern that repeated exposure of a susceptible or fragile child to multiple vaccines over the developmental period may produce atypical or nonspecific immune or nervous system injury that could lead to severe disability or death [(334)].

The study comparing vaccinated and unvaccinated will never be done: Even though no safety study exists, the Committee on the Assessment of Studies of Health Outcomes Related to the Recommended Childhood Immunisation Schedule supports the NVAC Safety Working Group statement that;

> *"the strongest study design, a prospective, randomised clinical trial that includes a study arm receiving no vaccine or vaccine not given according to the current recommended schedule, would be unethical and therefore cannot be done"* (NVAC, 2009, p.38) [(335)].

That gives me such confidence in vaccines, Heidi. A person with free will may ask why the Vaccine Confidence Project (VCP) doesn't just answer the question [(337)].

We could put this censored debate to bed once and for all: The enduring indoctrination of public health says 'vaccines save lives', 'the benefits outweigh the risks' and 'vaccines are safe'. Then enter Wakefield the 'quack' smokescreen to discount the body of studies showing legitimate links, and never mention the study that hasn't been done. Any parent of unvaccinated children knows the connection between vaccination and autoimmune disease is beyond doubt. In order to alleviate vaccine hesitancy or vaccine refusal, it is pertinent for the scientific community to address both healthcare worker (HCW) and public safety concerns surrounding the adverse effects of vaccines. Yet this study remains vetoed. This censored debate around vaccine safety could be put to bed once and for all by conducting a cohort study comparing the health outcomes [neurodevelopmental disorders (NDDs), inflammatory disease, autoimmune disease] of completely unvaccinated to completely vaccinated children. The study could be randomised, restricted, matched and adjusted for confounders. As discussed in Chapter 4, 'Vaccine Refusal and the Age of Censorship', instead, Heidi Larson's VCP trolls the internet, flagging and censoring vaccine safety concerns with the misguided aim to increase our confidence in vaccines. The VCP Thought Police's job is to never allow the truth to surface as the VCP knows the truth is more contagious than COVID.

Determining vaccine safety and efficacy: As previously discussed, observational studies determine vaccine effectiveness once the vaccine is in use. Observational studies are inherently at risk of confounding (events that may be associated but not necessarily causally related) and selection bias (people in the study are not representative of the population of interest). More robust observational study designs are needed to avoid the risk of confounding and selection bias [(636)]. Administering vaccines at the same time or in close succession increases the complexity of assessing vaccine safety. To date, no controlled trials and very few observational studies have determined the impact of vaccination schedules on overall health. The balance of the risks and benefits from mass vaccination, therefore, remains uncertain. To say 'the science is settled' is disingenuous. Many recent studies suggest links between multiple vaccinations and increased risk of diverse multisystem diseases such as allergies, infections, neuropsychiatric disorders or NDDs [(637)].

Too many shots, too hard to tell: A book by internationally recognised health law expert and bioethicist Efthimios Parasidis entitled *Recalibrating Vaccination Laws* discusses how to remedy the Vaccine Act that provides broad legal immunities for vaccine manufacturers. This legal immunity results in a lack of regulation and, embedded within this, presents complex legal hurdles in obtaining compensation. In his book, Parasidis gives an anecdotal report describing a situation whereby he called the FDA with a handful of vaccine lots from vaccines administered to his children to specify what adverse reactions (ADRs) had been reported for each specific lot. Parasidis goes on to describe that whilst the FDA agent was able to rapidly locate the vaccine lots in the FDA database, the FDA agent was unable to say confidently whether any reported ADRs were linked to vaccines from these specific lots. The FDA agent explained that, in accordance with the Centres for Disease Control and Prevention (CDC) schedule, children receive multiple vaccines during a single visit meaning that, even when ADRs are reported, the FDA is unable to determine which vaccine is associated with the ADR, and also unable to determine whether the vaccine administered is causally related to that ADR [(638)].

Establishing a causal relationship between a vaccine and an adverse reaction: It is important to understand that most causality assessments of adverse events following immunisations (AEFIs) will be put down to temporally (occurs at the same time) associated incidental illness. The boffins are currently putting ADRs following the COVID-19 vaccines down to temporally associated incidental illness. Additionally, as we see with COVID-19 linked myocarditis and blood clots, AEFIs are found to be 'extremely rare' when compared with those associated with the target diseases. The injured person has to prove the damage and the causal link between the vaccine and the disease [(639)]. This aside, causality has been established, liability determined, and no-fault compensation payouts have occurred [(640)]. In homeopathy, vaccine damage is called vaccinosis. I treat vaccinosis. From a naturopathic perspective, vaccine damage is caused by 'immune overload'. Immune overload is when the vaccine is the straw that breaks the camel's back in a susceptible individual. 'Immune overload' is recognised as a reason for holding vaccine safety concerns by Swiss physicians [(295)].

The Bradford Hill criteria: The Bradford Hill criteria are a group of nine principles that are used to determine epidemiological evidence of a causal relationship between a vaccine and an AEFIs. These criteria are widely used in public health research [(641)]. In the context of multiple antigens in vaccines, the Bradford Hill criteria that apply are the biological gradient or dose-dependent relationship [(642)]. An allergen is a particular type of antigen which causes an IgE antibody response [(643)]. Vaccines contain multiple antigens which are used to generate an immune response. Antigens are typically proteins, peptides, or polysaccharides [(644)]. Each vaccine in the childhood vaccination schedule has between 1 and 69 antigens. Thus, a child receiving recommended vaccines in the 2018 childhood immunisation schedule is exposed to up to 320 antigens by the time they are two years old [(645)]. As antigens are biological agents, the sheer number of antigens makes the Bradford Hill criteria difficult to apply.

Antigens are acknowledged to cause an immune response, so 320 antigens are likely to cause an exceptional immune response. Allergic disorders, including anaphylaxis, hay fever, eczema and asthma, now affect 25% of people in the developed world [(646)]. As previously discussed, when it comes to answering the question, does exposure to multiple antigens directly and permanently redirect or skew the immune system toward autoimmunity and allergic disease, the ISR hasn't got the foggiest. I am not suggesting that vaccines are the only cause for the rise in the following conditions, nonetheless, my unvaccinated children don't suffer from autoimmune or allergic disease.

Accurately assessing risk and benefit is impossible: Different countries have different reporting methods, and rates for AEFIs and underreporting is acknowledged [(647)]. It is impossible to accurately assess the risks versus benefits of vaccination as the risks are hugely underreported, and benefits are grossly overstated.

In the US, AEFIs are reported to the Vaccine Adverse Event Reporting System (VAERS). A study entitled 'Who is unlikely to report adverse events after vaccinations to the Vaccine Adverse Event Reporting System?' published in *Vaccine*, surveyed how HCWs reported adverse events to VAERS. The study authors noted that HCW awareness of, and practices regarding reporting these adverse reactions to vaccinations, are understudied. The survey found that only 71% of HCWs were aware of VAERS. 37% of HCWs had identified at least one AEFI, yet only 17% had ever reported this adverse reaction to VAERS. The HCWs were more likely to report serious events. Factors associated with not reporting AEFIs included HCWs not being familiar with filling in the VAERS report or not being aware of what was required of them to file a VAERS report [(648)]. In the US, a Harvard Pilgrim study reported that less than 1% of AEFIs are reported to VAERS, leaving more than 99% unreported [(649)].

In the UK, HCWs report suspected AEFIs through the UK Medicines and Healthcare products Regulatory Agency (MHRA) Yellow Card [(650)]. In Ireland, the Health Products Regulatory Authority (HPRA) receives reports from individuals from the Irish public on a voluntary basis about suspected AEFIs. The Health Service Executive (HSE) in Ireland also acknowledge that 99% of AEFIs go unreported [(651)]. Thus, when public health says the 'benefits outweigh the risks', the risks are grossly underreported.

Vaccines injury compensation payouts: Compensation claims are made for vaccine injury. Adverse events do not necessarily have a causal relationship with the vaccine. Payments are awarded for true reactions and temporally events (events occurring at the same time). The adverse event may be any unfavourable or unintended sign, abnormal laboratory finding, symptom or disease. In 2018, the World Health Organisation (WHO) revised the AEFI classification, and also changed their definition of 'causal association'. A causal association is now used only when there is "no other factor intervening in the processes". Therefore, if a child with underlying congenital heart disease (other factor), develops fever and cardiac decompensation (a clinical syndrome in which a structural or functional change in the heart leads to its inability to maintain an efficient circulation) after vaccination, the cardiac failure would not be considered causally related to the vaccine (642). Regarding US vaccine injury payouts, the National Childhood Vaccine Injury Act (NCVIA) of 1986 was passed by the US Congress, and the National Vaccine Injury Compensation Programme (VICP) created. The VICP began accepting petitions in 1988. Since the programme started accepting petitions, a total of US$4 billion in vaccine injury compensations have been paid. In 2019, there was US$46,146,803 in vaccine injury compensation payouts. The activity reported for 2019 was the lowest since 2007 (652). Vaccine injury compensation is discussed further in Chapter 16 'Criminality, Litigation and Zero Liability'.

Studies Comparing Vaccinated to Unvaccinated Populations

Parents who have completely avoided vaccinating their children are indeed rare. This makes recruitment and comparison studies of entirely unvaccinated children to completely vaccinated children according to the CDC schedule difficult. Studies that have supposedly proven 'vaccines are safe' have looked at one vaccine only, or a component of one vaccine, and have never compared the whole schedule to no schedule. There have however been useful comparisons studies whose conclusions warrant further studies.

PARSIFAL study: Asthma is an atopic or allergic disease. According to the latest World Health Organisation (WHO) estimates, asthma killed 383,000 people in 2015. This figure represents over three times the number of deaths from measles (653). The Prevention of Allergy-Risk Factors for Sensitisation in Children Related to Farming and Anthroposophic Lifestyle (PARSIFAL) study was conducted in five European countries (Austria,

Germany, the Netherlands, Sweden, and Switzerland) and included 14,893 children. Questionnaire responses indicated that 73% of children were vaccinated against measles, 20% had been infected with measles (including 11% of vaccinated children), and 14% had been neither vaccinated nor naturally infected. The study found an inverse association between measles infection and atopic sensitisation. Among the children who never had measles infection, vaccinated children were more likely to have nasal allergies. Further analysis showed that allergies were less likely in children who had measles but not in those who had been vaccinated against measles. This study used IgE, which is a reliable indicator of allergic disease (654, 655).

Mawson US homeschooling study: Another study exists that compared the health outcomes of completely unvaccinated and vaccinated children. The study was conducted by Professor of Epidemiology and Biostatistics at the School of Public Health at Jackson State University US, Andrew Mawson, in 2016. A cross-sectional study of mothers of homeschooled children was conducted in four US states; Florida, Louisiana, Mississippi and Oregon. Mothers completed an anonymous online questionnaire on their six to12 year old children regarding pregnancy-related factors, birth history, vaccinations, medically diagnosed illnesses, medications and health services. NDDs were defined as having one or more of the following closely related diagnoses: a learning disability, attention deficit hyperactivity disorder (ADHD), and autism spectrum disorder (ASD). The study found that the vaccinated children had a higher rate of allergies and NDDs than the unvaccinated children (656). The study upset the apple cart and was quickly retracted. Mawson was denigrated and vilified.

Hooker US paediatric medical practice study: A study entitled 'Analysis of health outcomes in vaccinated and unvaccinated children: Developmental delays, asthma, ear infections and gastrointestinal disorders' was published in *SAGE Open Medicine* in May 2020. Using data from three medical practices in the US, vaccinated children were compared to unvaccinated children during the first year of life for later incidence of developmental delays, asthma, ear infections and gastrointestinal disorders. The diagnosis was by International Classification of Diseases-9 and International Classification of Diseases-10 codes through medical chart review. The study concluded that a higher incidence of developmental delays, asthma, ear infections and gastrointestinal disorders were observed within the vaccinated versus unvaccinated group [657]. The study was also published in the *Journal of Translational Science* [658].

Vaccination and Allergic Disease

The American College of Allergy, Asthma and Immunology (ACAAI) states that allergic or immunoglobulin E (IgE)-mediated reaction to vaccines are more often caused by vaccine components than by the immunising agent itself. Aside from the antigens used to generate an immune response, allergenic vaccine components include, but are not limited to, gelatin, egg protein, yeast, latex (contained in vial stoppers or syringe plungers), neomycin (antibiotic) and thimerosal (mercury-based preservative) [659]. As previously mentioned, a child receiving the full schedule of vaccines receives 320 antigens by the age of two.

Vaccines and anaphylaxis: Vaccines are described as containing food proteins. Evidence existed as far back as 1913 that food proteins in vaccines cause the development of food allergies. In 1913, Charles Richet won the Nobel Prize in Physiology or Medicine for demonstrating that injecting a protein into animals or humans causes immune system sensitisation to that protein. In 1902, Richet used dog studies to demonstrate that after an initial low dose of a substance, another dose a few weeks later produced a severe reaction. Richet named this phenomenon anaphylaxis [660]. The results of these studies should have had important implications for understanding allergies and serious implications for vaccine policy.

Anaphylaxis after childhood vaccination: Anaphylaxis after vaccination is rare in all age groups. Anaphylactic reactions occur at about one per one million doses. The *Journal of Allergy and Clinical Immunology* reports that the risk of anaphylaxis after vaccination in children and adults is 1.31 per million vaccine doses [661]. Allergy to components in vaccines can be either an immediate or delayed reaction. In its 2011 report on vaccine adverse events, the IOM confirmed that many vaccines and injections contain food proteins. The IOM committee reviewed antigens in vaccines, e.g., hepatitis B surface antigen, toxoids, gelatin, ovalbumin, casamino acids, and adverse events in its 2011 report entitled *Adverse Effects of Vaccines: Evidence and Causality*. The IOM admitted that adverse events on their list are thought to be due to what is known as immediate IgE-mediated hypersensitivity reactions. The IOM concluded in its report that, whilst aforementioned antigens in the vaccines do not typically elicit an immediate hypersensitivity reaction as in anaphylaxis, these antigens do occasionally induce IgE-mediated sensitisation in some individuals, resulting in subsequent hypersensitivity reactions, including anaphylaxis [(662)]. IgE-mediated food allergy is a leading cause of anaphylaxis and food allergy [(663)].

An article published in the *Journal of Developing Drugs* in 2015 said that evidence exists that food proteins in vaccines cause food allergy. Since the 1940s, multiple studies have demonstrated that food proteins in vaccines cause sensitisation in humans. Allergens in vaccines are not fully disclosed, and no safe dosage levels for existing injected allergens have been established. No regulation exists at all for allergen quantities in vaccines and injections. It is recognised that only a tiny quantity of an allergen is needed to cause sensitisation. It is also recognised that many approved vaccines on the market have enough allergen in them to cause an anaphylactic reaction. Vaccine schedules today include 30-40 injections, and up to five injections may be simultaneously administered in one sitting. In addition to proteins, the adjuvants in vaccines, such as pertussis toxins and aluminium compounds, also predispose a child to allergy.

Many researchers are calling for the removal of food proteins from vaccines and a reevaluation of adjuvants in vaccines. Additionally, urgent action is needed to change vaccine policy surrounding vaccine specifications, manufacture, package insert requirements, the Vaccine Adverse Event Reporting System (VAERS) and the National Vaccine Injury Compensation programme (VICP) [(334)]. At the very least, parents should be warned that vaccines may cause food allergies so parents can weigh up the pros and cons. The current cause of the food allergy epidemic is not a $64,000 question. Allergy sufferers require lifelong steroids and EpiPens, and asthmatics require lifelong medication. The hypothesis is that food allergy is caused by different combinations of factors, including increased caesarean sections and decreased breastfeeding, the indiscriminate use of antipyretics and antibiotics, and the overuse of vaccines containing adjuvants and antigens, yet the scientific ethicists say it is 'unethical' to conduct the study to disprove the null hypothesis.

Food allergy is rising exponentially globally: Nationwide data on hospital admissions for food anaphylaxis or clinical history in combination with allergen-specific IgE measurement in population-based cohorts provide consistent evidence for the increasing prevalence of food allergy in high-income countries. Recent reports also show that children of East Asian or African ethnicity, who are raised in a western environment such as Australia and the US, have an increased risk of developing food allergy when compared with resident Caucasian children. This evidence suggests that food allergy might also increase across Asian and African countries as their economies grow and populations adopt a more westernised lifestyle (664).

EpiPens are not fit for purpose: Millions of allergy sufferers are using EpiPens that have fatal flaws. After investigating the death of Natasha Ednan-Laperouse (Ar dheis Dé go raibh a anam dílis), coroner Sean Cummings called on the MHRA to take action after he said the EpiPen's "inadequate dose of adrenaline for anaphylaxis and an inadequate length needle" raised serious safety concerns (665). The preferred needle length required to access the muscle is 25mm for adrenaline injectors. However, Cummings said that the EpiPen's needle length was 16mm, its standard length. Additionally, the standard emergency adrenaline dose is 500mcg; the EpiPen contains a 300mcg dose only (666).

CHAPTER TWELVE – PART II

VACCINATION & AUTOIMMUNE DISEASE

Vaccine-induced autoimmunity, and the mechanisms by which vaccines can cause autoimmune reactions are said to be, 'a hotly debated topic surrounded by controversy'; doublespeak for 'hotly censored' [(667)].

Vaccine-induced autoimmunity: Numerous studies have described vaccine-induced autoimmunity with a view to developing safer vaccines [(668-670)]. Reports have amassed of various autoimmune disorders, including idiopathic thrombocytopenia purpura, myopericarditis, primary ovarian failure and systemic lupus erythematosus (SLE) following vaccination [(668)]. This is like reading the list of adverse events following COVID-19 vaccination. Some studies conclude that, in relation to vaccine-induced autoimmunity, the 'benefits outweigh the risks'. However, the incidence and burden of autoimmune disease is rising, and public health specialists should be asking the difficult questions.

Seasonal H1N1 influenza vaccines have the potential to induce autoantibodies (antibodies that attack our own cells) in selected autoimmune inflammatory rheumatic disease (AIRD) patients and in healthy adults [(671)]. Guillain-Barré syndrome (GBS) is a severe demyelinating neurological disease. The swine influenza vaccine used in the US during a swine influenza outbreak in 1976 was linked to an increased risk of GBS due to an association with an immune-mediated demyelinating process [(672)]. Statistical data from hepatitis B vaccination programmes showed a significant correlation between the number of hepatitis B vaccinations performed and the onset of multiple sclerosis (MS) occurring between one and two years later. When Bradford and Hill's criteria were applied to these data, a correlation between the hepatitis B vaccine and MS was found, and it was concluded that this might be causal [(673)]. Narcolepsy is an autoimmune disorder [(674)]. After the Pandemrix vaccination campaign in 2009-2010, narcolepsy risk increased five to 14-fold in children and adolescents and two to sevenfold in adults. The risk remained elevated for two years after the Pandemrix vaccination [(675)]. The Pandemrix withdrawal is discussed later under historical vaccine scares and withdrawals and recalls below. An increased risk of narcolepsy was recently included in the spectrum of autoimmune/auto-inflammatory syndrome induced by adjuvants [(ASIA) discussed next], which has been associated with the human papillomavirus (HPV) vaccination [676]. Autoimmunity following hepatitis B vaccine as part of the spectrum of ASIA has also been recognised [677].

ADEM and ASIA: Acute disseminated encephalomyelitis (ADEM) is an inflammatory demyelinating disease of the central nervous system (CNS). ADEM is considered an autoinflammatory disorder and thought to be triggered by epigenetic (environmental) factors in genetically susceptible individuals [678]. ADEM often occurs in the post-infectious or post-vaccination environment. The immune adjuvants used to augment immune response have been found to be important in the development of post-vaccination CNS demyelination syndromes [679]. Autoimmune/autoinflammatory syndrome induced by adjuvants (ASIA) incorporates many autoimmune conditions induced by exposure to various adjuvants in vaccines [680]. Thus, using another adjuvant containing vaccine as a comparison product in vaccine trials instead of a placebo seriously affects trial validity.

Vaccine-induced escape mutants: When antibacterial and antiviral medicines are used, organisms continue to evolve and undergo mutations that can result in antimicrobial resistance (AMR). AMR includes antibiotic resistance and antiviral drug resistance. Frequent vaccination may also be a risk factor for escape mutants. Just as antimicrobials drive drug resistance, evidence of vaccine driven resistance also exists. An 'effective' vaccine drives the natural evolution of pathogens, allowing random mutations that cause the vaccine to lose effectiveness. Alternatively, vaccine driven pathogen evolution occurs when antigen survivors multiply, making pathogens less vulnerable to the vaccine [681]. Vaccines potentially impose strong selective pressure on microorganisms and promote vaccine-induced escape mutants (VEMs). VEMs are one cause of breakthrough infection (BI); when a vaccinated person becomes infected with the disease the vaccine is supposed to protect them from [682]. Vaccine-induced mutant strains of hepatitis B virus (HBV) are acknowledged to exist [683]. In an effort to bamboozle us with science jargon, the ability of vaccines to drive frequencies of nonvaccine strains is also known as vaccine-induced serotype replacement (VISR). VISR has occurred following pneumococcal vaccination and resulted in increased antibiotic-resistant *Streptococcus pneumoniae* (*S. pneumoniae*) strains [684].

Vaccine-induced antibiotic resistance: While some studies conclude the pneumococcal vaccine reduces AMR infections in children, other studies conclude that the pneumococcal vaccine can increase AMR frequencies among nonvaccine serotypes (microorganisms not covered by the vaccine) [685, 686]. Pneumonia causing infections are one of the leading causes of death in children under five globally. A rise in the prevalence of antibiotic-resistant *S. pneumoniae* strains was seen after the introduction of the children's pneumococcal conjugate vaccine (PCV7) vaccine in 2000. Antibiotic-resistant *S. pneumoniae* strains also rose after the introduction of the adult's PCV13 vaccine for pneumococcal disease in 2012 [687].

The Bill & Melinda Gates Foundation is trustee of the Wellcome Trust, that other great 'philanthropic organisation'. Nicholas Croucher, from the Wellcome Trust Sanger Institute, said,

> *"Different strains adapt to become resistant (to antibiotics); however, with vaccines, we see a decline in the prevalence of vaccine susceptible bacteria, thus allowing opportunistic bacteria to evade the vaccine and become the dominant strain"* [688].

A heptavalent 7-in-1 vaccine pneumococcal conjugate vaccine is already used in adults. This vaccine contains the cell capsule sugars of seven serotypes of the bacteria *S. pneumoniae* [689]. Pfizer already inject 13 types of bacteria at once in adults over 65. The 13-valent pneumococcal conjugate vaccine [Prevenar 13, Prevnar 13 (PCV13)] consists of 13 serotype-specific polysaccharides of *S. pneumoniae*, also called *pneumococcus*. Since the introduction of these 13-valent pneumococcal conjugate vaccines in children, there has been an emergence of three antibiotic-resistant strains of *S. pneumoniae* in children [690]. Moreover, the PCV13 vaccination has not been shown to reduce the incidence of community-acquired pneumonia (CAP), lower respiratory tract infections (LRTI) or LRTI-related antibiotic use or total antibiotic use in primary care in the elderly [691]. Yet the economist Jim O'Neill has informed the world that vaccines are the holy grail to address the global antibiotic apocalypse [692]. If 13-in-1 vaccines are not enough to bamboozle our immune system, have no fear, the old boy network is concocting endless possibilities. Evidence that vaccines may increase deaths from antibiotic-resistant *S. pneumoniae* is irrelevant, Gate's Wellcome Trust and an economist says vaccines are the solution to the antibiotic-resistant apocalypse.

Sicker than Ever

Bearing in mind we have already achieved massive gains in global vaccination uptake and moved towards the global vaccination policy, the fact remains that the human race has never been so unwell, nor so medicated. Evidence shows that life expectancy has peaked. The age at death of the world's oldest person has not increased since the 1990s [693, 694]. Medical error (iatrogenesis) is the third leading cause of death. In the US, iatrogenesis results in the deaths of between 250,000 and 450,000 people every year [351]. In an article published in *The BMJ*, Martin Makary and Michael Daniel of Johns Hopkins University School of Medicine say that better death certificate reporting is necessary to understand how widespread the problem of iatrogenesis is [695].

Non-communicable diseases have far exceeded deaths from infectious disease: Non-communicable diseases (NCDs) are the leading cause of death globally. The majority of NCDs are due to cardiovascular disease, cancer, chronic respiratory diseases or diabetes. According to a paper published in *Nature*, there were 36 million deaths from NCDs in 2008, totalling 63% of all deaths worldwide [696]. Mortality from many NCDs continues to increase worldwide, with a disproportionately larger impact in low-middle income countries (LMIs), where almost 75% of global deaths occur from these causes [697].

Autoimmune disease correlates with the rise in mass vaccination programmes: The incidence and prevalence of all autoimmune diseases have increased significantly over the last 30 years. These observations point to a stronger influence of epigenetics (environmental factors) as opposed to genetic factors on autoimmune disease development [698]. Presently, one in five people suffers from autoimmune disease [699]. Autoimmune disease is the leading cause of death in young and middle-aged women in the US [700]. The causes of autoimmune disease are multifactorial, but this rise has correlated (occurred simultaneously) with mass vaccination programmes that began in the mid-1950s. In the 1950s, the Public Health Service Hygienic Laboratory was reconstituted as the Division of Biologics Standards at the National Institute of Health (NIH). In 1972 these responsibilities were transferred to the FDA. By 1971, regulations had been established for more than 80 generic biological products used for passive and active immunisation. In the early 1950s, four vaccines were available; diphtheria, tetanus, pertussis and smallpox.

Vaccines for poliomyelitis, measles, mumps and rubella, adenovirus infections and meningococcal disease came shortly after (701). The rise in C-sections, a reduction in breastfeeding, and the overuse and abuse of antibacterials, antimicrobials, and antipyretics all correlate with a rise in autoimmune disease.

Autoimmune disease is not so rare in Africa. Conventional beliefs and some publications had in the past asserted that systemic autoimmune diseases such as inflammatory arthritis, connective tissue disorders and vasculitis were rare. Many of these reports, however, had been hospital-based and were not based on the American College of Rheumatology criteria. Rheumatoid arthritis was reported as being rare, especially among West Africans. SLE, scleroderma, inflammatory myopathies and vasculitis were also reported as rare. However, increased reports of these conditions indicate that these conditions do occur and are being underreported. As efforts are being made to overcome acute and chronic infections, chronic debilitating diseases may rear their head (702).

Our Children are Sicker than Ever

Although chronic health conditions are generally associated with adults, roughly 25% of children and adolescents in the US are affected with a chronic, degenerative medical condition requiring lifelong medication (703). According to the CDC, the prevalence of autism spectrum disorders (ASDs) increased from one in 150 in 2000 to one in 59 children in 2104 (704). During 2013-2014, a survey of American children and adolescents using US NHANES (National Health and Nutrition Examination Survey) found that approximately 20% of children and adolescents take at least one prescription medication. Disturbingly one in 12 of these children and adolescents took more than one prescription medication and were potentially at risk for major drug-drug interactions (705).

Allergy and inflammatory disease: An article published in the *Journal of Allergy and Clinical Immunology* described that the overall incidence of Accident and Emergency (A&E) department visits for anaphylaxis rose two to threefold between 2008 and 2016. The greatest increase was in children under the age of five (706). In addition, the CDC's National Centre for Health Statistics (NCHS) state the prevalence of allergy is increasing overall, describing significant increasing linear trends for food allergy, skin allergy and respiratory allergy. Rises are greatest in lower socioeconomic status (SES) households and communities [707].

Asthma compared to measles: The reduction in deaths from a successful measles vaccine has correlated with an increase in the incidence and prevalence of the allergic disease asthma. Asthma is currently a far more deadly disease than measles. In 2017 about 85% of the world's children received one dose of measles vaccine by their first birthday, and there were 110,000 measles deaths globally [708]. Putting things into perspective, asthma is a common chronic allergic disease affecting 300 million children and adults worldwide [709]. According to the latest WHO estimates, there were 383,000 deaths due to asthma in 2015 (653). This number of deaths is nearly four times the number of deaths from measles. Currently, 8.4% of persons in the US have asthma as compared with 4.3% of the population worldwide [710]. According to the CDC, one in 13 people in the US have asthma [711]. Scientists will argue that a successful measles vaccine is the reason for lower measles deaths than asthma deaths. however, the question remains; do vaccines cause asthma?

Strange, Rare and Fandangle Diseases in Children

Although children may be affected by any of the 80+ medically recognised autoimmune diseases, only a handful of these diseases are diagnosed relatively often in adolescents and children. Type 1 diabetes (T1D) in children was rare but well recognised before the introduction of insulin. Low incidence and prevalence rates were recorded in several countries between 1925 and 1955. There was no change in the incidence of childhood T1D over that period until a simultaneous upturn was documented in several countries around the 1950s, the same time as mass vaccination programmes were introduced. The overall pattern since then is one of linear increase. Dramatic rises in T1D in children under age five have been recently recorded [712]. T1D is one of the most prevalent chronic illnesses diagnosed in childhood and occurs in one in 400-600 children in the US, with 15-20% of all new diagnoses occurring in children under the age of five. The experts state that the reason for the increased incidence in this youngest age group is unknown [713]. The question remains; do vaccines cause T1D and autoimmune disease? I have seen and treated all of the following what I describe as 'strange, rare and fandangle diseases in children', in my practice.

Coeliac disease is an inflammatory bowel disease: Inflammatory bowel disease (IBD) is an inflammatory disease with an autoimmune component. Although there are few epidemiologic data from developing countries, the incidence and prevalence of IBD is increasing with time and in different regions around the world, indicating its emergence as a global disease [714]. Coeliac disease can develop at any age, however the incidence of coeliac disease is approximately one in 1000 children [715, 716].

Scleroderma and lupus: Scleroderma, also known as systemic sclerosis (SSc), is a chronic connective tissue disease classified as an autoimmune rheumatic disease. 5,000 to 7,000 children in the US have scleroderma [717]. The incidence of SSc is one per million children [718]. Both scleroderma and lupus are uncommon in children. The incidence of localised scleroderma (LS) in children is one to three per 100,000 children [718]. Lupus is another autoimmune disease. Systemic lupus erythematosus (SLE) is the most common lupus. Childhood-onset SLE (cSLE) has an incidence of 0.3-0.9 per 100,000 children. A higher incidence of cSLE is reported in Asians, African Americans, Hispanics and Native Americans. When compared to two more common childhood autoimmune diseases, juvenile idiopathic arthritis (JIA) and T1D, cSLE is around ten to 15 times less common in white children. In Asian children, however, cSLE is equally as common as JIA [719].

Juvenile idiopathic arthritis: JIA is the most common autoimmune disease affecting children [720]. Systemic-onset juvenile idiopathic arthritis (SJIA) is also called Still's disease. The prevalence of JIA is 44.7 per 100,000 children, with the peak incidence rate occurring in children aged 11-15 years. Juvenile dermatomyositis (JDM) and juvenile polymyositis (JPM) are rare childhood autoimmune myopathies (neuromuscular disorders). Population-based studies indicate JDM has an annual incidence ranging from 2-4 cases per one million children, with the peak incidence from five to ten years of age [721]. The incidence and prevalence of paediatric autoimmune neuropsychiatric disease associated with strep infection (PANDAS) is not known, although it is rare. In one prospective study, only ten cases were identified among 30,000 throat cultures (one in 3000) positive for group A streptococcus (group A strep) [722].

Historical Vaccine Scares and Withdrawals and Recalls

The CDC has a webpage entitled 'Historical Vaccine Safety Concerns' [723]. I've panned it out as it is somewhat thin in detail. What is important to highlight is that under normal circumstances vaccines found to cause injury or death are withdrawn. Currently, 22,000 post-COVID-19 vaccine deaths have been reported to Europe's EudraVigilance alone and the boosters are coming.

Cutter Incident: defective vaccine recall: The Cutter occurred in 1955 and involved a recall of a polio vaccine manufactured by the California-based family firm of Cutter Laboratories. More than 200,000 children in the US received a polio vaccine in which the manufacturing process inactivated the live virus and rendered the vaccine ineffective. Reports of paralysis occurred within days of the rollout, and the polio vaccine was withdrawn within a month of the first mass vaccination programme. A total of 40,000 cases of polio developed, leaving 200 children with varying degrees of paralysis and resulting in the deaths of ten children [(724)].

DTP vaccine litigation: Three manufacturers of diphtheria-tetanus-pertussis (DTP) vaccines indicated an alarming increase in the number of lawsuits filed against them alleging damage caused by the DTP vaccine, mainly pertussis vaccine, including encephalopathy and seizures. One such case was filed in 1978, whereas 73 were filed in 1984. During the seven year period from 1978 to 1984, the average amount claimed per suit rose from US$10 million to US$46.5 million. As a result, vaccine companies threatened to stop manufacturing vaccines which threatened to derail the vaccine programme. Thus the National Vaccine Injury Compensation Programme (VICP) was created, giving vaccine manufacturers the green light to injure without fault [(725)].

Simian Virus 40 (SV40) and human cancer: Between 1955 and 1963, it was estimated that between 10-30% of polio vaccines administered in the US were contaminated with simian virus 40 (SV40). SV40 comes from monkey kidney cell cultures that were used to make polio vaccines at that time. The contamination was found in both the inactivated polio vaccine (IPV) and the oral polio vaccine (OPV). After discovering the contamination, the US government established testing requirements to verify that all new lots of polio vaccines were free of SV40. Recent molecular biological experiments and epidemiological studies suggest that SV40 could transmit in humans by horizontal infection from the earlier administration of SV40-contaminated vaccines. SV40 in humans is associated with a higher prevalence of brain and bone tumours, mesotheliomas and lymphomas [(726)]. The boffins assure us that vaccines used today do not contain the SV40 virus. As explained in Chapter 13, 'COVID-19 Vaccines are Safe for Two Months', the ingredients in a vaccine "baffle" scientists.

Kulenkampff and pertussis vaccine: In 1974, Kulenkampff's findings were published in the *Archives of Disease in Childhood*. Kulenkampff noted that he had observed 36 children in the previous 11 years who were believed to have suffered from neurological complications of pertussis vaccination and that the clustering of complications within the first 24 hours after vaccination suggested a causal rather than a coincidental relation (727). An article from 1979, published in the *Journal of Epidemiology and Community Health,* discussed the pattern of reactions and sequence of events observed in the present study and published reports. The article suggested an association between certain reactions to pertussis vaccine and subsequent severe brain damage, the incidence of which appeared to be not less than one per 50,000 children vaccinated during the last 20 years of mass vaccination in the UK (728).

Swine influenza vaccine and Guillain-Barré syndrome: In 1976, a small increased risk of the neurological disorder Guillain-Barré syndrome (GBS) following the swine influenza vaccine occurred. The increased risk was approximately one additional GBS case for every 100,000 people who got the swine influenza vaccine. After over 40 million people were vaccinated against swine flu, federal health officials decided that the possibility of an association of GBS with the vaccine, however small, necessitated halting the immunisation programme until the connection could be further examined. The IOM conducted a thorough scientific review of this issue in 2003 and concluded that people who received the swine influenza vaccine between 1976 and 1977 had an 'unexplained' increased risk of GBS (729). Once again, there is an explanation.

Meningococcal conjugate vaccine and Guillain-Barré syndrome: Case reports of GBS began to be reported to the VAERS after the introduction of the new meningococcal conjugate vaccine (MCV4) in 2005. In 2006, the CDC and the FDA requested the evaluation of GBS risk after MCV4 vaccination and concluded that no confirmed cases of GBS occurred within six weeks after vaccination (730). According to the Vaccine Injury Table symptoms, whilst the symptoms of GBS after the influenza vaccine manifest between three and 42 days post-vaccination, it is still possible to file a successful claim if the onset of symptoms do not fall within this time frame [731]. The CDC and FDA six week cut-off for assessment for GBS exists for a reason.

Hepatitis B vaccination and the risk of multiple sclerosis: Since 1998, multiple studies have evaluated a possible relationship between the hepatitis B vaccination (HBV) and MS. A nested case-control study was published in *The New England Journal of Medicine* in 2001. The study was conducted in two large cohorts of nurses in the US; the Nurses 'Health Study, which followed 121,700 women since 1976, and the Nurses' Health Study II, which followed 116,671 women since 1989. The study concluded that the multivariate relative risk of developing MS was associated with exposure to the HBV vaccine [732].

Wakefield and MMR: Wakefield is a smokescreen for the body of data clearly linking vaccines to long-term injury and a cover-up for the definitive study that has not been done. In 1998, *The BMJ* published an article that suggested a causal link between the measles-mumps-rubella (MMR) vaccine and inflammatory bowel disease. This article stated that doctors at the Royal Free Hospital in London believed they uncovered what they described as a new bowel disease in children that may be linked to autism and triggered by the MMR vaccine. The claim followed controversial work from the same team [733]. Wakefield's 1998 retracted study published in *The Lancet* stemmed from the investigation of 12 children aged between three and ten years who were referred to the department of paediatric gastroenterology at the Royal Free Hospital London. After a significant period of normal development, these children were referred to the paediatric gastroenterology unit as they had regressed in their acquired skills and had developed gastrointestinal symptoms [734]. This censored topic is discussed in greater detail in Chapter 23, 'Measles Shmeezles and the Great Autism Cover-up'.

MMR vaccine withdrawal: In 1992, the UK Department of Health withdrew the two market-dominating MMR vaccines, produced by the pharmaceutical companies SmithKlineBeecham [now GlaxoSmithKline (GSK)] and Merieux, following reported links with mumps meningitis [735]. On June 25th 2012, *Pharmaceutical Technology* reported that Merck had recalled MMR vaccines from the US [736]. On March 19th 2006, the Biotech company Chiron recalled five million doses of MMR vaccine it called the

Morupar vaccine for developing countries. The company said it distributed about five million doses of the Morupar vaccine to developing countries in 2005. 450,000 doses were distributed in Italy [737]. Chiron recalled the vaccine after data suggested it may be associated with a higher rate of adverse events than other vaccines [738].

LYMErix withdrawal: In 1998, the FDA approved a new recombinant Lyme vaccine, LYMErix, by manufacturer SmithKline Beecham. LYMErix was reported to reduce new infections in vaccinated adults by nearly 80%. Just three years later, after repeated reports of vaccine side effects that resulted in declining sales, SmithKline Beecham withdrew its product from the market. Musculoskeletal complaints such as arthritis were the main adverse reactions reported [739].

Rotashield and intussusception: On August 31st 1998, Rotashield, manufactured by Wyeth-Lederle Laboratories, was licensed by the FDA for oral administration to infants at two, four and six months of age. Following reports to the VEARS of 15 infants who had received the rotavirus vaccine and developed intussusception (a type of bowel obstruction that occurs when the bowel folds in on itself), the vaccine was withdrawn in 1999. Intussusception was radiographically confirmed in all 15 infants. Eight infants required surgical reduction, and one required resection of 18 cm of the distal ileum and proximal colon [740].

Nigeria and oral polio vaccine: In 2003 five northern Nigerian states boycotted the oral polio vaccine (OPV) due to fears that it was unsafe. Soon after, the vaccination drive was brought to a halt in three countries after Islamic community leaders claimed that the vaccines were unsafe and requested that the vaccines be double-checked for safety. One community leader, president of Nigeria's Supreme Council for Sharia Law, doctor Datti Ahmed said,

> *"There were strong reasons to believe that the polio immunisation vaccines were contaminated with anti-fertility drugs, contaminated with certain viruses that cause HIV/AIDS, contaminated with Simian virus that is likely to cause cancer"*.

While continuing to assert that the vaccines were safe, the WHO eventually agreed to test the vaccines to confirm their safety, and the campaign was set back significantly [741]. Vaccines were used to forcibly sterilise women in Kenya. In November 2014, a UN vaccine programme in Kenya was denounced by doctors and Catholic bishops for purposefully sterilising millions of women. The Kenya Catholic Doctors Association ordered laboratory tests of WHO and UNICEF tetanus vaccines being administered in Kenya and discovered that the vaccine was laced with the anti-fertility drug human chorionic gonadotropin (hCG), (hormone essential to pregnancy), also known as a sterilising agent. The hCG found in the UN tetanus vaccines caused the women's bodies to develop antibodies to attack hCG, resulting in the unborn child's death and permanent sterility. The UN gave these vaccinations to Kenyan women under the guise of 'preventing neonatal tetanus'. The women were completely unaware and did not provide free, prior and informed consent [(742)]. Anti-fertility vaccines are also covered in Chapter 15, 'COVID-19 Vaccines and Pregnancy Safety Concerns'.

HIB vaccine contamination with bacteria withdrawal: In December 2007, pharmaceutical company Merck recalled 1.2 million doses of Haemophilus influenzae type b (Hib) vaccines due to concerns about potential contamination with bacteria called *Bacillus cereus* (*B. cereus*) [(743)].

Porcine circovirus and rotavirus vaccine withdrawal: Porcine circovirus (PCV) is a common virus found in pigs. In 2010, porcine circovirus type 1 (PCV1) material was unexpectedly detected in the oral live-attenuated human rotavirus (RV) vaccine, Rotarix (GSK Vaccines, Belgium). In 2010, both rotavirus vaccines licensed in the US, Rotarix and RotaTeq, were found to contain PCV type 1 [(744)].

Typhoid vaccine withdrawal: In 2012 Manufacturer Sanofi Pasteur [(MSD) MSD is known as Merck in the US and Canada] recalled 88% of its stock of its Typhim Vi (typhoid) vaccine. The BBC News reported that 729,606 people who had received the typhoid vaccine might not have had full protection as the batch was too weak. The UK MHRA stated that these 729,606 people were not fully immunised against typhoid [(745)].

Human papillomavirus vaccination withdrawal: On December 16th 2013, the manufacturer of Gardasil, Merck, informed the CDC that it was to recall one lot (lot J007354) of Gardasil (human papillomavirus quadrivalent types 6, 11, 16, and 18 vaccine) after it discovered that a small number of vials contained glass particles as a result of breakage during the manufacturing process. A total of 743,360 vials were in the affected lot. Merck reassured worried parents that if the vaccine contained glass particles that were tiny enough to fit through a needle, mild reactions routinely seen after vaccination were likely to occur [(746)].

HPV vaccine and postural orthostatic tachycardia chronic fatigue syndrome: A case report and literature review discussed a link between postural orthostatic tachycardia syndrome with chronic fatigue syndrome (POTSCFS) after human papillomavirus (HPV) vaccination as part of the autoimmune/auto-inflammatory syndrome induced by adjuvants (ASIA) [(747)]. A cluster of serious adverse event reports of POTSCFS after HPV vaccination in Danish girls and young women occurred between September 2009 and August 2017 [(748)]. The young Irish women affected are known as the 'Gardasil Girls' and their parents have to defend themselves from being called 'anti-vaxxers'. I could write a chapter on the HPV vaccine's purported success.

Dengvaxia withdrawal: On December 4th 2017, the Philippines ordered French pharmaceutical company, Sanofi Pasteur, to recall its dengue vaccine, Dengvaxia. Dengvaxia was the world's first vaccine for dengue. The request to recall the vaccine was made after it was found to pose health risks in people that had not previously been infected with dengue. Sanofi said that individuals who had never had a dengue infection were at a significantly higher risk of a more severe form of dengue and hospitalisations after Dengvaxia than if they had not received it Dengvaxia [(749)].

Pandemrix withdrawal: A link between GSK's Pandemrix (AS03-adjuvanted H1N1 pandemic swine influenza vaccine) and the sleeping disorder narcolepsy was first suspected in Sweden and Finland in 2010, following a number of reports in children and adolescents. Pandemrix was soon after withdrawn from use in most countries, including Ireland [(750)]. As aforementioned, after the Pandemrix vaccination campaign in 2009-2010, narcolepsy risk increased five to 14-fold in children and adolescents, and two to sevenfold in adults. Observational studies indicated that the risk of narcolepsy remained elevated for two years post-Pandemrix vaccination [(675)]. An investigation confirmed the crude association between Pandemrix vaccination and narcolepsy observed in Finland and Sweden. There is increasing evidence that narcolepsy is an autoimmune disorder [(674)].

Disturbingly the UK Department for Work and Pensions argued that the permanent disability of narcolepsy was not serious enough to warrant compensation n those damaged by this vaccine. Thankfully ministers lost their fight to stop payouts over the Pandemrix narcolepsy cases, thus allowing the affected children to be able to apply for compensation after the high court ruling [(751)].

A report by *The BMJ* in September 2017 suggested that greater safety concerns existed surrounding the Pandemrix vaccine, which neither GSK nor public health authorities had made known to the public. *The BMJ* examined several GSK-made internal safety reports that had been obtained through an ongoing lawsuit alleging a causal link between Pandemrix and narcolepsy. *The BMJ* found a large discrepancy in the rates of AEFIs reported that dated years back between Pandemrix and two other GSK pandemic vaccines. The article stated that by December 2nd 2009, for every million doses of vaccine administered, 76 cases of serious adverse events were reported in people who received Pandemrix, compared to eight serious adverse events reported for the unadjuvanted vaccine, Arepanrix and another unadjuvanted vaccine combined. *The BMJ* noted that this pattern continued for the next eight reports and that by the end of March 2010, the rate of serious events following Pandemrix was seven times higher than that for Arepanrix and the third vaccine combined [(752)]. Public health authorities suppress the truth.

Deaths of two Samoan children after MMR due to iatrogenesis: Samoa's measles outbreak in 2019 was blamed on low vaccination rates. These low vaccination rates were contributed to vaccine safety concerns after the deaths in July 2018 of two children given a wrongly mixed vaccine MMR vaccine. The deaths were later established to have been due to the nurses mixing the vaccine with an expired muscle relaxant instead of water. The two nurses pleaded guilty to manslaughter and were sentenced to five years in prison [(753)].

Deaths in Korea after influenza vaccine and influenza vaccine recall: In only October 2020, the CDC had been made aware of reports of 59 deaths in South Korea following these people receiving the influenza vaccines distributed in South Korea. The Ministry of Food and Drug Safety (MFDS), formerly known as the Korea Food and Drug Administration (KFDA), reported that most of these deaths involved people in their 70s and 80s.

After the MFDS investigated 46 of these deaths, it reported that it did not find evidence of a causal association with the influenza vaccination [(754)]. The daily propaganda originally reported that only 13 deaths had occurred after receiving the seasonal influenza vaccine. One of these deaths was of a 17 year old boy who died two days after receiving an influenza vaccine [(755)]. Eventually, a total of 108 people were reported to have died after receiving a seasonal influenza vaccine. Needless to say, South Korea's health agency concluded that the deaths had no direct causal relations with the vaccines [(756)]. On October 9th 2020, however, South Korea's MFDS said that it had ordered Korea Vaccine Company to recall 615,000 doses of its influenza vaccines. The MFDS said it had issued the recall after "white particles" were confirmed to be found in influenza vaccines in the public health centre in Yeongdeok. The ministry said the white particles appeared to be protein. It was believed that the efficacy and safety of vaccines were not compromised. The vaccine maker, Korea Vaccine however, decided to voluntarily recall them [(757)]. As described in Chapter 13, 'COVID-19 Vaccines are Safe for Two Months', proteins in vaccines have been linked to anaphylaxis as in complement activation-related pseudo-allergy (CARPA). Pseudoallergy is a serious threat to public health [(758)].

Influenza vaccine recall in Nova Scotia: On November 16th 2020, it was reported that Nova Scotia had recalled some influenza vaccines after 3 "adverse events" in New Brunswick. Symptoms had appeared within a week of receiving the Flulaval Tetra vaccine from lot number KX9F7 [(759)].

What the Experts Say To Increase our Confidence in Vaccines

Vaccine safety according to Bill Gates: On July 23rd 2020, Norah O'Donnell interviewed Bill Gates on CBS News. At 15 minutes 33 seconds, Norah questions Gates on the fact that after the second dose of the Moderna vaccine, 80% experience a systemic side effect ranging from mild to severe. Bear in mind 80% of people with COVID-19 are completely asymptomatic. Norah asks, "Are these vaccines safe?" Gates answers,

> *"Well the ahh...the FDA...not being pressured...will look hard at that. The FDA is the gold standard of regulators...ahh and their current guidance on this...if they stick with that is very, very appropriate...Ahh and you know the it, the, the side effects were not super severe...that is it didn't cause permanent health problems for ah the things that (illegible)".*

Note Mr no longer smirking can't even be bothered furnishing us with an answer. Norah says, *"The data shows that everybody with a high dose had a side effect"* Mr no-longer-smirking replies, *"Yeah but some of that is, is not dramatic...where, you know, it's just super painful"* (760). Super painful? Miss Larson, if I were the head of the Vaccine Confidence Project, I would censor Bill Gates, as his wishy-washy answers and abhorrent body language do not instil confidence in vaccines.

Vaccines are not safe, according to those who make them: On December 2nd 2019, at the Global Vaccine Safety Summit, the World Wealth Organisation and vaccine experts were caught on tape saying the following...Dr Heidi Director of the I'll censor all evidence of vaccine dangers so you have confidence in vaccines Larson says;

> *"There's a lot of safety science that's needed and um...without the good science we can't have good communication, so although I'm talking about all these other contextual issues and communication issues, it absolutely needs the good science as the backbone. You can't repurpose the same old science to make it sound better if you don't have the science that's relevant to the new problems so".*

Do these new problems include the rampant incidence of autoimmune disease and an exponential rise in neurological disease, *per se*?

Dr Soumya Swaminathan Chief Boffin at the WHO says;

> *"I think we cannot overemphasise the fact that we really don't have very good safety monitoring systems in many countries and this adds the...the miscommunications and apprehensions because we are not able to give clear cut answers when people ask questions about deaths...this always gets blown up in the media...one should be able to give a very factual account of what has happened and what the cause of the deaths are...in most cases, there's some obfuscation at that level, and therefore there is less and less trust then in the system".*

Obfuscation is the act of making something obscure, unclear, or unintelligible. Heidi is very good at her job.

Dr Martin Howell Friede coordinator and Initiative for Vaccine Research (IVR) at the WHO says;

"Every time there is an association be it temporal or not temporal, the first accusation is it is the adjuvant and yet without adjuvants, we are not going to have the next generation of vaccines, and many of the vaccines we do have ranging from tetanus through to HPV, require adjuvants in order for them to work. So the challenge we have in front of us is how do we build confidence in this. And the confidence comes from the regulatory agencies (he looks to his crony Marian) when we add an adjuvant, it's because it's essential...when we add them its adds to the complexity, and I give courses every year on...how do you develop vaccines how do you? And the first lesson is while you're making your vaccine, if you can avoid using an adjuvant, please do so. Lesson two is if you're going to use an adjuvant, use one that has a history of safety, and lesson 3 is if you're not going to do that, think very carefully".

Professor Stephen Evans. Professor of Pharmacoepidemiology says;

"It seems to me that adjuvants multiply the immunogenicity of the antigens that they are added to, and that is their intention. It seems to me that they (adjuvants) multiply the reactogenicity in many instances, and therefore, it seems to me that it's not unexpected if they multiply the incidence of adverse reactions that are associated with the antigens but may not have been detected through lack of statistical power in the original studies".

Dr Martin Howell Friede answers;

"You are correct. As we add more adjuvants, especially some of the more recent adjuvants...we do see increased local reactogenicity. The primary concern though usually is systemic adverse events rather than local adverse events and we tend to get in the phase II beyond the age 50 that have had the pleasure of having the shingles vaccine will know that this has quite significant local reactogenicity. This is not the major health concern. The major accusation is of long-term health effects, and again I point to regulators, it comes down to um ensuring that we conduct the phase II and phase III studies with adequate size and appropriate measurement".

David C. Kaslow, M.D. Chief Scientific Officer, Director of the PATH Centre for Vaccine Innovation and Access (CVIA) says;

"So in our clinical trials we are actually using relatively small sample sizes, and when we do that, we are at risk of tyranny of small numbers. Which is, you just need a single case of Wegener's granulomatosis, and your vaccine has to solve Walts...and how do you prove a null hypothesis? And that takes years and years to try and figure...that out. It's a real conundrum right?"

Dr Marion Gruber Director, Office of Vaccines Research and Review/Centre for Biologics Evaluation and Research (CBER) at FDA, says;

"One of the additional issues that complicates safety evaluation is if you look at the struggle with the length of follow-up that's in a let's say pre-licensure or even post-marketing study, if that's even possible, and as you mentioned, pre-licensure clinical trials may not be powered enough. It's also the subject population that you administer the adjuvant to because we've seen data presented to us where an adjuvant, a particular adjuvant added to a vaccine antigen, did really nothing when administered to a certain population and usually the elderly. You know compared to administering the same formulation (containing adjuvants) to younger aged strata so, so, these are the things which uh, need to be considered as well and further complicate safety and effectiveness evaluation of adjuvants combined with vaccine antigens".

Dr Bassey Okposen, Programme Manager National Emergency Routine Immunisation Coordinating Centre (NERICC), says;

"I cast back my mind to our situation in Nigeria, where at six weeks, ten weeks, 14 weeks, a child is being given different antigens, from different companies, and these vaccines have different adjuvants, different preservatives and so on, Something crosses my mind. Is there a possibility of these adjuvants, preservatives, cross-reacting among themselves? Has there ever been a study on the possibilities of cross-reactions?"

Dr Robert Chen Director of the Brighton Collaboration, answers;

"Now the only way to tease that out is if you have a large population database like the vaccine safety datalink as well as some of the other national databases that are coming to being worthy. Actual vaccine exposure is trapped down to that level of specificity of who is the

manufacturer. What is the lot number? Etc. and there's uh initiative to try to make the uh vaccine label information uh barcoded. So it included the level of information so that in the future when we do these type of studies, we are able to tease that out. And in order to be, and in each time you subdivide then the uh sample size gets...becomes more and more challenging. And that's what I said about earlier today, about that we're really only in the beginning of the era of large data sets where hopefully you can start to um kind of uh harmonise the databases from multiple studies. Um, and there is actually uh initiative underway..."

His nonsensical answer drags on..

"The other thing that's a trend and an issue is not just confidence in healthcare providers but confidence of healthcare providers. We have a very wobbly health professional frontline that is starting to question vaccines and the safety of vaccines. When the frontline uh professionals are starting to question, or they don't feel like they have enough confidence about the safety to stand up to it, to the person who is asking them the questions, I mean most medical school curriculums, even nursing curriculums, I mean in medical school you're lucky if you have half a day on vaccines never mind keeping up to date on all of this" (761).

That gives me so much confidence in vaccines, Heidi.

CHAPTER TWELVE – PART III

VACCINES DON'T ALWAYS WORK

"The most potent weapon of the oppressor is the mind of the oppressed".
Stephen Biko (762)

Even if COVID-19 vaccine candidates are effective and receive full licensure, vaccines can fail when the global experiment/rollout proceeds. The business model vaccine companies use, and the daily propaganda perpetuates when vaccines fail, is to blame 'failure to vaccinate'. Whilst natural infection to measles is lifelong, it is acknowledged that despite sustained high vaccine coverage, the reemergence of 'vaccine-preventable diseases' (VPDs), including measles and mumps, is linked to waning vaccine immunity (763, 764). Thus, the 'highly efficacious' COVID-19 vaccines will likely not be so efficacious in the real world.

Primary and secondary vaccine failure: The daily propaganda frequently reports on failure to vaccinate but neglects to report on both primary and secondary vaccine failure. Vaccine failure occurs for many reasons. Primary vaccine failure occurs when the immune system does not produce enough antibodies after vaccination. Secondary vaccine failure occurs when enough antibodies are produced after vaccination, but the levels wane (fall) over time, or due to a break in the cold chain production, storage and distribution (765). Vaccination recommendations and programmes are based on clinical trials performed in selected, healthy and primarily young populations. However, the population is increasingly ageing and increasingly unhealthy, and the efficiency of vaccines in these populations needs to be surveyed.

Primary vaccine failure in older adults: Immunosenescence describes the reduced response to vaccination observed in the elderly. The concept of immunosenescence is important for understanding vaccine responses in older adults. There is increasing evidence that immunosenescence is not universally or evenly experienced with biological ageing but is part of what contributes to the variability in susceptibility seen with frailty and an increasing burden of health conditions. Thus the story is more complex than simply older age resulting in immunosenescence. Frailty is increasingly understood to affect older adults' responses to vaccines for influenza, shingles and pneumococcus [(766)]. While the boffins tell us the world population is rapidly ageing and an ageing immune system is particularly susceptible to infectious disease, and preventing infectious diseases in the elderly is an important public health measure, current vaccines are designed for young and adult individuals and prove less protective in the older people.

Ideally, in vaccine effectiveness trials, we should see vaccines being tested in the population most at risk, and we need transparency on the health and age of vaccine trial participants. What happens is quite the opposite. Influenza vaccine effectiveness trials are conducted in younger people less susceptible to the detrimental effects of influenza infection, therefore it is difficult to determine the exact primary vaccine failure rate in older adults. Also, there are not many randomised controlled trials (RCTs) on influenza vaccine efficacy (VE) in older adults. Additionally, no RCTs on the prevention of influenza among elderly diabetics or institutional-ised elderly have been published at all, as a trial on mortality has been deemed ethically unacceptable [(767)]. There is that ethical excuse again.

Bias in vaccine studies in the elderly: Influenza vaccines are increasingly being recommended, yet controversy surrounds the benefits of the influenza vaccine in older adults, and there is no consensus on VE based on subsequent epidemiologic studies. Frailty selection bias in vaccine trials occurs through enrolling younger, healthier people more likely to achieve a positive result in the trial. All-cause mortality refers to the number of deaths from all causes and is a non-specific endpoint used in vaccine trials that can introduce bias.

A *Lancet Infectious Disease* study concluded that frailty selection bias and the use of all-cause mortality leads to cohort studies greatly exaggerating the effectiveness of the influenza vaccine. The use of all-cause mortality as an endpoint has introduced bias in a number of VE studies [(768)]. Andrew et al. noted in a letter to the editor published in *The Journal of Infectious Diseases* that among the study participants of influenza vaccine trials, information on frailty was missing in 44% of cases who took the influenza vaccine, compared to only 4% of controls who took a placebo [(769)].

Public health's motto is, if it doesn't work, give them more: Approaches to improving vaccine efficiency in the elderly include high-dose vaccines, booster vaccinations, different immunisation routes, and the use of new adjuvants [(770)]. Scientists achieve higher VE in the elderly by increasing doses of the antigen and adding more adjuvants. The adjuvant used in influenza vaccines to promote a 'better immune response' is shark liver squalene, also called MF59 [(771)]. The use of MF59-adjuvanted H1N1 influenza vaccines is associated with an increased incidence of local and systemic adverse events, and adjuvant use is a significant predictor of systemic adverse events [(772)]. Shark liver squalene is also used as an adjuvant in some COVID-19 vaccines [(773)]. In addition to increasing adjuvant levels, scientists also increase antigen levels. The Fluzone High-Dose Quadrivalent used in the elderly is a high-dose influenza vaccine that contains four times the amount of antigen as the standard-dose inactivated influenza vaccine [(774)]. Graphene oxide is a novel vaccine nano-adjuvant for robust stimulation of cellular immunity [(775)].

Primary vaccine failure in obese individuals: Obesity-induced chronic inflammation affects the immune system, and obese populations have been observed to respond poorly to vaccines [(776)]. Obesity has been shown to reduce vaccine immunogenicity, the ability to provoke an immune response, and increases the likelihood of a poor vaccine-induced immune response [(534)].

Primary vaccine failure in healthy individuals: Obesity and older age aside, approximately 2-10% of healthy individuals fail to mount antibody levels to routine vaccines and experience vaccine failure [(777)]. Vaccines do not work in up to 10% of healthy people!

Primary vaccine failure in children exposed to persistent organic pollutants: Many persistent organic pollutants (POPs) chemicals are immunotoxic and include toxic substances used as chemical warfare agents. A number of studies have indicated that increased exposure to polychlorinated biphenyls (PCBs) during pregnancy may result in reduced antibody responses to childhood vaccinations and primary vaccine failure. The clinical implications of insufficient antibody production emphasises the need to prevent immunotoxicant exposures where we can [(778)]. A prospective birth-cohort exposure study on exposure to POPs known as polyfluoroalkyl substances (PFAS) and responses to paediatric vaccines and immune-related health outcomes in children up to three years of age found that the higher the concentrations of the four PFAS, the lower the level of anti-rubella (German measles) antibodies in the children [779]. A study led by Grandjean found that children exposed to PFAS had significantly reduced antibody concentrations after tetanus and diphtheria vaccinations [780]. A certain type of PFAS called perfluorobutyrate (PFBA) accumulates in the lungs. Another study led by Grandjean found that elevated blood-PFBA concentrations were associated with an increased risk of a more severe course of COVID-19 disease [781]. Bear in mind a number of POPs are detected at high concentrations in blood samples of the US population and that this information can be extrapolated globally [782].

Genetic basis for measles primary vaccine failure: A US measles epidemic in 1989-1991 included a series of outbreaks, with the greatest proportion being due to primary vaccine failure. This study revealed that 10% of children vaccinated against measles lacked antibody on follow-up and that these vaccine failures clustered in families, indicating a genetic basis [783].

Secondary vaccine failure: Vaccine failure also occurs due to a break in the cold chain, which results in the vaccine not being kept at the correct temperatures and the vaccine spoiling. Cold chain management failures are caused by human error such as staff negligence, insufficient training, breaking established protocols and inefficient equipment use. An adult measles outbreak in the Federated States of Micronesia in 2014 was attributed to vaccine failure resulting from cold chain management failures [784].

The elderly, obese, polluted, genetically challenged and healthy people all experience vaccine failure. That's a large proportion of the population. Human error can result in vaccine failure. The evidence of vaccine efficacy, effectiveness and protection is irrelevant. Shut up! Obey! Take your shot!

Flawed Vaccine Trials say Vaccines are Safe and Effective

Non-publication and delayed publication of vaccine trials: The public believes vaccines are safe and effective because government policy on vaccines is not led by 'the science'; it's led by flawed science. The main flaws associated with vaccine trials include non-registration, nonreporting and misreporting.

The Health Research Authority is responsible for 'promoting research transparency': In the UK, an executive non-departmental public body of the Department of Health known as the Health Research Authority (HRA) exists to provide a unified national system for the governance of health research. Since 2014, the HRA has been explicitly tasked with 'promoting research transparency' as part of its objectives, but no significant change in transparency of health research has occurred.

UK/EU rules and guidelines on transparency regarding the publication of trial results: A new EU Clinical Trials Regulation is to supersede the current EU Clinical Trials Directive. The new directive set out to include new transparency requirements regarding publication of trial results and requires member states to lay down rules on and penalties for non-compliance. This was expected to occur in 2019 after the UK left the EU. Enter the global health security agenda for population control and zero likelihood of transparency in vaccine trials, and in fact, zero likelihood of full-length vaccine trials again. A range of UK and EU rules and guidelines are in force to improve clinical trials transparency. Despite these rules and guidelines to improve clinical trials transparency in tackling non-registration, nonreporting and misreporting, around half of all clinical trials are left unreported, clinical trial registration is not yet universal in the UK, and reported outcomes do not always align with the original study proposal.

According to the HRA, issues surrounding the best global practice in the publication of scientific trials are as follows;

Non-registration: In 2013, the HRA made it a condition of a trial receiving a 'favourable opinion' from a research ethics committee that the trial must be registered or deferred for specific reasons. The HRA's audit in 2017 found that 32% of 599 studies that received a 'favourable opinion' (and no agreed deferral) could not be found on a publicly accessible registry.

Nonreporting: Around half of trials go unreported. Since July 2014, the European Commission has required all trials on the EU Clinical Trials Register (trials of medicinal products) to post results to the registry within 12 months of completion, with a final compliance date of December 21st 2016. A study by Dr Goldacre and his team at the Evidence-Based Medicine

Data Lab in 2019 identified 7,274 trials where it could be verified that results were now due. Of these, just 49.5% had reported results.

Misreporting: A multi-journal initiative exists to ensure that the full results from trials are reported. The Consolidated Standards of Reporting Trials (CONSORT) statement, first published in 1996 and updated in 2010, sets out "a standard way for authors to prepare reports of trial findings, facilitating their complete and transparent reporting, and aiding their critical appraisal and interpretation".

A study of the work of the Hampshire Research Ethics Committee A, by Dr Kolstoe found that 57% of publications associated with trials approved by the committee showed "inconsistencies with the outcomes originally declared in the ethics application". The Medical Research Council (MRC) also reported that whilst reporting rates for the trials it funds were high, regarding its most recent audit of corresponding publications, "only half of these appeared to include the main trial results".

Public Health England withholds vaccine trials: The *EU Trials Trackerwebsite* (2019) set up by Dr Goldacre and colleagues at the Evidence-Based Medicine DataLab also reveals that Public Health England (PHE) has three overdue trials dating from 2010 -2016 relating to meningitis vaccines. PHE and a range of National Health Service (NHS) Foundation Trusts fail to report clinical trials results. NHS Trusts have high numbers of unreported clinical trials. According to the site, in 2019, the Manchester University NHS Foundation Trust had 13 overdue trials, NHS Greater Glasgow and Clyde had 12 overdue trials, and both Newcastle upon Tyne Hospitals NHS Foundation Trust and Hull and East Yorkshire Hospitals NHS Trust had 11 overdue trials. The HRA requested PHE to write to them with an explanation and the steps it will take to correct this [(785)].

The UK parliament Commons Select Committee and research integrity: The UK parliament Commons Select Committee in their *Research integrity: clinical trials transparency* report indicates that 50% of all clinical trial results are not published, thus posing a risk to public health. The Committee is concerned that selective non-publication, or publication bias, distorts the published evidence base and threatens research integrity. Committee witnesses indicate examples of 'publication bias' having led to wasted public expenditure in the UK and even patient deaths in other countries. One example included the government's decision to stockpile millions of pounds worth of Tamiflu in response to the H1N1 swine influenza pandemic in 2009.

The Committee heard that the government was, *"relying on a marketing spiel claiming successful trials of this drug rather than being able to consider the actual evidence of the drug efficacy for themselves"*. Sound familiar?

The Committee also recommends that;

- The government should ask the HRA to publish a detailed strategy for achieving full clinical trials transparency by December 2019.
- The HRA should be provided with funding to establish a national programme to audit clinical trials transparency, including the publication of a list of which UK trials have published results and those which are due to but have not.
- The HRA should introduce a system of sanctions to drive improvements in clinical trials transparency, such as withdrawing favourable ethical opinion or preventing further trials from taking place, and the government should consult specifically on whether to provide the HRA with the statutory power to fine sponsors for non-compliance [(786)].

The WHO statement on unpublished clinical vaccine trials: The WHO says vaccine trials are biased, and many remain unpublished, yet they influence government vaccination policy. The WHO has made it clear that researchers have an ethical imperative to make results publicly available from all clinical trials, including past trials. The WHO statement on Public Disclosure of Clinical Trial Results states:

- Results from clinical trials should be publicly reported within one year of the trial end date.
- Calls for results from previously unpublished trials to be made publicly available.
- Calls on organisations and governments to implement measures to achieve this [(787)].

Table 7 outlines the percentage of vaccine trials published on time according to the WHO [(788)]

Table 7: Tracking time to publication of vaccine trial results

Number of vaccine trials	Published time years	Percentage
154	1 (on time)	24%
90	2	14%
72	3	11%
42	4	7%
21	5	3%
61	6+	10%
193	unpublished	30%
633		

Industry-sponsored trials: Out of 890 vaccine trials in total, according to the WHO, 428 or 48% are industry-sponsored [(788)]. Many studies reveal pharmaceutical company-funded clinical drug trials influence drug trials in many ways to produce favourable results for company products more often than independent trials do. As many as half of all trials financed by pharmaceutical companies are never published. Findings included incomplete trial registration, constraints on publishing rights, withholding knowledge of adverse drug reactions, and the use of ghostwriters who the pharmaceutical companies supplied. Public access to trial protocols and results must be ensured. Moreover, more effort should be made to carry out drug trials independently, without the financial support of pharmaceutical companies [(789)]. The 890 vaccine trials registered is an indication of how many vaccines public health has in store for us.

Positive publication bias: The proportion of positive results in scientific literature increased between 1990/1991, reaching 70.2% and 85.9% in 2007, respectively. The average yearly increase was found to be 6%, with the effect constant across most disciplines and countries [(790)].

Leading academic medical centres withholding of trial results: An aggregate analysis of *ClinicalTrials.gov* database regarding the dissemination of clinical trial results across leading academic medical centres concluded that despite academic institutions' ethical mandate and expressed values and mission, poor performance and noticeable variations exist [791].

Results across academic medical centres of 4347 interventional clinical trials across 51 centres;

- 23% enrolled more than 100 patients.
- 28% were double-blind.
- 50% were phase II through IV, completely skipping phase I trials.
- Results were disseminated in 66% of trials, with 35.9% publishing results within 24 months of the study end date.
- Clinical trials results disseminated within 24 months of study end date ranged from 16.2%-55.3%.
- Clinical trials published within 24 months of study end date ranged from 10.8% to 40.3%. Results reporting on *ClinicalTrials.gov* ranged from 1.6%-40.7% [791].

A person with free will may question why vaccine trial results are withheld? Vaccines are not safe. There is no evidence showing that vaccines do not increase the risk of autoimmune, autoinflammatory and allergic disease. The concerns that repeated exposure to multiple vaccines in a susceptible child may produce atypical or nonspecific immune or nervous system injury that could lead to severe disability or death have not been allayed. Without a doubt, the Emergency Use Authorisation (EUA) unlicensed biological agent COVID-19 'vaccine' will be added to this schedule. Until the safety study is done and published according to best global practice, and indeed, until all vaccine trials are conducted according to international rules and regulations, vaccine mandates should be off the table. Heidi Larson's Vaccine Confidence Project and her peanut gallery of 'Fact-Checkers' are the Thought Police [338]. The Global Vaccine Safety Summit is a complete smokescreen. To trust public health officials, we need all the information and to have our personal liberty protected. Alternatively, we could continue to harken back to days of old public health and deem people unable to reason, then apply public health police powers to hold them down, beat them into submission and accomplish our task of universal vaccination [792].

CHAPTER THIRTEEN

COVID-19 VACCINES ARE SAFE FOR TWO MONTHS

"Those who do not move do not notice their chains".
Rosa Luxemburg [(793)]

When it comes to vaccine safety, the boffins' definition of 'safe' is, the 'benefits outweigh the risks'. I agree completely that the benefits for the Big Pharmaceutical Research and Manufacturers of America (PhRMA) are huge, and, seeing as they have no liability at all, the risks are zero. Regarding the benefits and risks posed to the consumer (us), the risks are massively underreported and rarely found to be caused by the vaccine, and the benefits are grossly overstated.

COVID-19 vaccines are not vaccines: First and foremost, the currently unlicensed coronavirus disease 2019 (COVID-19) vaccines are not vaccines. While the fact-wreckers say that the following is a 'conspiracy', Moderna and Pfizer-BioNTech do indeed call their products called an 'operating system' and 'biological agent' respectively. Moderna's operating system is said to transform the human body into a vaccine-making machine that uses RNA as a messenger inside our cells to produce an immune reaction [(794)]. The Moderna website says the operating system sets out to create a technology platform that functions as an operating system on a computer. It is designed so that it can plug and play interchangeably with different programmes. The programme is the man-made mRNA drug, the unique mRNA sequence that codes for a protein [(795)]. Moderna's is an operating system designed to programme humans. Pfizer calls their product an experimental biological agent [(796)]. These biological agents are being used in a continued biological attack on us. For the sake of congruency, I will call them vaccines.

COVID-19 vaccines have been issued under Emergency Use Authorisation (EUA) [(592)]. This means that the time required to assess safety and efficacy for each phase of clinical research from phase I to phase IV was massively reduced, resulting in the trials being too fast to gain adequate safety and efficacy data.

Operation Warp Speed and EUA

Overview of clinical trials when there is no 'emergency': Under normal circumstances, the clinical trials stages to get a vaccine to market include;

- **Preclinical trials**: Research using animals to find out if a drug, procedure, or treatment is likely to be useful. Provides information on dosing and toxicity, pharmacodynamics (how it works) and pharmacokinetics (how it is absorbed, distributed, metabolised and excreted).
- **Phase I:** Dose-ranging on human volunteers for safety.
- **Phase II:** Testing of drug on human volunteers to assess efficacy and side effects. Phase II trials recruit up to several hundred patients with the condition to take part. This phase typically lasts several months to two years.
- **Phase III:** Testing of a drug on human volunteers to assess efficacy and safety. The length of the phase III trials is normally one to four years.
- **Phase IV:** Post-marketing surveillance in public [(797)].

Operation Warp Speed: Operation Warp Speed is the US government's vaccine accelerator mechanism to develop a severe acute respiratory syndrome coronavirus 2 (SARS-CoV-2) vaccine using new technology, in a first of its kind human trial at break-neck speed [(798)]. Dublin-based pharmaceutical, biotechnology and medical device company ICON partnered on the implementation of the Pfizer-BioNTech COVID-19 vaccine trial. This information was only able to be released in January 2021 due to commercial reasons. ICON said the trial was conducted across 153 sites in the United States (US), Europe, South Africa and Latin America in what they described as, *"unprecedented trial timelines"* [(799)]. That gives me so much confidence in vaccines, Heidi.

Animal trials in the normal sense were bypassed: Animal trials occur in the pre-clinical stages, however in terms of study length and study outcomes, the animal trials for the COVID-19 vaccines were not in the normal sense. Pre-clinical stage animal trials normally last 1-2 years, so it is safe to say animal studies were bypassed. An article entitled 'Current global vaccine and drug efforts against COVID-19: Pros and cons of bypassing animal trials' published in the *Journal of Biosciences* in June 2020, confirms the biotech companies bypassed animal studies and moved to phase I clinical trials. The problem with the biotech companies bypassing animal studies and moving straight into phase I clinical trials is that human outcomes cannot be predicted in the absence of complete animal studies [800].

The animal preclinical tests for the COVID-19 vaccines were as follows: The Pfizer-BioNTech mRNA vaccine Comirnaty preclinical trial tested six rhesus macaque monkeys who were vaccinated and then exposed to the SARS-CoV-2 virus. The vaccinated monkeys were found to have less of the virus in their lower and upper respiratory tracts [801, 802]. Oxford University's original report based on the vaccination of six rhesus macaques showed that all the vaccinated monkeys became infected when challenged (deliberately infected with the virus) [803]. The vaccine did not work at all; no matter, on to the great apes. The Moderna COVID-19 vaccine study pushed the boat out by involving 24 rhesus macaques. Eight monkeys were used as controls, eight given a low dose of vaccine and eight given a high dose [804].

As previously explained in Chapter 7, 'Does SARS-CoV-2 Exist?', back in 2003, scientists used two monkeys to satisfy Koch's postulates for the original severe acute respiratory syndrome coronavirus (SARS-CoV). For SARS-CoV-2 however, scientists have not proved the 3rd of Koch's postulates which states, "*The microorganism (from the pure culture) should cause the disease when inoculated into a healthy organism*". Scientists have completely skipped this step in animals and therefore have not satisfied Koch's postulates to prove that SARS-CoV-2 causes COVID-19. Those zany scientists on Tik Tosser try to convince us (those of us who get our information from social media) that whilst the COVID-19 vaccine trials have happened at break-neck speed, they haven't skipped any steps and are 'safe and effective', what these in the pharmaceutical pocket scientific influencers don't explain is Emergency Use Authorisation (EUA) [805].

Emergency Use Authorisation; six monkeys, seven days, two months, seven billion: Under EUA, vaccine safety has been assessed after two months and vaccine efficacy after seven days. Under EUA, the Food and Drug Administration (FDA) state that COVID-19 vaccine candidates only require phase III data to include a median follow-up of at least two months after completion of the full vaccination regimen [592, 806]. As mentioned, preclinical animal trial length and thus study outcomes were inadequate.

Phase I trials were conducted concurrently with phase II. Phase II trial efficacy data showed the vaccine worked for seven days. Phase II trials typically last several months to two years. Phase III safety data showed the vaccine was safe for two months. Phase III trials typically last one to four years. The concern is that many adverse reactions (ADRs) to vaccines take much longer than two months to manifest. Six monkeys, seven days, two months, roll it out to seven billion human beings. You whacky scientists! Operation Warp Speed and EUA mean human beings are now the great apes in the global experiment.

The vaccine candidates may never get full licence: This is what is supposed to happen however, that was before COVID (BC) during the old normal. Now that the vaccines are being rolled out, there should be a genuine danger that the vaccine candidates will never get full licence. According to the FDA's Vaccines and Related Biological Products Advisory Committee (VRBPAC):

> *"Licensure of a COVID-19 vaccine will be based on a review of additional manufacturing, efficacy, and safety data, providing greater assurance of the comparability of the licensed product to product tested in the clinical trials, greater assurance of safety based on larger numbers of vaccine recipients who have been followed for a longer period of time, and additional information about efficacy that addresses, among other questions, the potential for waning of protection over time"*.

The VRBPAC document confirms that, *"the sponsor proposes that these participants will be unblinded upon request"* [807]. The pharmaceutical companies producing the COVID-19 vaccine candidates say they have an ethical obligation to unblind the trials. In December 2020, after their vaccine was awarded EUA, Pfizer sent a letter to its trial participants telling them they could learn whether they were in the placebo arm so that they could receive the vaccine [808]. Thus, as the rollout occurred, the trial participants were unblinded, and those receiving the placebo received the vaccine, even jumping the queue. Unblinding trial participants means it is now impossible to compare the health outcomes of the vaccinated to the health outcomes of those who received a placebo. In this way, the vaccine trials essentially ended. Thus vaccine manufacturers will not be able to produce the data necessary to achieve full approval and licence for their product [809]. By August 30th 2021, the FDA had approved the Pfizer vaccine even though Pfizer had confirmed immunity wanes after six months. It has become blatantly obvious that public health authorities will never compare vaccinated and unvaccinated health outcomes.

Former FDA Chief Boffin Jesse Goodman said,

> *"Vaccinating the people who received placebo injections, the trial's control arm, would end the ability to continue to compare the two groups after what would have been a short trial"*.

Goodman agreed that an early EUA might leave a manufacturer with too little data to persuade the FDA to issue a full licence. Marion Gruber, Director of the FDA's Office of Vaccine Research and Review, put the issue to VRBPAC members. Gruber said, "We are concerned about the risk that use of a vaccine under EUA would interfere with long-term assessment of safety and efficacy in ongoing trials and potentially even jeopardise product approval". Gruber continues to say, "and not only the first vaccine but maybe even follow-on vaccines". The acting chair of the committee, physician and epidemiologist at the University of Michigan School of Public Health, Arnold S. Monto, also stated that the COVID-19 vaccine manufacturers may not be able to generate enough additional data to apply for full licensure [(810)]. On January 14th 2021, the WHO Ad Hoc Expert Group on the Next Steps for COVID-19 Vaccine Evaluation wrote a letter to *The New England Journal of Medicine* stating that the relatively short follow-up in phase III trials, even in the event of vaccine efficacy appearing to be high, means that reliable information is needed on longer-term safety and duration of protection. Sir Richard Peto, Emeritus Professor of Medical Statistics and Epidemiology at the University of Oxford, said, *"If you're going to prioritise people to get vaccinated, the last people you should vaccinate are those who were in a placebo group in a trial"* [(811)].

Vaccine Ingredients: Many parents read their children's cereal ingredients, yet most parents do not consider vaccine ingredients. If we spoon-fed our children vaccine ingredients, we would be charged with poisoning. Additionally, many people avoid genetically modified (GM) foods yet are unconcerned that COVID-19 vaccines are genetically modifying 'gene vaccines' that contain GM ingredients. DNA and RNA-based gene vaccines are discussed in Chapter 20, 'The Future is Vaccines, Vaccines and More Vaccines'. Vaccines are not Halal, Kosher, vegan, or green. Vaccines are full of small amounts of known mutagenic (damages genetic material), carcinogenic (promotes cancer), teratogenic (damages the foetus), and neurotoxic (damages the brain) poisons. We are indoctrinated with the mantra, 'safe in small amounts', it is not difficult to understand however, that small amounts accumulate to large amounts, and we are bombarded daily with small amounts of poisons in our air, food and 'drinking' water. Applying science's precautionary approach; when in doubt, get it out.

In addition to weakened or killed disease antigens (viruses or bacteria), vaccines contain very small amounts of other ingredients called excipients. A table listing of vaccine excipients and media by excipient is published by the Institute for Vaccine Safety at Johns Hopkins University [(812)]. The FDA publishes excipients included in US vaccines [(813)]. Excipients include antibiotics, formaldehyde used to deactivate the virus, the mercury-based preservative thimerosal, the vaccine adjuvant aluminium etc. Adjuvants in vaccines are used to enhance immunogenicity. One adjuvant used in COVID-19 vaccines is called squalene or MF59. The chemical name is known as C30H50. As mentioned in Chapter 12, 'Vaccines aren't Described as Safe and don't Always Work', autoimmune and inflammatory disorders are associated with adjuvants. The condition known as autoimmune /inflammatory syndrome induced by adjuvants (ASIA) encompasses multiple autoimmune phenomena that are caused by exposure to adjuvants. ASIA is also known as Shoenfeld's syndrome [(814)].

The main substance associated with ASIA in the multisystem disorder known as Gulf War Syndrome was the adjuvant shark liver squalene [(815)]. According to the Committee on Veterans' Affairs, during the Gulf War, a number of squalene containing vaccines for cholera, meningitis, rabies, tetanus and typhoid were deployed to protect against potential exposures to biological threats [(816)]. Mounting evidence suggests that autoimmune mechanisms may underlie the chronic symptoms characteristic of Gulf War Syndrome [(817)]. Neither squalene, M59 or C30H50 is listed as an active ingredient in the COVID-19 vaccines. However, it is known that 19 of the 193 candidate COVID-19 vaccines use adjuvants, and five of those use shark-based squalene as an adjuvant. Specific vaccines were not identified [(773)]. Squalene is discussed further in Chapter 22, 'Vaccines are not Green'.

Comirnaty (Pfizer-BioNTech) vaccine ingredients: The active substance in the COVID-19 mRNA vaccine in mRNA. After dilution, the vial contains six doses of 0.3 ml with 30 micrograms mRNA each. The other ingredients are:

- ((4-hydroxybutyl)azanediyl)bis(hexane-6,1-diyl)bis(2-hexyldecanoate) (ALC-0315) [synthetic lipid]
- 2-[(polyethylene glycol)-2000]-N,N-ditetradecylacetamide (ALC-0159) [polyethylene glycol (PEG)/lipid conjugate, derived from petrol]
- 1,2-Distearoyl-sn-glycero-3-phosphocholine (DSPC) [Distearoylphosphatidylcholine is a phosphatidylcholine, a phospholipid]
- Cholesterol
- Potassium chloride
- Potassium dihydrogen phosphate
- Sodium chloride
- Disodium phosphate dehydrate
- Sucrose
- Water for injections [(818)]

Graphene oxide may be in the Pfizer COVID-19 vaccines: The fact-wreckers are fact-checking this, so chances are it holds true. Heidi Larson's peanut gallery says graphene oxide is not in the COVID-19 vaccines because it is not listed in the official list of ingredients according to the FDA and Centres for Disease Control and Prevention (CDC). A laboratory analysis conducted at the University of Almería in Spain claimed the Pfizer vaccine vial contains 99% graphene oxide. The university has distanced itself from the findings. The Vaccine Confidence Project (VCP) should refute such claims and instil confidence in vaccines by getting an independent researcher to examine the contents of a vial.

Is graphene bound to polyethylene glycol as a nano-adjuvant? Graphene oxide is used as a novel vaccine nano-adjuvant for robust stimulation of cellular immunity (775). An article published in *Nanoethics* in 2018 discussed the risk or not associated with graphene nanotechnology. Graphene is a nanomaterial with many promising and innovative applications, yet early studies indicated that graphene may pose risks to humans and the environment. One researcher said of graphene,

> *"It is not clear how toxic graphene can be. If you change graphene with molecules, it will be safe. If you insert graphene into your body, it might hurt you. But you don't insert it into the body"* [(819)].

Do we or don't we? Recently graphene and graphene-related materials (GRMs) have attracted huge attention due to their wide spectrum properties such as high surface area, high electrical mobility and conductivity, excellent mechanical, electrochemical, piezoelectric properties (can generate an electric charge in response to applied mechanical stress), and efficacy against microbes and viruses. These properties are being examined as potential graphene-based materials to combat COVID-19 [820]. Alum-functionalised graphene oxide nanocomplexes are used in addition to alum-based adjuvants to elicit further cellular immune responses in vaccines. Scientists have formulated novel AlO(OH)-modified (alum-modified) graphene oxide (GO) nanocomplexes [GO-AlO (OH)] to use in anticancer vaccines [821]. Aluminium-containing adjuvants have been used in vaccines since the 1930s.

ALC-0159 [polyethylene glycol (PEG)] is a listed ingredient in the Pfizer and Moderna vaccine. The association between PEG and post-vaccination anaphylaxis is discussed later in this chapter. PEG and polyethylenimine (PEI) are nanomaterials used for gene delivery. PEG is grafted with carboxylated graphene oxide as a novel interface modifier for polylactic acid/graphene nanocomposite known as GO-PEG. GO-PEG is a vaccine nano-adjuvant. Another novel vaccine nano-adjuvant is known as graphene oxide polyethylenimine (GO-PEI) [775, 822]. Whether the PEG in COVID-19 vaccines is GO-PEG is a possibility and should be investigated, not discounted as a conspiracy theory.

The contents of vaccines baffle scientists: A report entitled *New Quality-Control Investigations on Vaccines: Micro and Nanocontamination,* published in the *International Journal of Vaccine and Vaccinations,* examined 44 vaccine samples from Italy and France using a powerful environmental scanning electron microscope. Vaccines examined included diphtheria-tetanus-pertussis (DTP), hepatitis B, poliomyelitis, measles-mumps-rubella (MMR), chickenpox and meningitis. Researchers found lead, stainless steel, iron particles and other inorganic material in the vaccine samples. The authors said, *"The quantity of foreign bodies detected and, in some cases, their unusual chemical compositions baffled us".*

The findings surprised the authors so much so that they admit the undue presence of the inorganic material is "for the time being inexplicable" [823].

'Baffled' and 'inexplicable' are not words that inspire confidence in vaccines.

Moderna COVID-19 vaccine ingredients

- Messenger ribonucleic acid (mRNA)
- Lipids (SM-102)
- Polyethylene glycol [PEG]
- 2000 dimyristoyl glycerol [DMG]
- Cholesterol
- 1,2-distearoyl-sn-glycero-3-phosphocholine [DSPC]
- Tromethamine
- Tromethamine hydrochloride
- Acetic acid
- Sodium acetate trihydrate
- Sucrose [824]

SM-102: In the Moderna COVID-19 vaccine, the RNA is embedded in SM-102 lipid nanoparticles. A safety concern was circulating that the ingredient SM-102 in the Moderna vaccine is not for human or veterinary use. A warning exists on the Cayman webpage that "this product is not for human or veterinary use"; however, there is a link to 'Read our statement on SM-102 for research use only', which provides additional information. This information says Cayman develops and manufactures chemical compounds for research use only (RUO) and has a separate business producing small molecules as active pharmaceutical ingredients (API) for human and veterinary use [825]. I am not suggesting that this is not a genuine vaccine safety concern, but I believe these rumours are tactfully released so that fact-checkers can delegitimise even more pressing vaccine safety concerns.

Vaxzevria (Oxford-AstraZeneca) COVID-19 vaccine ingredients: One dose (0.5 ml) contains: COVID 19 Vaccine (ChAdOx1-S* recombinant) 5 × 10^10 viral particles. *Recombinant, replication-deficient chimpanzee adenovirus vector encoding the SARS-CoV-2 spike glycoprotein. Product is produced in genetically modified human embryonic kidney (HEK) 293 cells and contains genetically modified organisms (GMOs).

- L-histidine
- L-histidine hydrochloride monohydrate
- Magnesium chloride hexahydrate

- Polysorbate 80
- Ethanol
- Sucrose
- Sodium chloride
- Disodium edetate dehydrate
- Water for injections [826]

Janssen COVID-19 vaccine ingredients:
Recombinant, replication-incompetent adenovirus type 26 expressing the SARS-CoV-2 spike protein

- Citric acid monohydrate
- Trisodium citrate dihydrate
- Ethanol
- 2-hydroxypropyl-β-cyclodextrin (HBCD)
- Polysorbate-80
- Sodium chloride [827]

DART studies: Developmental and reproductive toxicity (DART) studies are discussed in Chapter 15, 'COVID-19 Vaccines and Pregnancy Safety Concerns'.

Assessing Safety
Assessing the safety of the COVID-19 vaccines is the same as assessing the safety of vaccines. It is important to note that causality is near impossible to prove, and the onus is on the person who received the vaccine to prove injury. Additionally, the risk and benefit are nigh impossible to assess as only 1% of adverse events following vaccination are reported, and observational studies used to describe the benefits are prone to bias and confounding. The difficulties surrounding accurate vaccine safety assessment were also covered in Chapter 12, 'Vaccines aren't Described as Safe and don't Always Work'.

Establishing a causal relationship between a vaccine and an adverse reaction: As previously mentioned, the Bradford Hill criteria are a group of nine principles that are used to determine epidemiological evidence of a causal relationship between a vaccine and an adverse drug reaction (ADR)[641]. The Bradford Hill criteria that apply when using multiple antigens altogether are the biological gradient or dose-dependent relationship [642].

An allergen is a special type of antigen which causes an IgE antibody response [643]. Vaccines contain multiple antigens. How many antigens are in the COVID-19 vaccine? We'll probably never know. I have seen the COVID-19 mRNA vaccine being described by the CDC as antigenic [828].

Accurately assessing risk and benefit is impossible: It is impossible to accurately assess the risks versus benefits of vaccination as adverse effects are hugely underreported. Reporting suspected ADRs after a vaccine is authorised allows for continued monitoring of the benefit to risk balance of the product. Different countries have different ADR reporting rates, and under-reporting is acknowledged [647]. In the US, adverse reactions following COVID-19 vaccines are reported to the Vaccine Adverse Event Reporting System (VAERS). Not all ADRs are reported, however, as many healthcare workers (HCWs) are not familiar with how or when to fill out a VAERS report [648]. HCWs report ADRs following COVID-19 vaccination through the UK Medicines and Healthcare products Regulatory Agency (MHRA) Yellow Card or through the new COVID-19 Yellow Card reporting site [650]. In Ireland, the Health Products Regulatory Authority's (HPRA) receives reports from individuals from the Irish public on a voluntary basis about suspected side effects from the vaccines. In Ireland, as of February 2021, 740 reports of suspected side effects had been sent to the HPRA [829]. By April 15th 2021, this number had increased to 6,616 [830].

By August 3rd 2021, the HPRA had received 13,529 reports of suspected side effects related to the COVID-19 vaccine. The Irish government is said to be finally working to establish a vaccination injury compensation scheme in Ireland to compensate people who suffer an injury caused by the State vaccination programme [831]. That is called closing the stable door after the horse has bolted.

Only 1% of adverse reactions are reported: In the US, a Harvard Pilgrim study reported that less than 1% of AEFIs are reported to VAERS [649]. The Health Service Executive (HSE) in Ireland also confirm that 99% of ADRs go unreported [651]. When public health says 'the benefits outweigh the risks', this is grossly misleading.

How adverse reactions to COVID-19 vaccines are reported: The UK's MHRA expected so many ADRs from the COVID-19 vaccines that *Tenders Electronic Daily* supplement to the *Official Journal of the EU* put out a tender for an artificial intelligence (AI) software tool to process the expected high volume of ADRs. This was to ensure that no details from the ADRs' reaction texts were missed. Once again, the fact-wreckers say this is false. However, the text continues;

> *"For reasons of extreme urgency under Regulation 32(2)(c) related to the release of a COVID-19 vaccine, MHRA has accelerated the sourcing and implementation of a vaccine-specific AI tool...it is not possible to retrofit the MHRA's legacy systems to handle the volume of ADRs that will be generated by a COVID-19 vaccine. Therefore, if the MHRA does not implement the AI tool, it will be unable to process these ADRs effectively. This will hinder its ability to rapidly identify any potential safety issues with the COVID-19 vaccine and represents a direct threat to patient life and public health"* (832).

That gives me so much confidence in vaccines, Heidi.

Note to Thought Police, the information I am about to provide is, according to the boffins, "suspected side effects, but which are not necessarily related to or caused by the medicine". If only the boffins applied the same rules to COVID-19 deaths.

UK reporting: A UK government report of systemic adverse events for the Oxford-AstraZeneca COVID-19 vaccine received between January 4th and March 14th 2021, included blood disorders such as immune thrombocytopenia (immune disorder in which the blood doesn't clot), cardiac disorders such as myocardial infarction (heart attack), endocrine disorders including acute adrenocortical insufficiency, immune system disorders such as anaphylaxis, infections such as COVID-19 (!), nervous system disorders such as trigeminal neuralgia, Guillain-Barré syndrome (GBS), narcolepsy, transverse myelitis and systemic inflammatory response syndrome (833). The UK MHRA publishes a weekly summary of Yellow Card reporting for COVID-19 vaccines. This report covers the period from December 9th 2020 to March 28th 2021. By April 8th 2021, the MHRA had received 302 reports of deaths after the Pfizer-BioNTech vaccine, 472 deaths reports for the Oxford-AstraZeneca vaccine and 12 deaths where the vaccine brand was unspecified, totalling 786 (834).

CHAPTER THIRTEEN – PART II

THE LANGUAGE OF ADVERSE REACTIONS

As previously mentioned, ADRs are also known as adverse events following immunisation (AEFIs). An ADR is a regulatory term defined by the Uppsala Monitoring Centre (UMC). ADRs are described as mild, moderate or severe in intensity. Fever, for example, is a relatively common, minor reaction that can be graded as mild, moderate or severe [(835)].

Mild ADRs: Minor ADRs occur within a few hours post-injection, are local, and self-resolve. Minor ADRs can be local or systemic.

- Local reactions include pain, swelling, redness at the injection site.
- Systemic reactions include fever, irritability, malaise and systemic symptoms, including muscle pain, headache or appetite loss [(836)].

Severe ADRs: Severe ADRs include;

- Fatal or life-threatening adverse event.
- Hospitalisation.
- Extended existing hospitalisation.
- Persistent or significant disability and/or incapacity.
- Congenital anomaly (birth defect).
- Requires intervention to prevent permanent damage or impairment.
- Serious unexpected ADRs include anaphylaxis, Bell's palsy, seizures, convulsion, encephalitis, GBS, neuritis, immune thrombocytopenic purpura (ITP), syncope, hyporesponsive episodes (HHE) and prolonged crying in infants [(837)].

Guillain-Barré syndrome added to the vaccine injury table: GBS and Bell's palsy were two serious adverse events (SAEs) picked up during the COVID-19 trials that will be surveyed in the great global experiment. In 2015, the Federal Register website issued a notice of proposed rulemaking (NPRM) by the National Vaccine Injury Compensation Programme (VICP) to make revisions to the Vaccine Injury Table. In 2015, GBS was added to the Vaccine Injury Table for seasonal influenza vaccines. The Institute of Medicine (IOM) committee stated that although evidence has not been adequate to accept or reject a causal relationship between the vaccine and the condition, researchers noted increased chances of contracting GBS with the 1992/93 and 1993/94 seasonal influenza vaccines [838].

Safety data summary COVID-19 vaccines: When reading these summaries, bear in mind that COVID-19 vaccine studies were subject to healthy vaccinee bias. Healthy vaccinee bias occurs when people enrolled in the trials are both in better health are more likely to follow recommendations than the general population, therefore results are not representative and generalisable to the population [611]. Additionally, people with previous allergic reactions to food or drugs were not excluded, however they were underrepresented [614]. Flaws in the vaccine trials were discussed in Chapter 11, 'Trial Protocols and Study Design Flaws'.

Brief Summary COVID-19 Vaccine Safety Trial Data Summary According to the FDA

Moderna COVID-19 Vaccine

- Injection site pain 91.6%
- Fatigue 68.5%
- Headache 63%
- Muscle pain 60%
- Joint pain 45%
- Chills 43%

0.2% to 9.7% experienced a severe adverse event (SAE), which were more frequent after the second dose than after the first dose. These were generally less frequent in participants ≥65 years of age when compared to younger participants. There were no anaphylactic or severe hypersensitivity reactions temporally associated with the vaccine. There were three reports of Bell's palsy in the vaccine group and one in the placebo group. Unsolicited adverse events of clinical interest, which may be possibly related to the vaccine, included lymphadenopathy (axillary swelling and tenderness of the vaccination group) (21.4%). A 72 year old vaccine recipient with Crohn's disease developed thrombocytopenia and acute kidney failure due to obstructive nephrolithiasis and died from multiorgan failure. As of December 3rd 2020, 13 deaths had been reported, six of these in the vaccine group and seven in the placebo.

Two deaths in the vaccine group were in participants >75 years of age with preexisting cardiac disease. An additional two vaccine recipients were found deceased at home; the cause of deaths was uncertain. These deaths represented events and rates that occur in the general population in these age groups. The most common SAEs occurring at higher rates in the vaccine group than in the placebo group were myocardial infarction (0.03%), cholecystitis (0.02%) and nephrolithiasis (0.02%) (839). Four non-COVID-19 deaths were reported across the studies, three in the placebo group and one in the vaccine group, all considered unrelated to the vaccine (840). The observation period of the trial was 28 days after injection (841, 842).

Pfizer-BioNTech COVID-19 Vaccine

- Injection site pain 84.1%
- Fatigue 62.9%
- Headache 55.1%
- Chills 31.9%
- Joint pain 23.6%
- Fever 14.2%
- Muscle pain 38.3%

SAEs occurred in 0.0% to 4.6% of participants, these events being more frequent after the second dose than after the first dose. These were generally less frequent in participants ≥55 years of age. There was a numerical imbalance of four cases of Bell's palsy in the vaccine group compared with zero cases in the placebo group. A total of six participants died, two in the vaccine group, four in the placebo group. The most common SAEs occurring at higher rates in the vaccine group than in the placebo group were appendicitis (0.04%), acute myocardial infarction (0.02%), and cerebrovascular accident (0.02%) (807, 843).

Janssen Ad26.COV2.S Vaccine for the Prevention of COVID-19

- Injection site pain 48.6%
- Fatigue 38.2%
- Headache 38.9%
- Nausea 14.2%

- Fever 9%
- Muscle pain 33.2%

A 25 year old male with no past medical history and no concurrent medications experienced a transverse sinus thrombosis on the 21st day post-vaccination. Reports of Bell's palsy were overall balanced between vaccine and placebo recipients, with two in the vaccine group and two in the placebo group. 0.7% and 1.8% of local and systemic solicited adverse reactions respectively in the vaccine and placebo group were reported as grade 3 SAEs. 19 deaths were reported, three in the vaccine group, 16 in the placebo group. Two deaths in the vaccine group were secondary to respiratory infections, not due to COVID-19. A 66 year old participant died of unknown causes after waking up with shortness of breath on Day 45. An update noted an additional six deaths. Of these six deaths, two occurred in the vaccine group, and four occurred in the placebo group. The proportions of participants who had at least one SAE reported by January 22nd 2021, were 0.4% in the vaccine group and 0.4% in the placebo group. The most commonly reported SAE was appendicitis occurring in six vaccine recipients and five placebo recipients. There were no significant numerical imbalances in SAEs between the two groups [844].

Brief summary Oxford-AstraZeneca COVID-19 vaccine safety data summary: Local and systemic reactions were found to be more common in participants in the vaccine group than in the placebo group. These reactions most frequently included injection site pain, chills and fever, myalgia and headache. These events were less common in adults aged ≥56 years than younger adults. Local reactions in people receiving two standard doses of the vaccine were reported in 88% of participants in the 18-55 years group, 73% of participants in the 56-69 years group, and 61% of participants in the 70 years and older group. Systemic reactions occurred in 86% of participants in the 18-55 years group, 77% of participants in the 56-69 years group, and 65% of participants in the 70 years and older group. 13 SAEs occurred during the study period [597]. Systemic reactions occurred in 86% of participants in the 18-55 years group!

Suspected adverse reactions reported during trials: In October 2020, pharmaceutical company Johnson & Johnson (J&J) temporarily paused its COVID-19 vaccine trial whilst an investigation was carried out into an 'unexplained illness' in a participant. No further details were provided about the illness or the health of the participant at the time [845]. The public was told the public is not privy to the patient's illness and must respect this participant's privacy [846]. In September 2020, the Oxford-AstraZeneca COVID-19 vaccine trial was paused because of a suspected adverse reaction in a UK patient believed to be transverse myelitis [847]. In September 2020, the Oxford-AstraZeneca COVID-19 vaccine trial was paused for the second time following a severe adverse event [848]. In December 2020, the National Institute of Health of Peru announced it had paused the clinical trials of the Chinese COVID-19 vaccine Sinopharm after detecting the autoimmune neurological disorder GBS in one volunteer [849].

Post COVID-19 Vaccine Rollout Adverse Reactions

As there is a complete media blackout on vaccine injury and deaths, the following describes how to search ADRs and/or deaths post-COVID-19 vaccines. The sites of use to monitor ADRs and deaths after COVID-19 vaccinations include, the US's VAERS, the WHO's VigiAccess and Europe's EudraVigilance.

US CDC Vaccine Adverse Event Reporting System (VAERS):

Go to the VAERS 'wonder CDC site'. Click 'I agree'. Click on the 'VAERS Data Search box' to start your search.

- Under 1 'organise table layout' and 'Group Results' choose 'Vaccine Type'.
- Under 2 'Select symptoms', select 'all symptoms'.
- Under 3 Select 'Vaccine characteristics' and under 'vaccine products' select 'COVID-19 (COVID-19 vaccine)'.
- Under 'vaccine manufacturer' select using control shift 'Moderna and Pfizer'.
- Under 4 Select 'location', select 'all location in US'.
- Under 5 Select 'other event characteristics', select 'death'.
- Leave all dates from the 1990s until present then hit 'send'.

As of February 28th 2021, Moderna deaths in the US alone reported to VEARS were 475. As of February 28th 2021, Pfizer-BioNTech deaths in the US alone reported to VEARS were 631. That represents a total of 1106 death reported to VAERS in the US as of February 28th 2021 [850]. As of February 19th 2020, VAERS had received 934 reports of death among people who received a COVID-19 vaccine representing 0.0018% of vaccine recipients [851].

6,000% increase in vaccine deaths reported to VAERS

As of May 10th 2021, I searched deaths from 'all vaccines'.

- Under 1 'organise table layout' and 'Group Results by' select 'all symptoms'.
- Under 2 Select 'Symptoms', select 'All'.
- Under 3, Select 'vaccine characteristics' under 'vaccine' select 'all'.
- Under 'vaccine manufacturer' select 'all'.
- Under 4 Select 'location, age, gender', select 'all locations'.
- Under 5 Select 'other event characteristics', select 'death'.
- Under 6 Search text fields, don't select anything.
- Under 7 Select 'report completed dates' and
- Under 8 Select 'report received dates' and
- Under 9 Select 'vaccination dates'.
- Under 10 Select 'adverse event onset date' and
- Under 11 Select 'death dates', select '2020' and then repeat for '2021'.
- Under 12 'Other options' leave 'show totals'.

In 2020, 94 vaccines deaths were reported to VAERS. For the year 2021, as of May 10th 3,225 deaths had been reported to VAERS. This represents a 3000% increase in deaths compared to the previous year. As May 10th is not yet halfway through the year, this will likely extrapolate to a 6000% increase in vaccine deaths reported to VAERS.

World Health Organisation's VigiAccess: VigiAccess is the World Health Organisation's (WHO's) global database for ADRs. VigiAccess is also called the Uppsala Monitoring Centre (UMC) database. This site can be used to search medications and view suspected ADRs [852]. The main disadvantage with this site is that you can only search using brand names. Many people do not know the name of the COVID-19 vaccines, each country has a different name for the COVID-19 vaccines, and many COVID-19 vaccines still have no official brand name.

Go to 'Vigiaccess' http://www.vigiaccess.org/ and 'accept terms' to search the database. Then go to 'enter trade name of drug'.

- On February 28th 2021, I entered 'Covishield' (India's AstraZeneca) then hit 'search'. Expand 'Adverse Drug Reactions (ADR)' then go to the expand 'general disorders and administration site conditions' scroll 19 places down to 'deaths':1585.
- On February 28th 2021, I entered 'Comirnaty' (Pfizer) then hit 'search'. Expand 'Adverse Drug Reactions (ADR)' then go to the expand 'general disorders and administration site conditions' scroll 19 places down to 'deaths':1585.

European Medicines Agency's EudraVigilance: The EMA's EudraVigilance is the European database of suspected drug ADRs reports to approved medicines. The website homepage says, 'To consult the reports for COVID-19 vaccines', follow this link, then click on the letter 'C' and scroll down until 'COVID-19'. Then click on the following individually to reveal the data. I emailed EudraVigilance to assist me in looking up deaths, and their answer, like their website, was designed to flummox. To find the deaths, you must place yourself in the mind of a HCW trained to be detached from death; death is a 'general disorder'!

EudraVigilance: Adverse Reactions

Moderna (CX-024414): As of April 13th 2021, the number of individual cases of ADRs post-COVID-19 vaccines identified in EudraVigilance for Moderna was 14,235 [(853)].

Pfizer-BioNTech (Tozinameran) now Comirnaty: As of April 13th 2021, the number of individual cases of ADRs post-COVID-19 vaccines identified in EudraVigilance for Pfizer-BioNTech was 138,321 [(854)].

Oxford-AstraZeneca, codenamed AZD1222 ChAdOx1 nCoV-19, now Vaxzevria: As of April 13th 2021, the number of individual cases of ADRs post-COVID-19 vaccines identified in EudraVigilance for AstraZeneca was 163,852 [(855)].

Janssen Ad26.COV2.S: As of April 13th 2021, the number of individual cases of ADRs post-COVID-19 vaccines identified in EudraVigilance for Janssen was 202 [(856)].

This represents a total of 316,610 reports of ADRs post these four COVID-19 vaccines by April 13th 2021.

EudraVigilance: Deaths

On April 20th 2021, I entered the following;

COVID-19 mRNA vaccine Moderna (CX-024414)

- Go to Tab 6 'Number of Individual cases for a selected Reaction'.
- On left in 'Reaction Groups & Reported Suspected Reaction'.
- Under 'Reaction Groups' scroll down choose 'Choose General disorders and administration site conditions'.
- Under 'Reported Suspected Reaction' scroll down choose 'death'.
- Then see 'Outcome' (lowest box on right) see 'Fatal' = 938.

COVID-19 mRNA Vaccine Pfizer-BioNTech (Tozinameran)

- Go to Tab 6 'Number of Individual cases for a selected Reaction'.
- On left in 'Reaction Groups & Reported Suspected Reaction'.
- Under 'Reaction Groups' scroll down choose 'Choose General disorders and administration site conditions'.
- Under 'Reported Suspected Reaction' scroll down choose 'death'.
- Then see 'Outcome' (lowest box on right) see 'Fatal' = 660.

COVID-19 Vaccine Oxford-AstraZeneca, codenamed AZD1222 ChAdOx1 nCoV-19

- Go to Tab 6 'Number of Individual cases for a selected Reaction'.
- On left in 'Reaction Groups & Reported Suspected Reaction'.
- Under 'Reaction Groups' scroll down choose 'Choose General disorders and administration site conditions'.
- Under 'Reported Suspected Reaction' scroll down choose 'death'.
- Then see 'Outcome' (lowest box on right) see 'Fatal' = 303.

COVID-19 Vaccine Janssen Ad26.COV2.S

- Go to Tab 6 'Number of Individual cases for a selected Reaction'.
- On left in 'Reaction Groups & Reported Suspected Reaction'.
- Under 'Reaction Groups' scroll down choose 'Choose General disorders and administration site conditions'.
- Under 'Reported Suspected Reaction' scroll down choose 'death'.
- Then see 'Outcome' (lowest box on right) see 'Fatal' = 7.

As of April 20th 2021, a total of 1910 suspected deaths (in Europe only) after COVID-19 vaccination had been reported to the European Medicines Agency's EudraVigilance. The COVID-19 Oxford-AstraZeneca was since given the name Vaxzevria. Vax everyone? This death figure rose to 22,000 by September 1st 2021.

Adverse Reactions after COVID-19 Vaccine Rollout

The mainstream media will not report vaccine injury or deaths. That is of course unless it happens to one of their own and they can't cover it up, such as the death post-vaccine of BBC radio presenter Lisa Shaw who died of brain haemorrhage caused by a blood clot, or *A Place in the Sun* star Laura Hamilton who was hospitalised with immune thrombocytopenic purpura (ITP) post second dose. Heidi Larson, the founder of the Vaccine Confidence Project (VCP), hunts viral rumours about 'real' viruses. According to Heidi, dispelling vaccine hesitancy means building trust and avoiding the term 'anti-vaxxer'. The VCP's mission is camouflage and doublespeak for, 'scour the internet for any vaccine safety concerns, censor it, then defame the author's character using libel (written defamation) and slander (spoken defamation)' [(857)].

The pandemic is over! 'Vaccinate the world': First and foremost, the 'cure' is entirely unnecessary as the pandemic is over. On June 9th 2021, the UK media reported the results of an analysis of a COVID-19 infection survey. Antibody and vaccination data was released showing that eight in ten people in Britain had antibodies to SARS-CoV-2 either through natural infection or vaccination. The analysis was produced in partnership with the University of Oxford, University of Manchester, Public Health England and the Wellcome Trust. This study was jointly led by the Office of National Statistics (ONS) and the Department for Health and Social Care (DHSC). This literally means that eight out of ten people cannot get or spread SARS-CoV-2 [(858)]. Previous herd immunity levels (HIL) to SARS-CoV-2 were estimated to be considerably lower than 60% [(859, 860)]. It is impossible for any virus to spread once the HIL is reached. This is the only proof we should require that the pandemonium is an audacious scam based on a PCR test set at a cycle threshold of greater than 25, which is literally diagnosing immune people as 'cases' to generate interest in and increase uptake of vaccines. Herd immunity is discussed in further detail in Chapter 18, 'Herd Immunity'.

83% get symptoms from the vaccine, 86% who get COVID have no symptoms as all: It is official that for the vast majority of the population that 'cure' is worse than the 'disease'. The vaccine causes symptoms in more people than the disease. Systemic symptoms typically include chills and fever, headache, fatigue, myalgia, and arthralgia, rash (textbook symptoms of COVID-19). 77.4% of Pfizer-BioNTech COVID-19 vaccine recipients 'asked' reported at least one systemic reaction. Systemic adverse events were greater in the younger recipients compared with the older age group (82.8% vs. 70.6%) (861). Most systemic reactions were classified as mild, not interfering with daily activity, or moderate, interfering with daily activity. Compare this to a study by University College London researchers collected for the ONS, which found that 86% of people who tested positive for COVID-19 had absolutely no symptoms of the virus at all. 83% will get symptoms from the vaccine, whilst 86% who contract the 'disease' won't experience any symptoms at all (862). Ireland's HSE website indicates that 80% of COVID-19 infections are mild or asymptomatic (863). Chinese data also supports this figure, describing that four-fifths (80%) of COVID-19 cases are asymptomatic (389). A longitudinal, population-level, cross-sectional study on anti-SARS-CoV-2 antibodies in Wuhan, published in *The Lancet* in March 2020, reported that more than 80% of people who had been infected were completely asymptomatic (864). WHO data shows that 80% of COVID-19 infections are mild or asymptomatic (865).

There are no two ways about it; the experts weighing up the risks and benefits of this vaccine have sold out. As I write, the Irish government is dictating that to go inside an Irish pub, we need to inject an unlicensed experimental biological agent that has an 83% chance of causing a systemic adverse reaction to prevent a disease that 86% of people will not even know they have had. Additionally, as herd immunity has been reached, continued vaccination has no benefit.

2.8% are unable to function as normal after the vaccine: The Advisory Committee on Immunisation Practices (ACIP), a committee within the US-CDC, stated that as of December 18th 2020, out of the 112,807 people who had received the COVID-19 vaccine, the V-safe Active Surveillance reported that 3,150 were unable to perform normal daily activities, unable to work and/or required care from a doctor or health care professional. That equates to 2.8% of recipients being unable to function as normal after receiving the vaccine (866).

European Healthcare workers told to stagger vaccines to avoid sickness absenteeism: Health authorities in some European countries are facing resistance to AstraZeneca's COVID-19 vaccine after side effects led hospital staff and other frontline workers to call in sick, putting extra strain on already stretched services. The French National Agency for Medicines and Health Products Safety said on February 11th 2021, that these side effects were "known and described" but should be subject to surveillance in regard to their intensity. The agency issued guidance to stagger vaccinations of frontline staff working in teams to minimise the risk of disruption to services (867).

Dropping like flies from anaphylaxis: As discussed in Chapter 12, 'Vaccines aren't Described as Safe and don't Always Work', anaphylaxis after vaccination is rare in all age groups, with anaphylactic reactions occurring at a rate of about one per one million doses (661). Due to the rates of underreporting as previously discussed, the following summary is likely the tip of the iceberg. Whilst Pfizer and Moderna's clinical vaccine trials were said to not find serious ADRs in tens of thousands of people with their COVID-19 vaccine, both studies excluded people with a history of allergies to components of the COVID-19 vaccines (587, 588). Pfizer also excluded those who previously had a severe adverse reaction to any vaccine (588). Whilst people with a history of allergic reactions to food or drugs were not excluded, they may have been underrepresented (614).

As of December 23rd 2020, 1,893,360 first doses of Pfizer-BioNTech COVID-19 vaccine had been administered in the US. There were 4,393 (0.2%) reports of adverse events submitted to the VAERS. Among these events reported, 175 case reports were identified for further review as possible cases of a severe allergic reaction, including anaphylaxis. Twenty-one cases were determined to be anaphylaxis, representing a rate of 11.1 cases per million doses. This represents 11 times the expected rates of anaphylaxis for other vaccines. The median time interval from vaccine receipt to symptom onset was 13 minutes, ranging between two and 150 minutes (868). The observation period after COVID-19 vaccination is either 15 or 30 minutes.

The following reports of anaphylaxis were soon suppressed hence I aim to document them here. In the first week of the vaccine rollout, Advocate Condell Medical Centre in Libertyville Illinois, US paused then restarted their COVID-19 vaccination programme after four employees experience reactions shortly after having received the vaccine. The immediate concern was that there was an issue with the particular batch the clinic had received. However, once the health department learned that the same vaccine batch was used at various other sites, their concerns were allayed in relation to the integrity of the vaccine and the rollout was continued (869). Simultaneously five Alaskan health care workers experienced adverse reactions after getting the COVID-19 vaccine, and health officials again continued to stress that such reactions are rare and treatable (870). On the eve of President Biden-his-time-until-Kamala-takes-over's '100 Million Vaccinations in the First 100 Days', a spanner was thrown in the works with California State Epidemiologist, Dr Erica Pan, recommending that California's COVID-19 vaccine rollout of the Moderna batch 041L20A be paused after an abnormally high amount of allergic reactions (871).

Why are they dropping like flies? Nanotechnology has helped propel novel candidate vaccines toward clinical testing at breakneck speed. Nanotechnology is used in inactivated vaccines and mRNA vaccines delivered by lipid nanoparticles (LNPs) (872). mRNA vaccine technology uses LNPs as a coating that prevents the mRNA from degrading too quickly to facilitate their entry into cells. As discussed above, a typical LNP contains four parts with polyethylene glycol (PEG) to promote stability. PEGs are petroleum-based compounds widely used in cosmetics as thickeners, solvents, softeners, cosmetic cream bases and pharmaceuticals. PEG is used as a LNP bubble stabiliser in both the Moderna and Pfizer-BioNTech COVID-19 vaccines (873).

CARPA is an allergy to polyethylene glycols: Polyethylene, also called polythene, is the most common plastic in use today. It is described as non-biodegradable. I personally wouldn't choose to ingest it, let alone inject it. PEGs were previously thought to be biologically non-immunogenic and non-antigenic inert substances, but a growing body of evidence suggests they are not (874). In 1999 Szebeni et al. described the mechanism of anaphylactoid reactions to nanoparticle-based medicines. The mechanism Szebeni described is a nonspecific immune response to nanoparticle-based medicines that often contain PEG. The authors termed the reactions a complement activation-related pseudoallergy (CARPA), a reaction whereby the immune system mistakenly recognises PEGs as viruses (614). Drugs and agents including Radiocontrast media, Doxil, Ambisome, DaunoXome and Taxol have been known to cause CARPA (758). Patients who suffered an anaphylactic reaction to PEG containing drugs had IgE antibodies to PEG rather than IgG and IgM (875). Pseudoallergy is not the only mechanism of allergy to PEGs. An analysis of preexisting IgG and IgM antibodies against PEG (anti-PEG Ab) in the general population found that up to 72% of people express at least some specific antibodies against PEG and that 7% had levels high enough to predispose them to anaphylaxis (876). 7% of the population have potentially enough antibodies to experience a life-threatening anaphylactic reaction requiring emergency medical treatment after being injected with either the Moderna or Pfizer-BioNTech COVID-19 vaccines.

Countries that suspended AstraZeneca (and others) due to blood clot link: The daily propaganda uses the term 'paused'; the actual term is 'suspended'. By March 5th 2021, Denmark, Norway, France, Italy, Germany, Spain, Iceland, Bulgaria, Ireland and the Netherlands had suspended the AstraZeneca COVID-19 vaccine after reporting cases of bleeding, blood clots and a low platelet count (877). On April 14th 2021, The National Immunisation Advisory Committee (NIAC) in Ireland changed its guidelines for AstraZeneca and withdrew its use in those under the age of 60, resulting in the cancellation of 15,000 vaccines (878). More than 12 countries followed suit, and, at the time of writing, a few countries had since resumed use after the European Medicines Agency (EMA) emphasised the 'benefits of the vaccine outweigh the risks' (624). On April 13th 2021, federal health agencies in the US recommended a pause in Johnson & Johnson's single-dose coronavirus vaccine rollout after it emerged that six recipients experienced a rare blood clotting disorder (879). Irish vaccine advisory group NIAC has since done a complete U-turn and is currently recommending the vaccine they withdrew in those under 60 to Irish children aged over 12.

Countries that completely withdrew, or nearly withdrew, AstraZeneca altogether: While Ireland and the UK are embracing AstraZeneca, on January 28th 2021, the German health ministry originally recommended that AstraZeneca's COVID-19 vaccine should only be given to people over 65 years old. Germany's vaccine committee later updated its vaccine recommendation, citing a lack of data to recommend its use in older age groups, "the AstraZeneca vaccine, unlike the mRNA vaccines, should only be offered to people aged 18-64 years at each stage" [622]. On February 3rd 2021, Switzerland announced it had banned the Oxford-AstraZeneca COVID-19 vaccine for all its citizens. The Swiss medical regulator claimed the lack of data on the efficacy of the COVID-19 vaccine meant they could not reach a conclusion [623]. On April 14th 2021, Denmark completely withdrew AstraZeneca from its COVID-19 vaccination programme, again citing a lack of data [624]. On October 23rd 2020, Peru rejected an AstraZeneca COVID-19 vaccine purchase deal. The Peruvian government said that it refused to sign a coronavirus vaccine purchase agreement with AstraZeneca PLC because it did not provide sufficient data from its studies [880].

Three named blood clots linked to COVID-19 vaccines: There are three named blood clots linked to COVID-19 vaccination. Scientists named one unusual prothrombotic syndrome reaction, vaccine-induced immune thrombotic thrombocytopenia (VITT) [881]. In an aim to bamboozle us with science jargon VITT is also called thrombosis with thrombocytopenia syndrome (TTS) and vaccine-induced prothrombotic immune thrombocytopenia (VIPIT) [882]. The second vaccine-associated blood clot is a clot in the vessels draining blood from the brain, known as cerebral venous sinus thrombosis (CVST). On April 2nd 2021, Oxford announced it had paused its COVID-19 vaccine study in children as it awaited more data on blood CVST after the AstraZeneca vaccine, Vaxevria [883]. Between March 2nd and April 21st 2021, case reports of CVST with thrombocytopenia were noted after Janssen COVID-19 vaccination [884]. A third named vaccine-associated blood clot is multiple blood clots in multiple blood vessels, which is known as disseminated intravascular coagulation (DIC). Contrary to popular belief, all COVID-19 vaccines are linked to blood clots. An Oxford University study found the number of people who report blood clots after receiving COVID-19 vaccines is approximately the same for those who received either the Pfizer, Moderna or the AstraZeneca vaccine [885].

A preprint Oxford Study recently determined that the risk of cerebral blood clots from COVID-19 disease is ten times that from COVID-19 vaccination [886]. The Oxford study is completely flawed and I suggest taking the results with a pinch of salt. The Oxford study compared blood clots in hospitalised COVID-19 patients only with blood clots in recipients of the COVID-19 vaccines. As obesity is the main risk factor for hospitalisation in COVID-19, hospitalised COVID-19 patients are statistically far more likely to be obese [887]. Being obese or overweight predisposes individuals to increased risk of thrombotic (clotting) disorders such as myocardial infarction (heart attack), stroke, and venous thromboembolism (a clot that moves) [888]. Sound science would compare blood clots in all COVID-19 populations, not just in those hospitalised. The reality is that a true comparison of the frequency of clots post COVID-19 infection with the frequency of clots post-COVID vaccination is a nigh impossible task given the difficulty in establishing baseline incidence [889]. A global perspective of COVID-19 epidemiology noted that the true total number of infections is likely >20 times greater than what is reported [890]. Regarding blood clot risk in the young, the UK Joint Committee on Vaccination and Immunisation (JCVI) recently recommended that people under 30 will be offered an alternative to the AstraZeneca COVID-19 vaccine [891]. In Ireland, as mentioned, adverse reactions after COVID-19 vaccines are reported to HPRA. By June 2021, the HPRA had received 18 reports of blood clots possibly associated with receiving the Oxford-AstraZeneca COVID-19 vaccine, Vaxzevria [892].

Myocarditis following COVID-19 vaccination: In August 2021, a case report published in *Radiology Case Reports* discussed myocarditis associated with the Pfizer-BioNTech and Moderna mRNA vaccines. This article noted that the Israeli Ministry of Health had received 62 reports of myocarditis in patients vaccinated for COVID-19 out of the five million people who had received vaccinations. Most cases had occurred after the second mRNA vaccines dose. The prevalence was found to be higher in men under the age of 30 years. Two of these 62 patients had died [893]. By June 2021, the CDC was investigating heart inflammation cases after Pfizer and Moderna COVID-19 vaccination. The CDC described the vaccine link to heart inflammation as being "stronger than previously thought". However, low and behold! In June 2021, the incidence of myocarditis and pericarditis after vaccination was already being reported as lower than the incidence of myocarditis and pericarditis after infection with SARS-CoV-2 [894]! Cardiologists have told parents to get our teenagers down to their general practitioners (GPs) for their 'shots'. Paediatric cardiologists have a message for us parents: COVID-19 should scare us a lot more, a whole lot more in fact, than the vaccine [895]. But it doesn't! My children had COVID-19 and got over it in a day. In fact my children have had COVID-19, COVID-20 and COVID-21. The science is wearing thin, and we know that paediatric cardiologists will be reluctant to vaccinate their young men against COVID-

19, a disease they are not at risk from. If you are concerned about your teenage son getting myocarditis after taking a COVID-19 vaccine, you are an anti-vaxxer! The science is settled! Shut up! Obey! Get your children shot!

UK JCVI does not recommend COVID-19 vaccines for children 12-15: In September 2021 the JCVI announced its decision not to recommend the COVID-19 vaccine to all healthy children was based on concern over what they describe as 'rare occurrences' of myocarditis and pericarditis following Pfizer and Moderna mRNA COVID-19 vaccinations. The JCVI say the benefit of vaccinating children is only marginal in terms of their health. This was after data from the US suggests there are 60 cases of the heart condition for every million second doses given to 12 to 17 year old boys (compared to eight in one million girls) (896). The JCVI determined the risk-benefit ratio was not favourable as they compared the 60 in one million risk of heart inflammation to the two in one million chance of dying. As previously mentioned, A University College London (UCL), Imperial College London and the universities of Bristol, York and Liverpool study published in July 2021, found that children with confirmed COVID-19 had a roughly one in 50,000 chance of being admitted to intensive care with COVID and a two in a million chance of dying (192). As previously mentioned also, Israel saw two deaths per 60 cases of myocarditis. The UK government don't listen to the experts at the JCVI, they are 'jabbing' the kids anyway.

Christian Eriksen died (and was revived) in front of the world on live TV: Denmark's footballer, Christian Eriksen, collapsed on the field during Denmark's Euro 2020 opener against Finland. It was confirmed he had no prior heart condition. Inter Milan Director Giuseppe Marotta dismissed suggestions that Eriksen had received the COVID-19 vaccine. Marotta said that "He didn't have COVID and wasn't vaccinated either". Marotta said Eriksen was under the guidance of the Danish medical staff, and it was for them to release this information but that Inter had been in touch with them. As of June 2021, the official line was that Eriksen's previous case of COVID-19 had caused scarring on his heart (897). Early reports taken from an Italian radio programme *Radio Sportiva*, said that the Inter Milan Chief medic and cardiologist confirmed that Christian Eriksen had received the Pfizer COVID-19 vaccine two weeks earlier on May 31st 2021. However, this was quickly debunked (possibly censored) by 'fact-checker' Politifact. In a curious twist, whilst Politifact were refuting that Eriksen had the vaccine,

Politifact said that the director of Eriksen's professional team said he hadn't received any COVID-19 vaccine or previously contracted the disease however, Eriksen's cardiologist, Sanjay Sharma, said that some players may have had mild or asymptomatic coronavirus infections, which may result in scarring of the heart (898). How mild or asymptomatic COVID-19 leads to scarring of the heart, I do not know. What is the truth? Did Eriksen have COVID-19? Did Eriksen have the COVID-19 vaccine? There is some explanation as to why this fit, young and healthy man collapsed and died (and was then revived) in front of the world. Eriksen will not be allowed to return to football until he has his implantable cardioverter-defibrillator (ICD) removed. Only Eriksen can speak his truth.

The mystery of the British Airways pilot deaths: British Airways (BA) announced on Twaddle that;

> *"Sadly four members of our pilot community passed away recently. Our thoughts are with their family and friends. However, there is no truth whatsoever in the claims on social media speculating that the four deaths are linked"* (899).

Top aviation and travel news magazine *Captain Jetson* confirmed that 85% of BA pilots had been vaccinated and questioned if, as this is due to the employer's requirement, is the employer therefore liable for subsequent adverse reactions and even fatalities (900)? I understand one of the pilots died after a 'long battle with COVID', however questions remain surrounding the untimely deaths of the other three pilots and why this news did not make mainstream media headlines.

A spate of deaths post COVID-19 vaccine rollout in America: Again, the following reports occurred shortly after vaccine rollout and were soon extinguished. Miami obstetrician Gregory Michael, aged 56, died on January 3rd 2021, 16 days after receiving the Pfizer COVID-19 vaccine. Dr Michael's wife Heidi Neckelmann, said he was, *"very healthy"* prior to receiving the shot and that, *"in my mind his death was 100% linked to the vaccine. There is no other explanation"*. Dr Michael succumbed to a stroke brought on by acute idiopathic thrombocytopenic purpura (ITP), an autoimmune blood disorder caused by a lack of platelets. The death was being investigated by the medical examiner's office in Miami, the Florida Department of Health and the CDC. Pfizer promptly replied that it was aware of the death but that Pfizer didn't think there was any direct connection to the vaccine [901]. ITP has in fact been previously connected with the MMR vaccine. An increased risk of ITP in children was identified to occur within six weeks post MMR vaccination [902]. Previous studies have also shown that ITP is associated with several other types of vaccination, including hepatitis A, varicella, and DTP vaccines in children and adolescents. As mentioned, autoimmune/inflammatory disorders, including ITP, are associated with adjuvants in vaccines that are used to enhance immunogenicity, a condition in which the exposure to adjuvants leads to an aberrant autoimmune response known as autoimmune/ inflammatory syndrome induced by adjuvants (ASIA) [814]. That gives me such confidence in vaccines, Heidi.

On January 29th 2021, the family of an Orange County man in the US who died within days of receiving his second dose of the Pfizer COVID-19 vaccine did not question that the potential that this man's death was caused by the vaccine. The man's family went on television to say they remained firm believers in vaccination, and rather than advising caution, they actively encouraged others to take the vaccine before having conclusive answers about his death [903]. On February 9th 2021, in New York, a 70 year old man collapsed and died 25 minutes after receiving his COVID-19 vaccine. It goes without saying that health officials did not attribute the death as being caused by the vaccine. They even went so far as to say that the man had exhibited no adverse reactions, nor did he have any allergic reaction to the vaccine during the required 15-minute observation period [904]. On February 14th 2021, a 28 year old HCW at SwedishAmerican Hospital, Sara Stickles from Beloit, Wisconsin, with no previous health conditions, suffered a brain aneurysm and died five days after receiving her second dose of the experimental Pfizer COVID-19 vaccination [905].

A spate of deaths post COVID-19 vaccine rollout in Portugal: On January 6th 2021, a Portuguese HCW died two days after receiving the Pfizer COVID-19 vaccine. The HCW had worked at the Portuguese Oncology Institute of Porto (IPO Porto) for more than ten years. The mother of two died suddenly in her home on New Year's Day, 48 hours after receiving the Pfizer COVID-19 vaccine [906]. The autopsy on the IPO Porto official concluded the very same day that the cause of death was not due to the vaccine, however the cause of death was not disclosed [907].

A spate of deaths post COVID-19 vaccine rollout in Israel: On December 30th 2021, at the beginning of the rollout in Israel, an 88 year old and a 75 year old Israeli died within hours of receiving the Pfizer-BioNTech COVID-19 vaccine. Medical professionals said both cases suffered from preexisting conditions and that they did not believe that the deaths were connected to the vaccines [(908)].

A spate of deaths post COVID-19 vaccine rollout in India: The vaccine used in India is the Covishield vaccine (AZD1222), another mRNA vaccine manufactured by the Serum Institute of India and developed by Oxford University and AstraZeneca. Covishield is called Comirnaty in the UK. On January 18th 2021, the first day of the Indian COVID-19 vaccine rollout, two deaths were reported. One was in a 52 year old male whose death was said to be unrelated to the vaccine, and the other occurred in a 43 year old male whose cause of death was already stated, although a post mortem hadn't been conducted. Also reported on the same day, a 46 year old public hospital male attendant died shortly after being vaccinated. The Indian Health Ministry said 580 adverse events had been reported since mass vaccinations began [(909, 910)]. On January 31st 2021, it was reported that 13 deaths had occurred within two weeks of receiving their COVID-19 vaccination. The 13 deaths took place within a few hours and five days after receiving the vaccine. The deaths were not in the elderly. Whilst Indian's Director of Public Health and Pharmaceutical Welfare in Telangana stated the deaths were not due to COVID-19 vaccination, a group of concerned doctors and public health researchers asked the Union Health Ministry to urgently investigate these deaths and share the information in the public domain [(911)].

Disclaimer of sorts: In regards to fatal outcomes post-vaccination, it is appropriate to note that I am not saying that the vaccine caused these deaths. What is important is that public health should survey these events and ensure they are reported and investigated. In considering whether these deaths were caused by the COVID-19 vaccine or COVID-19 disease, one must bear in mind that 6.6% of the people receiving the Pfizer-BioNTech COVID- 19 vaccine in Israel tested positive for COVID-19 [(237)]. It is not uncommon for people to test positive for COVID-19 long after recovery, with studies showing that people still tested positive 91 days after recovery [(912)]. Given the known sensitivities of the PCR test, it is far too convenient without an autopsy to say these vaccinated residents died of COVID-19.

A spate of deaths post COVID-19 vaccine rollout in nursing homes: Dr Kelly Moore, Associate Director of the US Immunisation Action Coalition, said,

> *"One of the things we want to make sure people understand is that they should not be unnecessarily alarmed if there are reports, once we start vaccinating, of someone or multiple people dying within a day or two of their vaccination who are residents of a long-term care facility"* (913).

Dr pushing-vaccines is saying; do not be unnecessarily alarmed; the shot will never cause the deaths. Shut up! Obey! Get your elderly shot! I have documented these accounts as the initial numerous global media reports of care homes being struck by COVID-19 post-vaccine rollout, and of people dying within days of the vaccine rollout, were soon after quashed.

A spate of deaths post COVID-19 vaccine rollout in nursing homes in Ireland: In Ireland, 81% of all coronavirus related deaths have occurred in nursing homes, and the median age of people dying is greater than life expectancy, yet we were all locked up. In Ireland, the vaccination rollout began in Dublin's residential care facilities on January 8th and was ramped on January 11th 2021 (914). At the beginning of February 2021, Irish news reported that a total of 1,543 people had died due to COVID-19 in nursing homes, with 369 of those having occurred in January 2021 alone (915). Rather than investigating a potential causal link between the vaccine and deaths in nursing homes, the deaths were blamed on the Irish public who had gone nowhere near nursing homes for having fun at Christmas. The rise in nursing home deaths that coincided with the start of the vaccine rollout in Ireland was so alarming that Health Freedom Ireland sent a letter to the Irish government saying that this could represent a serious adverse reaction to the vaccine and asked for the potential link to be investigated (916). Bewilderment aside, this is truly unbearable to write about.

On January 22nd 2021, the HSE recorded thirteen deaths during a 'COVID-19 outbreak' at a North County Dublin nursing home with a 'significant number' of residents and staff infected. Some 11 of the deaths at the HSE-run Lusk Community Nursing Unit were among residents who had been confirmed as having the coronavirus disease. The HSE said the first round of COVID-19 Pfizer-BioNTech vaccines had been administered within the Lusk nursing home, despite the outbreak at the care facility. "All residents and staff who consented and were deemed medically fit were vaccinated on the day". The HSE said that almost half of the residents at the 50-bed facility were vaccinated. The HSE spokesperson said,

"The remainder of the residents did not receive their vaccinations for a variety of reasons, including being COVID-19 positive, awaiting a COVID-19 test result, being medically unfit or unsuitable to receive a vaccine, or not consenting to receive the vaccine" (917).

A person with free will may ask how many of those vaccinated, compared to those unvaccinated, died? Public health's job is to survey. Perhaps also, they weren't all as 'medically fit' to be vaccinated as pre-determined.

On January 28th 2021, it was reported that a COVID-19 outbreak in a Dundalk nursing home had claimed six lives. The first dose of the Pfizer-BioNTech vaccine was administered to residents and staff on January 19th 2021, including to one resident who tested positive for COVID-19 in the days afterwards. It goes without saying that the deaths were not blamed on the vaccination. Instead, it was reported that the vaccine's benefits do not start to be felt until 12 days after administration. The nursing home manager sent an email to relatives saying that vaccinators would return on February 15th 2021 to give residents who received the first dose their second 'top-up' dose (918). I am confident that the manager didn't inform families that the side effects of the second dose are much more severe. Also on January 28th 2020, a County Laois nursing home reported the deaths of 17 residents in 20 days. The deaths were described as being due to a "post-Christmas COVID-19 outbreak" (919). On February 1st 2021, a Galway nursing home was reported as being hit by a 'tidal wave' of COVID-19 after 12 residents died from the virus. This article explained that three out of four residents who died in the past 24 hours had received their first dose of the COVID-19 vaccine. Out of 49 residents in Galway's Greenpark Nursing Home, 35 tested positive for the virus, while 12 died (920). On February 18th 2021, it was reported that up to 25 residents at a 51-bed nursing home in Upper Glanmire, Cork had died since the start of a 'significant' COVID-19 outbreak (921). Again the Irish COVID-19 vaccine rollout in nursing homes started on January 7th 2021, when it was reported that some 3,000 residents and staff were vaccinated (922).

A spate of deaths post COVID-19 vaccine rollout in nursing homes in the UK: The Pfizer-BioNTech vaccine, now known as Comirnaty, was approved for emergency use in the UK on December 2nd 2020. By January 19th 2021, the daily propaganda was reporting that coronavirus-related deaths in English care homes had risen by 46% after the vaccine rollout [923]. The daily propaganda attributed these deaths to a more transmissible form of COVID-19 variant or explained that the first shot did not offer enough protection. This contradicted the latest evidence at the time which stated that the first shot is very effective. On February 28th 2021, data from Israel published in *The Lancet* indicated that the Pfizer COVID-19 vaccine was 85% effective in offering protection after a single dose. Additionally, it was also announced that the Pfizer COVID-19 vaccine miraculously longer needed ultra-cold storage [924]. It is a contradiction in terms to report that the elderly are dying after one shot because it doesn't offer enough protection. The ONS UK site is where to search care home resident deaths registered in England and Wales. I checked the figures, and indeed, there was a sharp rise in deaths in care homes after the vaccine rollout. Deaths in care homes in the UK are normally approximately 1370 a month; this increased to 2175 between the dates January 8th and February 5th 2021, representing a 59% increase [925]. A 59% increase that the COVID-19 vaccine may have caused, yet our elderly are being lined up for their 3rd booster shot.

On January 28th 2021, it was reported that two Avery Healthcare care homes experienced a spate of deaths in the same month of the vaccine rollout. Again the Pfizer-BioNTech vaccine was approved for use on December 2nd 2020. The deaths were attributed to an outbreak of COVID-19. Twenty-four residents died in a Pemberley House care home, Basingstoke Hampshire. In addition, nine died in a second care home in the Midlands. The residents at Pemberley House were reported to have died in the weeks following the 'COVID-19 outbreak' in early January. Nine elderly residents died at Seagrave House care home in Corby, Northamptonshire, and dozens more were fighting infection at the time (or side effects of the vaccine?). An MHRA spokesperson, Dr Maurice Price, emphasised that there was no suggestion the deaths were linked to the vaccine, however, a photo widely circulated at the time showed Dr Price administering the Pfizer-BioNTech COVID-19 vaccine to Shrewsbury care home resident Beryl Humphreys on January 20th 2020. I wonder if Beryl made it. Nontransparently, Avery Healthcare did not confirm if residents at the home had received their first dose of the COVID-19 vaccine [926]. Avery Healthcare and MHRA should be surveying deaths post-vaccination by comparing deaths in those who received the vaccine with deaths in those who did not receive the vaccine, then determining if this is statistically significant. 'Wear a mask to save your Granny'; Granny died after she had her COVID shot; don't worry, Granny was old and frail and going to die anyway. Conscience is said to keep more people awake than cocaine.

On January 23rd 2021, British Prime Minister BoJo the clown ordered that the second dose be delayed by up to 12 weeks, stating that they wanted more people to have their first dose. I thought at the time that, as the adverse effects after the second dose are far worse, that BoJo's drug lords were afraid of the consequences of giving elderly, frail people that second dose. At the same time however, care home chiefs and doctors called on the UK government to cut the gap between first and second dose to six weeks because *"dozens of care home residents have died with COVID after the jab"* (927). I couldn't make it up.

Nursing homes deaths post rollout resulted in Norway pulling the Pfizer vaccine: Early into the rollout, Norway launched an investigation into the deaths of two nursing home residents after they received Pfizer's COVID-19 vaccine. On January 7th 2021, the Norwegian Medicines Agency said that the deaths had occurred "a few days" after they were administered the shot (928). Pfizer-BioNTech promptly responded by saying, "Serious adverse events, including deaths that are unrelated to the vaccine, are unfortunately likely to occur at a similar rate as they would in the general population…". The Swiss medical authorities promptly dismissed the possibility that the BioNTech-Pfizer COVID-19 vaccine resulted in the deaths and that the death certificate would list the previous illnesses as the person's "natural cause of death" (929).

Not long after, however, Norway U-turned to become the first European health authority to say that COVID-19 vaccines may be too risky for the very old and terminally ill. The Norwegian Institute of Public Health said, "For those with the most severe frailty, even relatively mild vaccine side effects can have serious consequences". The Institute also said, "For those who have a very short remaining life span anyway, the benefit of the vaccine may be marginal or irrelevant" (930). As of January 17th 2020, the number of suspected adverse drug reactions with fatal outcomes after the administration of the Pfizer-BioNTech vaccine reported to the Norwegian Medicines Agency increased to 33. As a result, the Norwegian health officials changed their COVID-19 vaccine recommendations not to vaccinate the terminally ill (Clinical Frailty Scale 8 or higher), as the vaccine's side effects posed too much risk (931). A Norwegian Medicines Agency review discussed in *The BMJ* in May 2021, looked into the cause of the first 100 reported deaths of nursing home residents who had received the Pfizer-BioNTech vaccine and found that the vaccine was "likely" responsible for the deaths of some elderly patients (932).

A spate of deaths post COVID-19 vaccine rollout in nursing homes in France: On January 20th 2021, it was reported that investigations were continuing in France after five people died within days of receiving the COVID-19 vaccine. Reports stated that there was no proven link and, yet again that all the vaccinated resident deaths were due to preexisting conditions in what they described as "bad timing" (933).

A spate of deaths post COVID-19 vaccine rollout in nursing homes in Spain: On February 2nd 2021, 78 residents of a nursing home in Madrid, Spain, were reported to have tested positive for COVID-19 after being given their first dose of the Pfizer-BioNTech vaccine on January 13th 2021, and that seven of those who had tested positive died. It goes without saying that those who "succumbed to the virus" had preexisting conditions (934).

A spate of deaths post COVID-19 vaccine rollout in nursing homes in the US: On January 30th 2021, it was reported that 257 deaths had occurred "in the last week" in congregate-care facilities. In an interview, Adam Sholar, the president and CEO of the North Carolina Health Care Facilities Association, stated that 95% of nursing homes in the states had administered the first dose. It goes without saying that the deaths were reported as being because the nursing home residents had not received their second dose or that other popular narrative, the greatest threat to global health, security and humanity; 'vaccine hesitancy' (935).

Look on the bright side: In November 2020, The UK government reported it had saved £600m on state pension payments due to 'COVID-19 deaths'. The fiscal watchdog reported that the number of excess pensioner deaths had increased by 45% (936).

Risk of Iatrogenesis: Iatrogenesis is medical errors in diagnosis, intervention or negligence that results in disease or harmful complications, including death. The Pfizer vaccine needs to be thawed and diluted with saline before injection. This physical dilution may lead to an increased risk of human error and a risk of either under-dilution or over-dilution. Unlike the Pfizer vaccine, the Moderna vaccine does not require dilution. Looking at the instructions entitled 'Preparation of Pfizer-BioNTech COVID-19 Vaccine (BNT162b2) Syringes for Administration', the 'procedure to remove the vaccines from original carton' includes no less than nine instructions. The 'dilution' instructions include 16 instructions. The 'withdrawal into syringes' contains 11 instructions [937]. There is no mention of adverse reactions. Reading these instructions, one would be reminded of purchasing a flat-packed item from a well-known Swedish furniture company known to be emotional torture.

On December 19th 2020, eight care workers at a residential home in Germany were accidentally given five times the recommended dose of the vaccine, resulting in four being hospitalised after developing flu-like symptoms [938]. In the first days of the Pfizer COVID-19 vaccine rollout, labelling confusion led to one dose per vial being completely wasted. Whilst the vaccine itself comes in vials labelled as containing five doses, pharmacists found that, upon thawing and diluting each vial with saline that in fact, each vial contained six vaccine doses. The final dose had to be discarded as explicit approval to use it had not been received from the manufacturer [939].

On January 18th 2021, a Wisconsin hospital pharmacist was arrested after being accused of intentionally removing more than 500 doses of COVID-19 vaccine from refrigeration on the understanding that the vaccines would be rendered ineffective if they became room temperature. The hospital pharmacist motives were described as being that recipients would mistakenly think they would be protected from COVID-19 disease [940]. Healthcare workers are only human. There are 1,500 cases of foreign bodies being left behind during surgical procedures in the US every year [941]. Between 1970 and 2006, a total of 90 criminal prosecutions of healthcare providers met the inclusion criteria for serial murder of their patients [942].

CHAPTER THIRTEEN – PART III

POTENTIAL ADVERSE REACTIONS FOLLOWING COVID-19 VACCINES

Vaccine-driven resistance: As mentioned in Chapter 12, 'Vaccines aren't Described as Safe and don't Always Work', just as antimicrobials drive antimicrobial resistance, so to can vaccines drive resistance. The natural evolution of pathogens occurs when random mutations of the virus cause the vaccine to lose effectiveness. Alternatively, vaccine driven pathogen evolution occurs when antigen survivors multiply, making pathogens less vulnerable to the vaccine [(681)]. Vaccines have the potential to impose strong selective pressure on microorganisms, promoting vaccine-induced escape mutants (VEMs) [(682)]. VEMs are one potential cause of breakthrough infection (BI) that is never discussed in the daily propaganda.

Specialists in viral resistance to vaccines, David A. Kennedy and Andrew F. Read of Pennsylvania State University, discussed the potential for COVID-19 vaccines to drive vaccine resistance and result in VEMs in an article published in *PLoS Biology* in November 2021. The authors stated that the potential exists for, rather than the vaccines putting an end to the pandemic, the vaccines driving new evolutionary change. The authors suggested that vaccine makers could use the results of nasal swabs taken from volunteers during trials to look for any genetic changes in the virus. If vaccine recipients had changes in the virus that were not seen in those who received the placebo, that would indicate the potential for resistance to evolve and is something researchers should monitor [(943)]. Now they have unblinded the trials, it is impossible for vaccine makers to monitor the potential for vaccine escape mutants. Outbreaks of the new vaccine-resistant strains will be blamed on failure to vaccinate, and new vaccines will be manufactured to combat these vaccine-resistant strains that may drive further mutations. However, Kennedy and Read argue that samples already collected as part of the clinical trials could be repurposed to determine which vaccine does not have this potential and could be prioritised.

The WHO now finally admit the booster could drive VEMs: On September 11th 2021 the WHO admitted it was concerned that the boosters would drive mutations and make the situation a lot worse. Whilst not admitting that the vaccines may have driven the emergence of the current mutant variants of concern (VOCs), the WHO is now saying that vaccine boosters could drive the emergence of new variants in the future. WHO Chief Boffin Dr Soumya Swaminathan said, *"I'm afraid that this (booster recommendation) will only lead to more variants...And perhaps we're heading into an even more dire situation"* [944]. The WHO doesn't listen to their own experts.

Antibody-dependent enhancement and COVID-19 vaccines: Bear in mind, regarding the current generation of COVID-19 vaccines, that safety has been assessed for a two month follow-up period only. During the continuing global experiment, scientists will monitor those receiving the vaccines for any ADRs. Again, they should compare this data to people who have not received the vaccine, however the trials have been unblinded, and the unvaccinated controls are rapidly dwindling [807]. Scientists will be (or should be) on the lookout for is a condition known as antibody-dependent enhancement (ADE). ADE is also called immune enhancement or, when associated with vaccines, is called vaccine-associated disease enhancement (VADE) [945]. ADE describes a phenomenon whereby the virus itself binds to suboptimal antibodies (non-neutralising) and enhances the entry of the virus into the host cells. In simple terms, the potential exists for vaccine-induced antibodies to, rather than prevent infection, make it easier for the virus to enter the cells, thereby making the virus more virulent and increasing mortality. Past vaccine candidates that targeted coronaviruses, respiratory syncytial virus (RSV) and dengue virus have resulted in VADE, and as a result, the trials were terminated [946]. VADE has been observed in mice vaccinated with whole killed SARS-CoV or recombinant (artificially produced) SARS-CoV spike proteins [947, 948]. Despite eliciting a neutralising and protective immune response in rodents studies, VADE has been observed in human B cell lines with a SARS-CoV vaccine candidate based on recombinant, full-length SARS-CoV spike-protein trimers (3 proteins) [949].

What the experts say about vaccine-associated disease enhancement: Nobel Laureate Luc Montagnier gave an interview in French exposing the dangers of COVID-19 vaccines, saying the vaccine will drive mutation, which will escape the effect of the vaccine. In the interview, Montagnier says that ADE would lead to much stronger infection by variants in vaccinated people. Montagnier says, "the new variants are created by the selection of the antibodies produced by the vaccination". Montagnier also says, *"This is a huge mistake; it is a scientific error and inexplicable medical malpractice. History will one day take stock of all this because it was indeed the vaccination that created the variant"*. Montagnier did not say vaccinated people would die in two years, as has been reported [950, 951]. Again I believe the Thought Police tactfully release these statements as a smokescreen to what is actually said.

Back in March 2020, speaking in relation to ADE, the Dean of the National School of Tropical Medicine at Baylor College of Medicine, CNN star, Dr Peter Hotez said, *"I understand the importance of accelerating timelines for vaccines in general, but from everything I know, this is not the vaccine to be doing it with"*. Dr Hotez said that the way to reduce that risk of immune enhancement is to prove that it does not occur in laboratory animals [952]. The minimal animal studies that were conducted did not test for immune enhancement. With the absence of animal studies, outcomes in humans can never be predicted [800]. The bottom line is that we do not know, and will likely never know if these experimental biological agents lead to ADE. What is 100% certain is that should worsening outbreaks occur due to VEMs or ADE, these will be blamed on failure to vaccinate and not vaccine failure. In a video posted on *BitChute* entitled *'Why people will start dying a few months after the first mRNA vaccination'*, Professor Dolores Cahill of the UCD School of Medicine begins by discussing a paper entitled 'Immunisation with SARS Coronavirus Vaccines Leads to Pulmonary Immunopathology on Challenge with the SARS Virus'. Cahill says:

> *"The issue when you inject messenger RNA, say if it had a protein from the virus, say the spike protein, this plus positive RNA can go into our cells. The spike protein from the virus is expressed in our cells and may be exposed to the immune system when those cells die, and the body starts mounting an immune response, including an antibody response. But then, so say if that happens in December...within two or three weeks that process would start...but if in February, March, April, another coronavirus is circulating naturally in 2021, that would be like a challenge with the natural...SARS coronaviruses...or it could even be the common cold. What happened is, the animal models, after being challenged (animals) got very sick, and some of them died. The abstract says caution in proceeding in humans is indicated, and so the*

name of this thing is an antibody-dependent response or cytokine storm or immune-priming or immune super priming. This is why there has been no vaccine for decades licensed for coronavirus".

Professor Cahill continues to mention another study on RSV from 1969 that tragically resulted in the deaths of two babies out of 35 who received the RSV vaccination that then became infected with the RSV virus. One baby was 14 months of age, and the second was 16 months of age... the conclusion was that the disease was enhanced by the prior vaccination [(953)].

In a video posted on *BitChute* entitled 'How Many Who've Had the Covid Jab Will Still be Alive Next Christmas?' Doctor Vernon Coleman also discusses potential deaths from vaccines.

"Ignorant, sanctimonious, spineless millions who that think they can live forever if they wear two facemasks with as stocking on top over their face...If you don't fight to preserve your identity and freedom and rights...despite all their false promises, you will ever again go to a sporting event, travel abroad, have a job...unless you agree to have regular unnecessary injections with an experimental poison...that government figures show is more likely to kill you or cause a serious injury than the disease known as COVID-19 and the experimental poison will almost certainly also dramatically increase your chances of dying of infection or cancer, or heaven knows what else in five, ten years time...When the death total rises in autumn, the authorities will blame new strains of the virus, they won't blame the lockdowns ...the deadly masks or dangerous vaccines. Remember, just under 3% of those who've had one of the vaccines will die or have a serious side effect. That's an official figure, and the same officials admit that only a tiny percentage of deaths and side effects caused by vaccines are actually reported...For anyone healthy and under 70, it's a truly absurd risk to take...The Gatesian myth makers...will all tell you that no one's died of the vaccine... Healthy people die within minutes of injections...But terminally ill patients that die with 28 or 60 days of a positive but unreliable test died not of their illness but of the universal COVID-19. When deaths go up...they'll tell the half-witted and tremulous that they must have more injections and wear more masks, and that's what people will do" [(954)].

Not practising what they preach: Project Veritas announced that Fascistbook whistleblowers leaked documents detailing the effort to secretly censor vaccine concerns on a global scale. The whistleblower states that within Facebook, there is a 'Health integrity team' that looks to find 'barriers to vaccination' on the Facebook site. From 12 minutes and 47 seconds, Zuckerberg violates his own policy by sharing his concerns about the vaccine's safety. Zuckerberg says (in reference to the COVID-19 vaccines) *"but I do just want to make sure that I share some caution on this because we just don't know the long-term side effects of basically modifying people's DNA and RNA"* (345). Zuckerberg is currently mandating gene vaccines for his employees.

An article published in the *Journal.ie* on April 25th 2020, debunks that Irish Professor of Biochemistry in the School of Biochemistry and Immunology at Trinity College Dublin, Luke O'Neill said he refused the COVID-19 vaccine during a programme on RTÉ. What Professor Lukey Kooky actually said is that he, "had not had a vaccine yet, though he had been offered one". One would wonder why he didn't jump for the opportunity to practice what he preaches and take the jab? Apparently, O'Neill refused because he is altruistic. "I don't work in the hospital", O'Neill replied.

> *"My lab is on Pearse Street. We have our COVID centre in Trinity, three people in my lab go to the hospital to get samples; they got vaccinated, the rest of us said no. We were offered a vaccine, but we said no because we're not on the front line"* (955).

Perhaps Professor Lukey Kooky had not received the news that Europe just ordered another 1.8 billion doses and there is plenty to go around. O'Neill also said on *The Pat Kenny Show*, an Irish radio programme back in August 2020, that there was "no way" he would take the Russian Sputnik COVID-19 vaccine if it was offered to him. O'Neill said,

> *"We're worried about that one because that clearly hasn't gone through all the rigorous safety analysis that the vaccines are going through at the moment".*

Professor Lukey Kooky is happy for the rest of us plebs to take it.

Graphical representation of COVID-19 vaccinations on mortality: There is (or was) a very telling video worth watching on You-will-obey-Tube entitled 'Impact of COVID-19 Vaccinations on Mortality', posted by Joel Smalley showing global mortality from COVID-19 before and after the introduction of COVID-19 vaccines (956).

Self-disseminating vaccines: The technology exists to develop vaccines that spread between human to human. It's not called shedding. I believe the concept of 'shedding' has been tactfully released so the 'fact-checkers' can detract from the potential reality. The fact-checkers cannot refute self-disseminating vaccines. Self-disseminating vaccines were described in an article published in *Expert Review of Vaccines* in 2015. It is the hope that self-disseminating vaccines can address emerging infectious diseases (EIDs). Self-disseminating vaccines are engineered to express target antigens from the EID pathogen. Self-disseminating vaccines can spread from vaccinated to non-vaccinated animals to result in the coordinated spread of artificial induced EID-specific vaccine immunity throughout the targeted population [(957)].

In an aim to bewilder us with science jargon, 'self-disseminating vaccines' are also known as 'transmissible vaccines', 'self-propagating vaccines' or even called 'transferable vaccines'. The technology for developing transmissible vaccines exists, as yet however, it is purported that researchers have not developed experimental self-spreading vaccines in humans. They are hoping to vaccinate animals to protect us. Previous field trials using disseminating vaccines to protect wild rabbits from a viral haemorrhagic fever have shown promising results. This radical technology involves the insertion of a small piece of the genome of the infectious disease agent into a benign virus that spreads naturally through the animal population. This transmissible vaccine spreads from animal to animal and immunises them against the target infectious disease. This is said to hugely increase immunity in the animal population and thereby reduce the risk of transmission to humans. Efforts are now underway to develop prototypes for the human pathogens, Lassa and Ebola viruses [(958)]. The hope is that transmissible and transferable vaccines can be given to a bat, which can then vaccinate other bats to prevent coronavirus transmission in humans. Scientists describe this process as 'infectiously vaccinated' [(959)]. The 'Global Citizens' are currently suffering from this now.

Shedding is very possibly what Pfizer call an occupational hazard: 'Shedding' refers to the transmission of the protein from a vaccinated to an unvaccinated person resulting in symptoms induced in the latter. Of course, SARS-CoV-2 sheds! That is how it can transfer from one human to another. A study published in *medRxiv* in January 2021 found that shedding of viral spike protein occurs in about 25% of confirmed

COVID-19 patients [960]. Shedding of SARS-CoV-2 spike proteins has been shown to occur in faeces and urine [961]. Contrary to the fact-wreckers claims, it is not totally implausible that the spike proteins created as a result of vaccination, shed. Shedding after vaccines is quite possibly referred to by Pfizer as an 'occupational hazard'. An article published in the *International Journal of Vaccine Theory, Practice, and Research* in May 2021 reviewed the possible unintended consequences of the COVID-19 mRNA vaccines. The article reviewed both vaccines components and their intended biological response, including the production of the spike protein itself and their potential relationship to a wide range of both acute and long-term induced pathologies. The authors' conclusion supported the potential for spike protein 'shedding' transmission [962].

A safety data sheet on the Pfizer-BioNTech COVID-19 vaccine refers to 'other hazards', including occupational exposure. Pfizer acknowledges that values have been established for one or more of the ingredients for which there is a reporting system, Occupational Exposure Band (B-OEB), and an acceptable daily intake (ADI) range for the vaccine components. This list of ingredients includes the RNA-lipid nanoparticles, for which the mutant viral spike protein of SARS-CoV-2 is encapsulated [963]. Pfizer says that Occupational exposure occurs when a person receives unplanned direct contact with the study intervention (vaccine), which may or may not lead to the occurrence of an adverse event. The investigator should report occupational exposure to Pfizer Safety within 24 hours of the investigator becoming aware, regardless of whether there is an associated serious adverse event (SAE), using the Vaccine SAE Report Form. Occupation exposure appears under Section 7: Handling and Storage. As expected, anyone handling the vaccine may be exposed to it [964]. Occupational exposure, as also expected, appears under an unexpected pregnancy or breastfeeding. Not so expected however, is that Pfizer reports that other people who may be exposed include healthcare providers, other roles involved in the trial participant's care, and family members and participants not enrolled in the study. The Pfizer trial protocol says occupational exposure includes those *"exposed to the vaccine by inhalation or skin exposure"* [588]. The question remains; how does a participant not enrolled in the study, such as a family member or other close contact become exposed to the 'study intervention' (vaccine) by inhalation or skin contact?

The first autopsy of a COVID-19 vaccine death: The first post-mortem study of a patient vaccinated against COVID-19 was published in June 2021 in the *International Journal of Infectious Diseases*. The autopsy was conducted on an 86 year old man who had received a single dose of the SARS-CoV-2 vaccine but passed away one month later. The patient did not present with any specific symptoms to COVID-19 but tested positive for SARS-CoV-2 before he died. The cause of death was put down as being due to acute bronchopneumonia and tubular failure, however the study authors did not observe any characteristic morphological features of COVID-19. These results indicated that the patient developed immunogenicity, but not sterile immunity. Spike proteins were created, and an immune response elicited, however neutralising antibodies that confer sterilising immunity (when the immune system stops the virus from entering cells and replicating) were not made [965]. As a result, spike proteins were found in all organs examined.

New Safety Concerns

Mix and match, no worries: When it comes to the new COVID-19 vaccines, it appears anything goes. In early January 2020, Public Health England (PHE) COVID guidelines were updated to allow the COVID-19 vaccines to be mixed and matched. The guidelines stated, "(If) the same vaccine is not available, or if the first product received is unknown, it is reasonable to offer one dose of the locally available product to complete the schedule" [966]. The main safety concerns with changing the dosing regimens are that the vaccines use completely different technology. The Oxford-AstraZeneca vaccine is a recombinant DNA vaccine. The Pfizer-BioNTech vaccine is an mRNA vaccine. Mixing and matching these vaccines has not been trialled at the time, therefore the advice to mix these technologies was unscientific [967]. This advice also contradicted the previous advice given by the CDC, which said, in reference to the interchangeability of the Pfizer-BioNTech and Moderna COVID-19 vaccines, that mRNA COVID-19 vaccines are not interchangeable with each other or with other COVID-19 vaccine products [218]. If the advice was that mRNA COVID-19 vaccines are not interchangeable with each other, how is it that mRNA vaccines can suddenly be interchangeable with recombinant DNA vaccines? The difference between DNA vaccines (which Big Media aims to suppress by calling them viral vector vaccines) and mRNA vaccines is covered further in Chapter 20, 'The Future is Vaccines, Vaccines and More Vaccines'.

One dose only, no worries: On February 2nd 2021, the French National Authority for Health, Haute Autorité de Santé (HAS), recommended that people who have previously contracted COVID-19 need only receive one dose of the vaccine. The HAS was the first health authority in the world to issue such a recommendation. The HAS released a statement that current data suggests "people who have already been infected retain an immune memory" whether their disease was either symptomatic or asymptomatic [(968)]. The evidence of immunity is irrelevant. Shut up! Obey! Take at least one shot!

Miscellaneous; the Australian COVID-19 vaccine gave you AIDS: The production of the University of Queensland and global biotech company CSL vaccine was halted after the vaccine was found to cause 'false positive' HIV tests in trial participants. The vaccine was an experimental molecular clamp COVID-19 vaccine. A molecular clamp is a polypeptide used to maintain the shape of proteins in experimental vaccines. This particular vaccine used parts of a HIV protein [(969)]. The vaccine production was stopped after discovering the antibodies produced to this vaccine were picked up in a range of HIV tests, potentially leading to people believing they were HIV positive [(970)]. How ironic that PCR inventor Kary Mullis argued that he could not find proof that testing positive for HIV using PCR caused AIDS.

Spanish influenza and experimental vaccines: A lesson from history. The Spanish influenza was never Spanish; the Spaniards had the finger pointed at them because they were honest. On a side note, in an attempt to address existing rumours surrounding who really died during the Spanish influenza, the following discusses experimental vaccines used by 'pioneering doctors' during the Spanish influenza outbreak. An article published in *Clinical Oncology News* in 2020 entitled 'Astonishing Numbers: Vaccine Efforts In the 1918 Flu Pandemic', discussed that German physician and bacteriologist Richard Pfeiffer had been searching for the cause of influenza since the 1889-1890 pandemic. In 1852, Pfeiffer discovered a bacterium in the nose of influenza patients in "astonishing numbers" and declared this bacterium to be the cause of influenza. Pfeiffer worked with Robert Koch of the German public health institute, the Koch Institute, to develop the concept and proved the existence of endotoxins and their roles in infectious diseases. Endotoxins are found on Gram-negative bacteria. Pfeiffer had previously pioneered the typhoid vaccination. Not everyone accepted the idea that bacteria caused influenza, however some accepted this theory as bacteria had already been shown to be the cause of anthrax, cholera and plague. During the Spanish influenza, pharmaceutical companies promoted vaccines already available for other diseases. Doctors manufactured large batches of these 'vaccines', which used, on the most part, inactivate microorganisms, then they distributed these vaccines to other doctors to inject in their patients or to be used in asylums and orphanages [(971)]. Needless to say, these concoctions did not treat bacterial influenza. Pfeiffer made claims of success, but these trials were neither regulated nor used a control group. The US surgeon general and the American Medical Association (AMA) were sceptical about the claims, and numerous articles about vaccines appeared in the medical literature in 1918, including one published in *JAMA* by George McCoy, of the US Public Health Service, entitled 'The Failure of a Bacterial Vaccine as a Prophylactic Against Influenza' [(972)]. It was not until 1933 that scientists isolated the influenza A virus from ferrets. In 2021, lessons from history have not been learned.

CHAPTER FOURTEEN

COVID-19 VACCINES ARE EFFECTIVE FOR SEVEN DAYS

"And the truth shall set you free". The Bible, John 8:32 [973]

Whilst the daily propaganda is currently working overtime, desperately trying to convince us that coronavirus disease 2019 (COVID-19) vaccines prevent transmission of severe acute respiratory syndrome coronavirus 2 (SARS-CoV-2); they don't. The summer of 2021 will have seen European countries open up to fully vaccinated people and outbreaks of COVID-19 in the 'double-jabbed'. When Australia and New Zealand finally open up after they have coerced most Antipodeans to shut up, obey and take their shot, the world will see what happens in the global control. The daily propaganda will do what they are paid to do, that is to blame failure to vaccinate, not vaccine failure. Reasons why vaccines fail were discussed in Chapter 12, 'Vaccines aren't Described as Safe and don't Always Work'.

UK's SAGES/ SPI said the vaccine is causing 3rd wave of hospitalisations and deaths: Data from one of the world's most vaccinated countries, the United Kingdom (UK), provided proof that the COVID-19 vaccines are ineffective. In April 2021, the UK Scientific Pandemic Influenza Group on Modelling, Operational sub-group (SPI-M-O), for the Scientific Advisory Group for Emergencies (SAGE) acknowledged that 60-70% of the deaths and hospitalisations in the UK's 3rd wave were occurring in people who had both doses of the COVID-19 vaccine. Page 10 says,
"The resurgence in both hospitalisations and deaths is dominated by those that have received two doses of the vaccine, comprising around 60%-70% of the wave, respectively" [422].

43% of COVID deaths in England are in the 'double-jabbed': The authors of the following article referred to are a behavioural psychologist and a statistician who say it is normal that the fully vaccinated are dying from COVID-19. 'No vaccine is 100% effective', yada yada. Proletariat, shut up! Obey! Take your shot! But it isn't normal. A vaccine should prevent infection or, at the very least, prevent deaths. On June 27th 2021, *The*

Guardian ran an article entitled 'Why most people who now die with COVID-19 in England have had a vaccination'. The article described two recent Public Health England (PHE) technical briefings. The first briefing occurred on June 13th 2021 and stated that 29% of COVID-19 deaths were in people that had received both vaccinations. The second released on June 25th 2021, revealed that this figure had risen, with 43% of COVID-19 deaths being in people who had been 'double-jabbed' and 60% of COVID-19 deaths being in people who had received at least one dose [(974)].

A drop in testing, not an effective vaccine, is the reason for decreased infections: The daily propaganda credits the COVID-19 vaccine rollout with a decrease in cases and purports this is proof that the vaccines prevent the spread of infection. The daily propaganda wilfully neglects to report that as people feel protected after having had the COVID-19 vaccine, they are less likely to get a COVID-19 test. In the US, there has been a dramatic decrease in the number of tests conducted. Between January and March 2021, testing for the virus dropped by a third [(975)]. One need not be a mathematical modeller to work out that cases dropped by a third.

Emergency Use Authorisation for vaccines explained: As previously mentioned, COVID-19 vaccines were found to be effective for seven days and safe for two months. The Food and Drug Administration (FDA) expects an Emergency Use Authorisation (EUA) submission for COVID-19 vaccines to include all safety data accumulated from phase I and phase II studies conducted, with an expectation that phase III data will include a median follow-up of at least two months (the exact requirement is that at least half of vaccine recipients in phase III clinical trials have at least two months of follow-up), and efficacy is assessed seven days after the second dose [(592)]. Seven whole days.

In the beginning, expectations weren't so stratospheric: The FDA had said that once a vaccine is shown to be safe and at least 50% effective, it would be authorised for use in the US. In May 2020, Professor Adrian Hill, Director of Oxford University's Jenner Institute, said the Oxford-AstraZeneca's coronavirus vaccine was given only a 50% chance of working. The reason Hill gave was that cases in the UK were declining so rapidly [(976)]. Master Mason Fauci of the National Institute of Health and Infectious Disease (NIAID), doublespeak for the 'National Institute to Destroy Health and Increase Infectious Disease' said his realistic expectations were for an efficiency rate of 50% or 60% [977]. COVID-19 vaccines are 95% effective! Hallelujah! We are saved!

COVID-19 vaccines are not 'effective'; they have shown high 'efficacy': Assessments of efficacy compare a vaccinated group with a placebo group and describe the degree to which a vaccine prevents disease (and possibly transmission) in these controlled circumstances. On the other hand, effectiveness refers to how well the vaccine performs in the real world [978]. The daily propaganda may lead one to believe that phase III studies revealed that COVID-19 vaccines are successful in keeping people from getting very sick and dying from COVID-19 and that COVID-19 vaccines prevent the spread of infection. As demonstrated in Chapter 11, 'Trial Protocols and Study Design Flaws', death, hospitalisations and prevention of transmission were not endpoints in the COVID-19 vaccine studies.

Effective at what exactly? The endpoints of the COVID-19 vaccine trials were mild COVID-19 disease prevention only. None of the COVID-19 vaccine trials were designed to determine a reduction in serious outcomes such as hospital admissions, intensive care admissions or deaths. The primary endpoint definitions in the COVID-19 phase III trials were infections with mild symptoms only. Additionally, the trials did not address the question of whether vaccines reduce transmission. Only a few trials considered whether the vaccine benefited the most vulnerable to COVID-19 disease, such as the elderly and immunocompromised. The COVID-19 vaccines were found to be '95% effective' at reducing mild symptoms of COVID-19, seven days after the second dose. Their definition of effective is not at all what most people will think it means [979]. Pfizer's exact terminology is *"in each case measured from seven days after the second dose"*, *"met all of the study's primary efficacy endpoints"*, trial endpoints being *"COVID-19 infections with mild symptoms only"*. What the trials did and did not determine was again discussed in Chapter 11, 'Trial Protocols and Study Design Flaws'.

95 % efficacy does not mean that 95 in 100 people are protected! Statisticians originally concocted the statistical analyses conducted today over a century ago. Statisticians use scientific language to bamboozle us so that we worship at the altar of science. 95% efficacy, for example, does not mean that 95 out of 100 people are protected. In statistics, there is a difference between what is known as absolute risk and relative risk. Simply put, researchers vaccinate some participants, and the others are given a placebo. A certain time elapses (in this case, seven days only after the second dose) until assessing if participants got sick, then researchers establish how many of those experiencing illnesses were from each group [980]. If no one got COVID-19 in the vaccinated group, the efficacy would be 100%. Efficacy is derived from the relative difference between those two fractions. This is where the 95% figure comes from. This 95% figure represents relative risk reduction (RRR), not absolute risk reduction (ARR) [608]. ARR is a more accurate yet far less impressive reduction in risk to report as it takes into account population heterogeneity (population diversity, we aren't all susceptible).

The absolute risk reduction of a COVID-19 vaccine is less than 1%: According to data published in the *New England Journal of Medicine*, of the 43,448 that received injections, 21,720 with Pfizer-BioNTech COVID-19 vaccine and 21,728 with placebo, 8 cases of COVID-19 (mild, severe or moderate) occurred with onset at least seven days after the second dose among participants that received the vaccine, and 162 cases of COVID-19 occurred among those assigned to placebo. This represents infection rates of 0.04% and 0.75%, respectively [981]. This results in a COVID-19 attack rate of 0.0004 in the vaccine group and 0.007 in the placebo group (8/21,720 x100 and 162/21,728 x 100). RRR for vaccination; 0.0004 divided by 0.007 = 0.057, which translates into a "vaccine effectiveness" of 94% [100 (1-0.057) = 100 (0.943)]. Thus the relative efficacy is 94%, meaning 94% of confirmed infections occurred in the placebo group. When reported as RRR, the relative efficacy sounds impressive, but the ARR for an individual is less than 1%, at 0.7% (0.007-0.0004= 0.007). The Number Needed To Vaccinate (NNTV) =143 (1/0.007= 142.85). Ultimately, this means that to prevent just one case of COVID-19 disease, a total of 143 individuals need to be vaccinated. All other 142 individuals derive no benefit whatsoever yet are placed at risk of serious adverse events following immunisation (AEFIs) [982].

A study published in *The Lancet Microbe*, in April 2021, after I had calculated the above ARRs, reiterates what I describe in relation to vaccine efficacy (VE) being reported in terms of RRR, and confirms my ARR calculations. Study authors reported RRRs being 95% for the Pfizer-BioNTech, 94% for the Moderna-US National Institutes of Health (NIH), 91% for the Gamaleya (GamCovidVac [Sputnik V] vaccine), 67% for the

Johnson & Johnson (J&J), and 67% for the Oxford-AstraZeneca vaccines. Study authors noted that RRR does not account for population heterogeneity (population diversity, we aren't all susceptible) and the difference between the risk of being infected with and without a COVID-19 vaccine and the risk of becoming ill with COVID-19 in different populations over a period of time. Whilst the ARR considers the population heterogeneity, these statistics are generally ignored as they are much less impressive. The study authors calculate the ARR as 0.84% for the Pfizer-BioNTech,1.3% for the Oxford-AstraZeneca, 1.2% for the Moderna-NIH, 1.2% for the J&J and 0.93% for the Sputnik V, now called Gamaleya (983).

There is a difference between immunisation & vaccination: Immunisation describes the process whereby people are protected against illness caused by microorganism infection. Vaccination refers to the act of giving a vaccine to a person (984). The COVID-19 vaccine does not immunise. Anyone using the word immunisation in relation to COVID-19 vaccines is spreading misinformation. This is why the boffins call them 'jabs' and 'shots'. In January 2021, the World Wealth Organisation's Chief Boffin Dr Soumya Swaminathan said there is a lack of evidence that COVID-19 vaccines prevent transmission and warned that vaccinated travellers should still quarantine, wear a mask and maintain social distancing (595). Deputy Chief Medical Officer Jonathon Van-Tam wrote in *The Sunday Telegraph* that *"Even after you have had both doses of the vaccine, you may still give COVID-19 to someone else, and the chains of transmission will then continue"* (985). The UK's National Health Service (NHS) say on their website about COVID-19 vaccines under the section 'How well do the COVID-19 vaccines work?' that there is a chance you might still get or spread COVID-19 even if you have a vaccine, so it's important to continue to follow all social distancing guidance (986). The COVID-19 vaccines trials tracked only how many vaccinated people became sick with COVID-19. In December 2020, the biotech companies Pfizer and Moderna had so much confidence in their COVID-19 vaccines that they said that even after you've had the COVID-19 vaccine, you still have to wear a mask (987). That all changed when Biden-his-time-until-Kamala-takes-over, emerged from his cave, took his mask off, and then took off his second mask.

COVID-19 vaccines don't prevent transmission of SARS-CoV-2: An article published in *Otolaryngology-Head and Neck Surgery* on February 21st 2021, said that the current COVID-19 vaccines are administered by injection, and that systemic vaccines may not prevent nasal SARS-CoV-2 infection and asymptomatic transmission. The article stated there is little evidence regarding mucosal immunity following vaccination and recommended that otolaryngologists (ear, nose, throat doctors) maintain viral transmission-based precautions in vulnerable patients who exhibit incomplete vaccine efficacy or waning vaccine-induced immunity [(219)]. The University of Hong Kong and coronavirus expert John Nicholls said the current range of COVID-19 vaccines undergoing trials will reduce cases of severe pneumonia but will not stop transmission of the disease. Vaccinated individuals exposed to the virus can still transmit the disease to high-risk populations, while they themselves are protected from developing severe disease. Nicholls said, "That's why the vaccine has to be put in together with social distancing". Nicholls said a nasal spray vaccine, such as is used for some influenza vaccines, would prevent transmission as it would cause the immune system to produce an intranasal antibody that stays in the nasal passages to intercept viruses and stop transmission [(619)].

Poor study designs show vaccines purportedly 'prevent infection': After looking at Israeli data, Pfizer issued a press release making claims that the vaccine offers 94% protection against asymptomatic infection [(988)]. Caution needs to be taken with these numbers as the study design used is poor. An article published in the *New England Journal of Medicine* discussed vaccine effectiveness (VE) and the need for VE to be assessed for a range of outcomes across diverse populations in a non-controlled setting. The authors noted that so far, VE studies, including those in Israel, only tested symptomatic participants instead of a more robust study designed to systematically test all study participants, so the findings as to how effective the vaccine is at reducing transmission could be overly optimistic [(989)].

The evidence to prevent transmission is irrelevant. Shut up! Obey! Take your shot! The trial to prove if COVID-19 vaccines prevent transmission was stalled in December 2020. The US 20 college campus study that intended to answer the question 'do the new COVID-19 vaccines stop the virus from spreading, in addition to protecting individuals from getting sick', was shelved due to lack of interest. The researchers weren't able to secure federal funding for the trial. The boffins can't say the COVID-19 vaccines 'likely' prevent transmission of SAR-CoV-2 if they know it definitively doesn't [(599)].

Domestic vaccine certificates on the table: As previously discussed in Chapter 3, 'Coercive Control' domestic vaccine certificates are on the table. They say listen to the WHO as they are the authority, however we don't listen to the WHO, we listen to Tony weapons of mass distraction Blair. Blair is now the expert in pulling the wool over our eyes in relation to the need for international vaccine certificates and UK domestic vaccine certificates. Tony's Vaccination Credential Initiative is a coalition of Big Tech and healthcare companies, including Gate's Microsoft, who want to create a "trustworthy, traceable, verifiable, and universally recognised digital record of vaccination status" that would allow people to "safely return to work, school, events, and travel" [(247)]. Get back in your cave Tony, and Gates, you need to learn that denial is not a river in Egypt. As of today, September 12th 2021, Tony's proposed UK domestic vaccine certificate has been scrapped thanks to the protestors!

Alpha to Lambda: Over time, the viral genome on any virus naturally accumulates mutations as it passes through its human hosts. This is a common evolutionary mechanism found in all microorganisms. 'Variants of Concern (VOC)' in times of pandemonium, is doublespeak for, 'increasing the vaccine-induced herd immunity level and the requirement for a booster shot'. At the time of writing, the WHO had renamed variants using Greek letters as naming them after their place of first detection created stigma that led to racism; doublespeak for, 'may lead people to realise that the variants came from the exact places where the trials were conducted' [(990)]. The UK variant (B.1.1.7) is now Alpha, the South African variant (B.1.351) is now Beta, the Brazilian variant (P.1) is now Gamma, and the Indian variant (B.1.617.2) is now Delta [(991)]. Coincidently the COVID-19 vaccine trials were conducted in the UK (Kent likely), South Africa, Brazil and India. Did the vaccines drive the variants in these places? Nobel winning scientist Luc Montagnier says they did [(950)]. To be able to say for sure, as previously mentioned, scientists would have to compare nasopharyngeal samples in the unvaccinated and the vaccinated [(943)]. Unfortunately, we are running out of unvaccinated people. New kids on the block; Zeta, Eta, Theta, Kappa, Epsilon, Iota and Lambda [(992)]. Each Greek letter potentially represents another lockdown and outbreaks being blamed on the unvaccinated. Just when you thought it was safe to go back into the pub, ...enter the Columbian Mu variant (B.1.621).

COVID-19 vaccines don't work against variants: As a result of Israel's aggressive vaccination campaign, Israel has the highest rates of vaccination in the world, so there is good data in relation to the vaccine's efficiency. The daily propaganda won't say that COVID-19 vaccines can result in the recipient of that vaccine testing positive for COVID-19, although 12,400 people in Israel tested positive after receiving the COVID-19 vaccine. After testing 189,000 people, Israel's health ministry has determined that 6.6 % of the vaccine recipients tested positive for COVID-19. Earlier, Nachman Ash, Israel's vaccine Czar and national coordinator on the pandemic, said that the Pfizer vaccine was, *"less effective than we had thought"* (237). Enter valid excuse; VOC. A *Lancet* study published in June 2021 noted that both increased age and time since the second dose of Pfizer-BioNTech COVID-19 vaccine significantly correlated with decreased neutralising antibody (NAb) activity against the Beta/South African variant, and the Delta/Indian variant and recommended further booster immunisations of Joint Committee on Vaccination and Immunisation (JCVI) Priority Groups in the UK and similar groups in other countries (993). A preprint article published in *MedRxiv* explained that the breakthrough infections in fully-vaccinated Israelis are also predominantly in those VOCs identified as Alpha/UK variant and again the Beta variant (994). Israel, of course, went back into lockdown in June 2021. It appears the vaccine does not work against the variants, most likely because the vaccine has created the variants. Nasal swabs from vaccinated and unvaccinated would prove or disprove this. However, it will never be done unless we demand it. Pfizer and Moderna both now say their vaccine works for six months and recommend a booster shot, Fauci, the FDA and the CDC say no (not yet) (995). The WHO also says not until we've achieved 'critical mass' of vaccination in low- and middle-income countries.

The new South African COVID-19 mutant strain: The South African variant carries a mutation called E484K, which works to change the receptor-binding domain, a key component of the spike protein that the virus uses to gain entry to human cells. This is an important site for neutralising antibodies, which, as opposed to non-neutralising antibodies, bind to a virus in a manner that blocks infection. Laboratory studies show that the change in the receptor-binding domain may make people's antibodies less effective at neutralising the virus, potentially rendering the vaccine less effective or ineffective (996). By January 4th 2021, it was thought that both the Moderna and Pfizer COVID-19 vaccines would be ineffective against the novel South African strain. These concerns were reported by anonymous UK government advisers to the UK broadcaster ITV. The now ex-UK Monster-of-Health Matt Hancock called it a "very significant problem" and said that he was "incredibly worried". John Bell, Regius Professor of Medicine at Oxford University, said that it might take a month or six weeks to get a new vaccine [(997)]. A month? That inspires such confidence in vaccines, Heidi. While all COVID-19 vaccines were described as 'largely effective' against the Alpha/UK (B.1.1.7) variant that emerged in February 2021, J&J, Novavax and then Oxford-AstraZeneca said their COVID-19 vaccines were less effective against the N501Y mutation in the Beta/South African (B.1.351) variant. A randomised, double-blind study in 2000 healthy vaccines (people receiving vaccines) conducted on the blood of those vaccinated found the vaccine showed significantly reduced efficacy against the Beta/South African variant. In February 2021, South Africa halted the rollout of the AstraZeneca vaccine saying the vaccine offered "minimal protection" against mild and moderate cases of COVID-19 [(998, 999)].

The new Brazilian COVID-19 mutant strain: In January 2021, a third new strain of coronavirus was identified after mutating in Manaus, Brazil. This variant is known as the Gamma/Brazilian (P.1) variant. This variant has been shown to reinfect people who have already had the virus, therefore experts are expecting the COVID-19 vaccines to be less effective or ineffective [(1000)]. Brazil Manaus variant is similar to the variant from South Africa and also contains mutations that are believed to increase transmissibility [(1001)]. It does not matter if the vaccine works against variants, when vaccines fail the daily propaganda will blame the 'pandemic of the unvaccinated'.

Fully vaccinated carry as much Delta virus as unvaccinated: As of August 19th 2021, the idea of reaching their precious vaccine-induced artificial herd immunity looks highly unlikely. A study not yet published, conducted by Oxford University researchers in partnership with the Office for National Statistics (ONS) and the Department of Health and Social Care (DHSC), showed the Delta variant wipes out the viral load reduction in vaccinated people. The study compared the results of 2.6 million nose and throat swabs results taken from more than 384,500 adults between December 2020 and mid-May 2021, and more than 811,600 test results from 358,983 adults between mid-May and August 1st 2021 (the period of Delta's domination). Researchers found that fully vaccinated adults can harbour virus levels as high as unvaccinated people if infected with the Delta variant [(1002)]. Sarah Walker, Professor of Medical Statistics and Epidemiology at the University of Oxford and chief investigator of the survey turned the results on their head by saying,

> *"But the fact that they (the vaccinated) can have high levels of virus suggests that people who aren't yet vaccinated may not be as protected from the Delta variant as we hoped. This means it is essential for as many people as possible to get vaccinated, both in the UK and worldwide."*

How Professor Walker can interpret her results showing that the vaccinated are not protected into the unvaccinated are not protected is beyond reason, particularly in light that eight out of ten people are immune (protected) to the SARS-CoV-2 and do not need a vaccine [(858, 1003)].

Israelis with natural immunity are more protected against Delta than vaccinated: Professor Walker is incorrect. People who aren't yet vaccinated but have been naturally infected are in fact more protected than the vaccinated. A large Israeli study proved that natural immune protection that develops after a SARS-CoV-2 infection offers considerably more protection against the Delta variant of the coronavirus pandemic than two doses of the Pfizer-BioNTech vaccine. The study demonstrates the power of the human immune system [(1004)]. Evidence of natural immunity against variants is irrelevant. Shut up! Obey! Take your shot!

Vaccinated are twice as likely to die from the delta variant than unvaccinated: A technical briefing entitled 'SARS-CoV-2 variants of concern and variants under investigation in England' was released in July 2021 by PHE. I got the briefing from the *LifeSite News* website, although I worked out my figures differently. I also took the first dose into account, as *Lancet* data from Israel suggested the vaccine is 85% effective after the first dose [(924)]. Table 8 compares deaths between that vaccinated and unvaccinated from the Delta variant and shows that the deaths from the delta variant in the vaccinated (>21 days post at least one dose vaccine) are twice that seen in the unvaccinated. 36/17,642 (=0.002) / 34/35,521 (=9.6) = 2. At the time this report was released, 85% of the adult population in the UK had been vaccinated [(992)].

Near-total vaccinated Israel, Iceland and Seychelles all went back in lockdown: Near total-vaccinated Iceland, Israel, and Seychelles are experiencing surges in COVID-19 cases and hospitalisation and are back in lockdown. Iceland, Israel and Seychelles have COVID-19 vaccination rates of over 95% and are described as near-total vaccinated [(1005-1007)]. Try as our drug-lords may, it is disingenuous to describe these outbreaks as being due to a 'pandemic of the unvaccinated'. It is also disingenuous to say this means the vaccines are working! So much for Iceland, Israel and Seychelles being 'the most vaccinated country in the world' and for 'leading the world in COVID-19 vaccinations'. These countries have led the world in tyranny. These are the nations that our governments are putting on a pedestal and want to identify as. If we wanted to identify as Israelis, we would move to Israel. Our governments are leading us up the garden path and back into lockdown if we don't stand. The latest 'vaccine success' back in lockdown is 90% double-jabbed Guam.

Table 8: Delta variant death in vaccinated and unvaccinated

	Unvaccinated	**< 21 days post 1st dose**	**> than 21 days post 1st dose**	**> than 14 days post 2nd dose**	**Total vaccinated**
Delta cases	35,521	4,094	9,461	4,087	17,642
Deaths	34	1	10	26	
Death rate	0.0957				0.2097

Breakthrough infection in the US: Again, I document these reports as they were soon censored. No vaccine is 100% effective against any viral disease, yada yada. Cases of breakthrough infection are seen with all vaccines. A breakthrough infection is when someone tests positive for COVID-19 at least 14 days after completing their vaccine series. On April 29th 2021, it was reported that a 75 year old man in the US tested positive and died from COVID-19 more than two weeks after his second vaccine dose. This man had caught the virus from one of his friends who tested positive for COVID-19. Officials in Illinois at this time said at least 97 fully vaccinated people had been hospitalised, and 32 had died. Out of nearly four million people fully vaccinated in Illinois at the time, this represented a breakthrough infection figure of less than 1/100 or 1% [(1008)]. In April 2021, it was reported that 246 fully vaccinated Michigan residents tested positive for COVID-19 and that three of those had died from COVID-19. The daily propaganda rolled out Michigan's top medical executive Dr Joneigh Khaldun to say that even if an individual tests positive for COVID-19 after getting the vaccine, it's highly unlikely that they would be hospitalised or die. Khaldun said,

> *"It is not a failure at all if someone does get COVID-19 after they've had the vaccine. They're likely gonna be not as sick, and they're also likely gonna not pass it to other people who can also get very sick".*

'Likely' and 'gonna'. That gives me so much confidence in vaccines, Heidi. The top medical 'expert' failed to explain why fully vaccinated people who contract COVID-19 after receiving both doses of the COVID-19 vaccine die [(1009)].

The CDC website discusses COVID-19 breakthrough case investigations and reporting. The CDC notes that, like with other vaccines, symptomatic vaccine breakthrough cases occur and that infections among vaccinated people occur. The CDC states, "there is *some* evidence that vaccination *may* make illness less severe". Those two words again; 'some' and 'may' that inspire such confidence in vaccines, Heidi. The CDC continues to say that whilst current data suggests that COVID-19 vaccines offer protection against most circulating SARS-CoV-2 variants, the variants will be responsible for some of these vaccine breakthrough cases. As of April 26th 2021, 95 million people in the US had been fully vaccinated with a COVID-19 vaccine. At this time, the CDC had received reports of breakthrough infections from 46 US states and territories. The total number of vaccine breakthrough infections reported to CDC were, at this time, 9,245. The total number of vaccine breakthrough deaths reported to CDC stood at 132. Isn't it ironic that on May 14th 2020, literally, the day that Biden announced medical apartheid in the US and that the vaxxed could go unmasked, the very next news report was one of an outbreak of COVID-19 among fully vaccinated baseball players and team staff. Major League Baseball team the New York Yankees reported that eight members had tested positive for coronavirus after receiving the one-shot does all Johnson & Johnson (J&J) COVID-19 vaccine. Those infected included coaches, staff members and a player [(1010)]. It goes without saying that the CDC continues on to say; 'Vaccines work'. 'When vaccines don't work, it's because they work'. Shut up! Obey! Take your shot!

Breakthrough infection in India: According to the Indian Council of Medical Research (ICMR) about 11 million recipients received the Covaxin COVID-19 vaccine. Covaxin is India's first indigenous COVID-19 vaccine. Of the 11 million people having received the vaccine, a minimum of 4,208 (0.04%) tested positive for the virus compared with only 695 (0.006%) people testing positive after the second dose. Regarding the Oxford-AstraZeneca's Covishield vaccine, of the 116 million people vaccinated, 17,145 (0.014%) tested positive for the virus after receiving the first dose and 5,014 (0.004%) tested positive after receiving the second dose (1011).

Breakthrough infection in Seychelles: On May 5th 2021, Seychelles announced that even with a 'successful' COVID-19 vaccination rollout, that had seen over 70% of the population receiving one dose and 63% being fully vaccinated against COVID-19, the archipelago with a population close to 100,000 people recorded near to 500 new cases in the three days to May 1st 2021 and had about 1,000 active cases. As the vaccination is not stopping the spread of infection, Seychelles had to bring back restrictions for their residents (1012). A third of the active cases were being seen in people who had received two doses of the vaccine. The remaining cases were occurring in those who had either a single dose of the vaccine or were unvaccinated. The vaccines used in Seychelles are the Chinese-made Sinopharm, the Oxford-AstraZeneca that was produced in India under the name Covishield, and the Russian Sputnik V vaccine (1013).

I premonisce (no crystal ball needed) there will be a new variant every year and a new booster shot (hint, the WHO's new labelling system goes from Alpha to Omega). Queue propaganda reports of the new strain evading natural immunity to previous strains, even though cross-reactive immunity to other coronaviruses is documented, and the recommendation for a booster shot for every man, woman, person, and child on the planet every year. Isn't this new mRNA vaccine technology dandy!

Natural immunity to COVID-19 is far more superior: Comparing this with literally six medically documented cases of reinfection with COVID-19 after natural infection on the whole planet, which can be counted on one hand, and bear in mind, it remains unclear whether true reinfection occurs (1014).

- 25 year old male, US (1015, 1016)
- 33 year old male, Hong Kong (1017)

- 51 year old female, Belgium [1018]
- 46 year old male, Ecuador [1019]
- 20 year old woman, Israel [1020]

Natural immunity is superior to artificially induced vaccine immunity, however 'the science is settled'. Shut up! Obey! Take your shot! Natural immunity is covered in Chapter 17, 'Natural Immunity'.

Earlier reports of flops: In January 2021, Big Pharmaceutical Research and Manufacturers of America (PhRMA) Merck announced that it had ceased developing two of its experimental COVID-19 vaccines after early trial data indicated that the vaccines failed to generate comparable immune responses to either natural infection or other vaccines [1021]. Merck had the bar set too high and will need to redesign its trial protocol accordingly to achieve more positive results. On January 29th 2021, J&J reported its recombinant vector-based COVID-19 vaccine (Ad26.COV2.S) was 66% effective overall in protecting against moderate to severe COVID-19, 28 days after a single dose. The vaccine was tested in a phase III trial involving nearly 44,000 participants in the US, Latin America and South Africa [1022].

A coronavirus vaccine developed by Beijing-based biopharmaceutical company Sinovac Life Sciences CoronaVac was found to be 50.4% effective in Brazilian clinical trials, which is barely over the 50% efficacy required to gain EUA. Several countries, including Brazil, Indonesia, Turkey and Singapore, placed orders for the vaccine. Sinovac is an inactivated vaccine and works by using killed viral particles to expose the body's immune system to the virus 'without risking a serious disease response' [1023]. In October 2020, a day after Brazil's Monster-of-Health, Eduardo Pazuello said Sinovac would be added to the immunisation programme, Brazilian President Jair Bolsonaro said Brazil would not buy the Chinese-made COVID-19 vaccine. The president said the vaccine had not yet finished its trials and that the federal government had reached a deal with São Paulo state to buy 46 million doses of the vaccine CoronaVac, being tested by the Butantan Institute, Brazil's biologic research centre. The CoronaVac vaccine still needs to be approved by the health regulator to be used in the population. Bolsonaro said, "the Brazilian people will not be anyone's guinea pig" [1024]. Whatever vaccine the Brazilian president negotiates, Brazilians will not be 'guinea pigs'; they will be great apes in the global experiment.

CHAPTER FIFTEEN

COVID-19 VACCINES & PREGNANCY SAFETY CONCERNS

"Nature knows no indecencies; man invents them".

Mark Twain (1025)

Pregnant women were excluded from all COVID-19 vaccine trials, so how exactly they know COVID-19 vaccines are safe in pregnancy is beyond the realms of possibility. All the coronavirus disease 2019 (COVID-19) vaccine candidate trials excluded pregnant and lactating, the boffins call them 'individuals'. I respect a person's decision to do whatever they like to their bodies, however I object to pregnant women now having to be referred to as 'pregnant persons' or 'pregnant individuals'. I was a pregnant woman. Virtually all clinical trials exclude pregnant and lactating women from participating. Not including pregnant women in trials is called the 'pregnant person paradox'. That gives me so much confidence in vaccines, Heidi.

The elephant in the room: The term 'expectant mothers' "may offend intersex men and trans men". I can't put it any better myself, Conservative MP Philip Davies said, "If you can't call a pregnant woman an expectant mother, then what is the world coming to?" (1026). In the document entitled 'A guide to effective communication inclusive language in the workplace' published by the British Medical Association (BMA), under 'Pregnancy and Maternity' it states,

> *"Gender inequality is reflected in traditional ideas about the roles of women and men. Though they have shifted over time, the assumptions and stereotypes that underpin those ideas are often deeply rooted. A large majority of people that have been pregnant or have given birth identify as women. We can include intersex men and transmen who may get pregnant by saying 'pregnant people' instead of 'expectant mothers"* (1027).

It is evident to me that transgender men and nonbinary people who can carry a pregnancy can identify as pregnant trans men, pregnant nonbinary, pregnant intersex, etc., and women can identify as pregnant women. Just because a term may offend someone is no reason to trample on the rights of a woman to call herself a woman or be referred to as a woman. No one has a problem discriminating against and offending people with a pro-natural immunity stance. This is all part of the World Economic Forum (WEF) agenda. According to Global Market Insights, Inc. the Sex Reassignment Surgery Market is to hit US$1.5 billion by 2026 [(1028)]. The puberty blocker drug Leuprolide Acetate, trade name Lupron market, is worth US$9.3 billion by 2025. That is enough money to get you into the WEF's old boy network and their Davos A-gender 201 [(1029)].

Obey pregnant women and take your shot: The only division is between rich and poor. We are all equally threatened with mandatory vaccination and the potential negative health consequences. If I were a pregnant woman or pregnant transman, pregnant nonbinary, pregnant intersex or thinking about becoming pregnant, I wouldn't need any expert or authority for me to know there is no way on God's green earth that I would take any vaccine, let alone an unlicensed, experimental biological agent under Emergency Use Authorisation (EUA). The fact-wreckers via GSKoogle will tell you that the COVID-19 vaccine is not called a 'biological agent'. They are correct. As discussed in Chapter 13, 'COVID-19 Vaccines are Safe for Two Months', Pfizer calls their product an 'experimental biological agent' [(796)]. Indeed the Moderna vaccine is not called a 'biological agent'. The Moderna website describes their product as an 'operating system', like an operating system on a computer, however an operating system designed to programme humans [(795)]. The terms 'biological agent' or 'operating system' do not bode well for a developing foetus.

A pregnant woman is not vulnerable! If you're going to have a baby, never let anyone tell you or treat you like you have a condition! As a mother, what really irks me the most about this novel virus and pregnancy is, since when did pregnant women become vulnerable? When I was pregnant, my children came down with the 2005 H1N5 bird flu in Phuket. With three degrees in Complementary and Alternative Medicine (CAM), I don't take my children to doctors unless they get hit by a bus. I was seven months pregnant at the time, and looking back on it, at no stage did I feel 'vulnerable'. I don't need any scientist or authority to tell me that my immune system is highly primed during pregnancy. The concept that pregnancy is associated with immune suppression is a myth. Pregnant women have 50% more blood within which circulates immune components

[1030]. The fundamental feature of a woman's immune system is to protect her foetus from pathogens, and our bodies adapt to do the job nature intends. Pregnancy is not a one-sided effort either. During pregnancy, the maternal immune system is reinforced by a network of recognition, communication, trafficking and repair that, when under attack, will raise the alarm to protect the mother and foetus. The foetus, as a developing active immune system, modifies its mother's response to the environment. A pregnant women's immune system is modulated, not suppressed [1031]. The daily propaganda is lying in an attempt to generate interest in and increase the uptake of vaccines.

All vaccine clinical trials exclude pregnant women: All the COVID-19 vaccine trials, like virtually all clinical trials, excluded pregnant and lactating women from participating [1032]. A *Lancet Global Health Study* published in December 2020 identified 155 COVID-19 therapeutic treatment (not vaccines) studies until April 2020 and found that 80% specifically excluded pregnant women [1033]. God forbid you apply logic, instinct and gut to question if these vaccines are safe for you and your baby in pregnancy or breastfeeding and chose natural medicine. Regardless of the fact that there is limited experience with the use of the Pfizer-BioNTech messenger ribonucleic acid (mRNA) vaccine Comirnaty, and COVID-19 Vaccine Moderna in pregnant or breastfeeding women, the boffin's advice was, until they changed their advice, as this is a new vaccine, as we proceed with the global rollout and include pregnant and breastfeeding women, we will learn about the safety of the COVID-19 vaccine in pregnancy and breastfeeding.

Previous WHO and EMA advice was don't offer COVID-19 vaccines in pregnancy: As the safety of COVID-19 vaccines currently available under EUA has not been tested in pregnant women, no safety data exists specific to use in pregnancy. Initially, global experts and authorities all said do not routinely recommend the COVID-19 vaccines to pregnant women. In January 2021, the WHO recommended against pregnant women receiving COVID-19 mRNA vaccines due to the exclusion of pregnant women and the resulting lack of data on how mRNA vaccines may impact women and their pregnancies [1034]. Regarding the Pfizer-BioNTech vaccine and COVID-19 Moderna vaccine, in June 2021, the European Medicines Agency (EMA) reiterated that there is limited experience with the use of these vaccines in pregnant women; thus the data on the use of these vaccines during pregnancy is insufficient. The EMA continued to say animal studies do not show direct or indirect harmful effects in regard to pregnancy, embryo/foetal development, parturition or postnatal development and recommend the use in pregnant or breastfeeding women [1035]. These agencies did not mention the DNA viral vector COVID-19 vaccines (Oxford-AstraZeneca, Janssen and Sputnik V) and safety in pregnancy.

There were no animal pregnancy studies available at this time to make this recommendation. What the EMA was referring to are called reproductive toxicology studies. Regarding Developmental and Reproductive Toxicity (DART) studies for the Pfizer-BioNTech COVID-19 vaccine, in January 2021, whilst animal data was said to be forthcoming, a verbal report of the data had not indicated any safety signals, and clinical studies in pregnancy were being planned [1036]. In March 2021, an article published in *Obstetrics and Gynaecology* reported that some vaccine manufacturers were expected to conduct clinical trials in pregnant women after DART studies were completed. Up until this time, pregnant women were being advised to consult their obstetricians to weigh the benefits and risks of COVID-19 vaccines using available data. As additional information from clinical trials and data collected on vaccinated pregnant women becomes available, the official advice was that obstetricians must keep up to date with this information [1037].

Flip-flop pregnancy advice; offer the COVID-19 vaccine at any stage of pregnancy: Whilst the monkeys are waiting for the scientific data revealed from quality human trials, the advice for our species is wishy-washy. In January 2021, Ireland's National Immunisation Advisory Committee (NIAC) and the National Public Health Emergency Team (NPHET) said that, although the available safety data did not indicate any safety concern or harm to pregnancy, there was insufficient evidence to recommend routine use of COVID-19 mRNA vaccines during pregnancy. Recommendations in January 2021 were that the administration of the Comirnaty or Moderna COVID-19 vaccine in pregnancy should only be considered when the potential benefits outweigh any potential risks for the mother and foetus. NIAC recommended the Pfizer-BioNTech mRNA vaccine Comirnaty and COVID-19 Moderna vaccine, where it is decided that the risk/benefit ratio is favourable. The advice was that the two-dose schedule should not commence before 14 weeks gestation and should be completed by 33 weeks gestation [1038]. Enter a scientific U-turn. In September 2021, NIAC flip-flopped to recommend that COVID-19 mRNA vaccines be offered to women at "any stage of pregnancy".

Enter another scientific U-turn by other global vaccination agencies, with the 'science' now saying offer any COVID-19 vaccine to women at any stage of pregnancy. Big Pharmaceutical Research and Manufacturers of America (PhRMA) employees, the American College of Obstetricians and Gynaecologists (ACOG) professional association now recommends that COVID-19 vaccines should not be withheld from pregnant women and should be offered to lactating women [(1039)]. On June 9th 2021, the Royal Australian and New Zealand College of Obstetricians and Gynaecologists (RANZCOG) and the Australian Technical Advisory Group on Immunisation (ATAGI), whilst acknowledging that the large majority of pregnant women infected with COVID-19 will experience only mild or moderate cold/flu-like symptoms, they recommended that pregnant women be routinely offered the Pfizer mRNA vaccine Comirnaty at any stage of pregnancy. This recommendation was made because the risk of 'severe outcomes' from COVID-19 is significantly higher for pregnant women and their unborn babies, even though as they stated simultaneously, the large majority of pregnant women infected with COVID-19 will experience only mild or moderate cold/flu-like symptoms [(1040)].

Great apes: Have confidence in vaccines! The animal studies do not indicate harmful effects in pregnancy! An article entitled 'Current global vaccine and drug efforts against COVID-19: Pros and cons of bypassing animal trials' in the *Journal of Biosciences* stated that that human outcomes cannot be predicted in the absence of animal studies [(800)]. Humans are a sub-group of primates known as the great apes; therefore we are officially the great apes in the global experiment. The Pfizer-BioNTech mRNA vaccine Comirnaty preclinical trials tested six rhesus macaques monkeys who were vaccinated and then exposed to the severe acute respiratory syndrome coronavirus 2 (SARS-CoV-2) virus, and those vaccinated were found to have less of the virus in their lower and upper respiratory tracts [(801, 802)]. No mention here of the monkeys being pregnant. The original Oxford University report was based on the vaccination of six rhesus macaques, and the vaccinated monkeys became infected when challenged (deliberately infected with the virus) [(803)]. No mention here of the monkeys being pregnant. The Moderna COVID-19 vaccine trial involved 24 rhesus macaques. Eight monkeys were used as controls, eight given a low dose of vaccine and eight given a high dose [804]. No mention here of the monkeys being pregnant. Pregnant women are being told the 'benefits outweigh the risks'. Pregnant women are not being told their data is being stored by Big PhRMA as the pregnant primates in the great global experiment.

Developmental and reproductive toxicity studies: When the boffins say the COVID-19 vaccines are safe in pregnancy, they are referring to developmental and reproductive toxicity (DART) studies in rats that Moderna conducted that "didn't uncover anything worrisome" [1032]. DART studies are conducted in rodents (mice or rats) and rabbits. Conducting DART studies in each species has advantages, disadvantages and limitations. The following information refers to the Pfizer-BioNTech mRNA vaccine Comirnaty. In February 2021, after already administering its COVID-19 vaccines to countless, unsuspecting pregnant women, Pfizer announced a global clinical trial to evaluate its COVID-19 vaccine in pregnant women. Prior to conducting their COVID-19 vaccine clinical trial in pregnant women, regulatory authorities required Pfizer-BioNTech to complete a DART study [1041]. The decision to evaluate the COVID-19 vaccine in pregnant women was on consideration that the safety and efficacy profile of the vaccine in pregnancy would be similar to that observed in non-pregnant individuals. However, DART study results showed that vaccine ingredients accumulate in ovaries and testes, which has not been publicly disclosed.

Reproductive targets in biodistribution: Pharmacokinetics refers to drug absorption, biodistribution, metabolism and excretion. Biodistribution refers to where the drug goes in the body. Research showed the Pfizer vaccine components, including the lipid nanoparticle (LNP) packaged mRNA accumulates in high concentrations in the female ovary. Canadian immunologist and vaccine researcher, Byram Bridle, gained access to Pfizer's biodistribution study through the Japanese regulatory agency [1042]. This study is referred to as the 'Pfizer ovaries study in English'. The 'Pfizer ovaries study in English' states that when the LNP packaged mRNA vaccines are injected intramuscularly, the concentration is at the highest value at the administration site and distributes widely throughout the body, including blood, plasma, brain, adrenals, bone, lung, uterus etc. The highest values aside from the injection site are in the liver, spleen, adrenals and ovaries. RNA encapsulated LNP also accumulate in the male testes

[1043]. As previously mentioned in Chapter 13, 'COVID-19 Vaccines are Safe for Two Months', polyethylene glycol (PEG) is a polyether compound derived from petroleum and the potential exists that graphene is bound to PEG. Polyethylene is the most common form of plastic, and when combined with glycol, it becomes a thick and sticky liquid [1044].

Table 9 and Table 10 show Pfizer's biodistribution data for RNA encapsulated LNP accumulating in the female ovaries and male testes. The long-term effects of which remain unknown.

Table 9: Total lipid concentration (µg lipid equivalent/g [or ml]) Ovaries

Time	0.25 h	1 h	2 h	4 h	8 h	24 h	48 h
µg /g	0.104	1.34	1.64	2.34	3.09	5.24	12.4

Table 10: Total lipid concentration (µg lipid equivalent/g [or ml]) Testes

Time	0.25 h	1 h	2 h	4 h	8 h	24 h	48 h
µg /g	0.031	0.042	0.79	0.129	0.146	0.304	0.320

European Medicines Agency study contradicts Pfizer's biodistribution study: An EMA pharmacokinetics study assessed the biodistribution of the two novel lipids, ALC-0315 (aminolipid) and ALC-0159 (PEG-lipid) in rats, a LNP-formulated surrogate luciferase RNA in mice, and a [3H]-labelled LNP-mRNA formulation in rats. The EMA study concluded that no evidence of vaccine-related macroscopic or microscopic findings was found in the ovaries in the repeat-dose toxicity studies, and no effects on fertility were identified in the DART study [1045]. These results contradict Pfizer's biodistribution study and are a cause for alarm.

The luciferase protein: mRNA SARS-CoV-2 vaccines are encapsulated in lipid nanoparticles. These novel lipids open new avenues for mRNA vaccines in general and for COVID-19 vaccines in particular. Rather than work directly with the virus (perhaps because it hasn't been isolated?), COVID-19 vaccine researchers manufactured pseudotyped viral particles. These manufactured pseudotyped viral particles typically carry a reporter plasmid, which is very likely known as firefly luciferase (FLuc) [1046]. A preprint article published in *bioRxiv* in October 2020 described the SARS-CoV-2 vaccine as an *"LNP-encapsulated luciferase mRNA vaccine"*. This article concluded that further research is required to examine how the luciferase protein is expressed in various tissues and organs; doublespeak for 'the boffins need a billion in 'research grants' to conclude that 'more research is warranted!' (1047)

'Conspiracy' about COVID-19 vaccines causing infertility: I have discovered that if a 'fact-checker' is checking a 'conspiracy theory', more often than not, the 'conspiracy theory' has legs and is an agenda (a plan). I found this with the information surrounding COVID-19 vaccines causing infertility which should warrant further study prior to vaccinating pregnant women. It goes without saying that the fact-wreckers say there is no evidence the Pfizer COVID-19 vaccine affects women's fertility. What they fail is to say is there is no evidence to the contrary. Fact-checker funding and conflict of interest was discussed in Chapter 4, 'Vaccine Refusal and the Age of Censorship'. The cause for concern is that the SARS-CoV spike protein and syncytin 1of the placenta is structurally similar. Therefore the potential exists for the antibodies made to attack the spike protein to attack syncytin 1. The fact-checkers say this is not likely, not because the possibility has been studied in women, but because "only two very small parts of these proteins look the same...and the body's immune system is not likely to confuse the two, and attack syncytin-1 rather than the spike protein on SARS-CoV-2 and stop a placenta forming" (1048). There are those words again; 'not likely'. My confidence in vaccines has skyrocketed. It must be known that 20% of the population, or one in five people, have an autoimmune disease (699). In Ireland, there was a spate of stillbirths in the first few months of 2021 that clinicians linked to SARS-CoV-2 infections. Keelin O'Donoghue, an obstetrician at Cork University Maternal Hospital, described the placentas as being extensively damaged. "The placentas look completely burnt out, just incredibly necrotic and damaged" (1049). If SARS-CoV-2 infection can cause this placental damage, it is possible that vaccine-generated spike proteins could also result in the same injury. This hypothesis should be investigated, not discounted.

All about syncytin: Syncytin 1 is a new gene from an endogenous retrovirus (HERV) in the human genome and is implicated in placental development, specifically in syncytiotrophoblast (SynT) development, the outermost layer of the placenta (1050). The syncytiotrophoblast is directly exposed to the maternal blood and is the main site of gas exchange and the transfer of nutrients and waste products between maternal and foetal blood [1051]. The SARS coronavirus (SARS-CoV) spike protein and syncytin 1and are homologous, meaning structurally similar. The two heptad repeat regions (NHR and CHR) of SARS-CoV are homologous to, that is similar in size and shape to, the two heptad repeat regions (NHR and CHR) in syncytin [1052]. When molecules are similar in size and shape, the immune system, particularly a naïve immune system unexposed to infectious disease due to modern-day living, may be unable to tell these cells apart. This inability to differentiate cells is called molecular mimicry and is due to the hygiene hypothesis, which science has not disproved. Molecular mimicry and the hygiene hypothesis are explained in greater detail in Chapter 17, 'Natural Immunity'. If, after vaccination, or indeed after natural infection, the body makes antibodies to the SARS-CoV spike protein (antigen), because of structural similarity, the immune system of a naïve individual may be unable to differentiate between SARS-CoV-2 spike protein and syncytin 1. Thus a genuine potential exists for autoimmunity and for a woman's body to attack her own placenta. This needs proper investigation prior to an indiscriminate global rollout.

Forced sterilisation: It is a cover-up, not a conspiracy, that Big PhRMA makes vaccines that attack human chorionic gonadotropin (hCG), the hormone essential to pregnancy. Further work is currently being undertaken to study the efficacy of these vaccines in humans for preventing pregnancy. Anti-fertility vaccines were used to forcibly sterilise Kenyan women. In November 2014, doctors and Catholic bishops denounced a United Nations (UN) vaccine programme in Kenya for purposefully sterilising millions of women. The Kenya Catholic Doctors Association ordered laboratory tests of WHO and UNICEF tetanus vaccines being administered in Kenya and discovered that the vaccine was laced with the anti-fertility drug hCG, otherwise known as a sterilising agent. The hCG found in the UN tetanus vaccines caused the women's bodies to develop antibodies to attack hCG, resulting in the death of the unborn child in the womb. These vaccinations were given to Kenyan women under the guise of 'preventing neonatal tetanus' and resulted in permanent sterility. The women were completely unaware and did not provide free, prior and informed consent [742]. In 1995, a priest (name not listed) and president of Human Life International (HLI) asked Congress to investigate reports of women in developing countries unknowingly receiving a tetanus vaccine laced with the anti-fertility drug hCG. If it was found to be true, the priest wanted the United States (US) Congress to publicly condemn the mass vaccinations and to cut off funding to UN agencies and other organisations involved in administering anti-fertility vaccines using hCG. These organisations include the usual list of 'population control' advocates, which is doublespeak for 'depopulation advocates'; the WHO, UN Population Fund, UN Development Programme, World Bank, Population Council, Rockefeller Foundation, US National Institute of Child Health and Human Development, All India Institute of Medical Sciences, and Uppsala, Helsinki, and Ohio State universities (61).

Between 1996 and 2000, during the Fujimori regime, more than 200,000 women in Peru were sterilised without providing free, prior and informed consent. A paper published in *Global Public Health* in 2020 attempted to understand the policies that legitimised the violation of women's rights through forcible sterilisation. These policies were due to the precarious structures occurring during a dictatorial regime and the narratives around sterilisation and reproduction produced by policymakers, political and religious leaders and healthcare workers during the time of the regime (73). We all live under the dictatorial regime called emergency COVID laws.

Anti-fertility/sterilising vaccines in animals: The principle of anti-hCG vaccines is to induce antibodies that can bind to hCG and render it biologically inactive. Other anti-fertility vaccines work against other hormones that regulate fertility. These anti-fertility vaccines 'react against', in other words, produce a bioeffective antibody response that attacks follicle-stimulating hormone (FSH), luteinising hormone (LH) and gonadotropin-releasing hormone (GnRH). Intratesticular injection of the Bacillus Calmette-Guerin (BCG), or tuberculosis vaccine, is used in animals to cause the degeneration of the blood-testes barrier, which leads to reversible azoospermia (semen containing no sperm) (1053).

Anti-fertility/sterilising vaccines in humans: As far back as 1989, anti-fertility vaccines inducing antibodies against the hCG had gone through phase I human trials. A vaccine producing a bioeffective antibody response to attack GnRH was, at the time, ready for phase I/II clinical trials in human prostate carcinoma patients. Vaccines that react against FSH and LH were also in the pipeline. Anti-hCG vaccines included beta-hCG linked to the tetanus toxoid, cholera toxin and the diphtheria toxoid vaccines. These vaccines had, at the time, shown efficiency in controlling fertility in baboons, and indeed, the beta-hCG- tetanus toxoid vaccine was shown to produce anti-hCG antibodies in 61 of 63 women tested. As far back as 1989, scientists were saying that the use of recombinant DNA techniques could potentially accelerate the development of male and female anti-fertility vaccines in humans [(1054)]. Janssen, Sputnik V, and Oxford-AstraZeneca COVID-19 vaccines are recombinant DNA vaccines, although the boffins prefer us to call them viral vector vaccines [(1055)]. The boffins would also prefer we believe that anti-fertility vaccines in humans are a conspiracy theory.

By 1990, a study published in *Contraception*, entitled 'Phase I clinical trials with three formulations of anti-human chorionic gonadotropin vaccine' discussed the clinical trials that were being conducted at the National Institute of Immunology in New Delhi, India, to control male and female fertility in humans. A total of 116 tubal ligated (tubes tied) female volunteers were enrolled in the study, and 101 subjects were followed up for one year or more until the antibody titres declined to near-zero levels. This anti-fertility vaccine was combined with tetanus toxoid vaccines. Every woman who received the vaccine produced anti-hCG and anti-tetanus antibodies [(1056)]. As previously mentioned, these anti-hCG vaccines are also effective when combined with cholera and diphtheria toxoid vaccines. Moving forward 30 years to 2017, a study published in *Frontiers in Bioscience* (*Elite edition*) discussed phase I clinical trials that had been conducted in India, Finland, Sweden, Chile and Brazil that proved the ability of vaccines to induce antibodies against hCG and their reversibility and safety. The authors noted that utilising a hetero-species dimer linked to tetanus toxoid enhanced the vaccine's 'immunogenicity', in other words, its sterilising effect. Phase II clinical trials showed that anti-hCG vaccines prevented pregnancy of sexually active fertile women without disturbing ovulation or menstrual regularity. When these anti-hCG antibodies waned, women were able to conceive again and give birth to a healthy child. A genetically engineered vaccine consisting of beta hCG linked to E. coli has been made. The National Review Committee on Genetic Manipulation and Drugs Controller General of India cleared this vaccine to prevent pregnancy for human clinical trials [(1057)].

As discussed further in Chapter 21, 'Chips, Dots and Bots', Gates wants to control our fertility with his big remote control. The Gates Foundation gave a grant of US$2 million to Microchips Biotech Inc. for the 'Purpose: to develop a personal system that enables women to regulate their fertility'

[1058]. This is a microchip-based implant that is able to be wirelessly controlled for the purposes of birth control [1059].

First data on COVID-19 vaccines in pregnancy: There was some talk that the abortion rates were 83% in women receiving their COVID-19 vaccine in the first trimester from a study by Shimabukuro, et al. published in the *New England Journal of Medicine* in 2021, regarding the mRNA vaccines only. I had a look at that data, and thankfully, this is not what I noted. The data from the v-safe pregnancy registry and the Vaccine Adverse Event Reporting System (VAERS) examined live birth, stillbirth, induced abortion and ectopic pregnancy in women who had received a COVID-19 vaccine and compared this with the general population before COVID (BC). The registry enrolled 3958 participants with vaccination from December 14th 2020 to February 28th 2021. Among 827 participants who had a completed pregnancy, the pregnancy resulted in a live birth in 712 women, meaning 125 women lost their babies. 125 abortions out of 827 completed pregnancies equates to a 15% abortion rate. The estimated frequency of spontaneous abortion BC was between 12% and 24% of all clinically identified pregnancies [1060]. Although the results are preliminary, I don't see a difference between the spontaneous abortion rates in COVID-19 vaccinated pregnant women and the normal rate of spontaneous abortion. Two things concern me about this study. Firstly, proper science would compare abortion rates in vaccinated women to completely unvaccinated women. Secondly, authors contradict themselves by saying women are encouraged to report congenital anomalies (birth defects) to VAERS, then they note that, as is the requirement under the EUA, no congenital anomalies are allowed to be reported to the VAERS [1061]. That gives me so much confidence in vaccines, Heidi.

Men matter: It takes two to tango. At present, the effects of COVID-19 vaccines on sperm are completely undetermined. There is currently an ongoing prospective case study whereby men scheduled to receive the COVID-19 vaccine will have the effect on semen evaluated for six months post-vaccination [1062].

Babies: Newborn babies are not susceptible to SARS-CoV-2 infection! Babies are born with antibodies against SARS-CoV-2 and protected from COVID-19. This is covered in Chapter 17, 'Natural Immunity'.

CHAPTER SIXTEEN

CRIMINALITY, LITIGATION AND ZERO LIABILITY

"This is a unique situation where we as a company simply cannot take the risk if in...four years the vaccine is showing side effects".

AstraZeneca senior executive Ruud Dobber [1063]

Criminality, corruption and dubious connections: I could write a book on drug company corruption, however I have chosen to use New York-based drug giant Pfizer as an example because they are the King of Corrupt. The coronavirus disease 2019 (COVID-19) vaccine manufacturer Pfizer is a criminal. Do you score your drugs from a criminal then inject your children with the drug produced by that criminal? That's exactly what parents are doing. We had the bank bailouts; now we have the pharmaceutical bailout. Pfizer's projected earnings from COVID-19 vaccine sales were US$15 billion-plus [1064]. This has since doubled to US$33.5 billion. The courts describe Pfizer as a *"habitual offender, persistently engaging in illegal and corrupt marketing practices, bribing physicians and suppressing adverse trial results"*.

Since 2002, Pfizer and its subsidiaries have paid out US$3 billion in criminal convictions, civil penalties and jury awards. In September 2009, Pfizer agreed to a record US$2.3 billion to settle civil and criminal allegations that it improperly marketed 13 medicines [1065]. This record-setting by Pfizer is not like setting a new Olympic record. We shouldn't be giving them a golden hand-shake. The US$2.3 billion payout was to settle claims of off-label promotion of the cyclooxygenase 2 (COX-2) inhibitor Bextra (Valdecoxib), a nonsteroidal anti-inflammatory drug used to treat osteoarthritis, rheumatoid arthritis and period pain. Valdecoxib was withdrawn in 2005 after it was found to increase the risk of cardiovascular disease, and there were reports of serious and potentially life-threatening skin reactions [1066]. Pfizer also faced a cluster of lawsuits after evidence showed that the drug Lipitor (atorvastatin) increased a women's risk of developing diabetes by as much as 700%. Why people trust that Pfizer is not now illegally marketing their Comirnaty COVID-19 mRNA vaccine is beyond reason.

COVID-colonialism is alive and kicking: In 2007, *The BMJ* wrote that Nigeria filed civil and criminal charges against Pfizer for its role in the deaths and disabilities of Nigerian children treated with an experimental drug during a meningitis epidemic back in 1996 (1067). Our vaccine saviour Pfizer tested this new drug on Nigerian children without obtaining prior official approval or free and informed consent. Pfizer admitted that local ethics approval given to conduct the trial may not have been properly documented. Europe withdrew the drug licence due to links with liver toxicity and 'some' deaths (1068). Why people believe that Pfizer cares about our children is beyond reason.

Why we are bailing out Pfizer: Money talks. According to Open Secrets The Centre for Responsive Politics, a United States (US) research and government transparency group that tracks money in politics and how this helps determine the outcome of elections, Pfizer made a contribution of US$3,782,466, ranking 175 out of 21,464 contributors, and spent $US11 million lobbying America politicians in the US in 2020 alone. The largest recipient was, as you may have guessed, President Biden-his-time-until-Kamala-takes-over (1069).

Vaccine injury: As discussed previously, adverse reactions (ADRs) following vaccination are also known as adverse events following immunisation (AEFI). The adverse event may be any unfavourable or unintended sign, abnormal laboratory finding, symptom or disease. Compensation claims are made for AEFI and vaccine injury. Payments are awarded for what is determined as either a 'true reaction' or a 'temporally coincidental event'. Adverse events do not necessarily have a causal relationship with the vaccine. The World Health Organisation (WHO) recently revised the AEFI classification in which the definition of 'causal association' was changed. Causal association is now only used when there is "no other factor intervening in the processes" (642). For example, if a person has an underlying condition that worsens after a vaccine, then that is not seen as causally related. Vaccine injury was explained in Chapter 12, 'Vaccines aren't Described as Safe and don't Always Work'.

All gain, no pain: COVID-19 vaccines manufacturers won't agree to procurement contracts or ship vaccines without liability protection. An AstraZeneca executive explained the company's bilateral contracts grant protection against all legal claims arising from the use of its AstraZeneca

COVID-19 vaccine since it "cannot take the risk" of liability [1070]. After the United Kingdom (UK) approval of the Pfizer COVID-19 vaccine, the UK state underwrote COVID-19 vaccine companies in a bid to 'reassure' the UK population. The UK government agreed to indemnify five pharmaceutical companies manufacturing COVID-19 vaccines against any liabilities from vaccine injury during the UK COVID-19 vaccine rollout [1071]. My government underwriting a vaccine company's liability 'reassures' me and increases my confidence in vaccines, Heidi.

The money is in autoimmune disease: The incidence and prevalence of non-communicable autoimmune diseases are rising fast every year. The global autoimmune disease diagnosis and therapeutic market is one of the fastest-growing and is expected to reach US$14 billion per year by 2025. Rheumatic disease such as rheumatoid arthritis is increasing by 7% per year, endocrine disease such as type 1 diabetes is increasing by 6.3% per year, neurological disease such as multiple sclerosis (MS) is increasing by 3.7% a year, coeliac disease is increasing by 4-9% a year. Autoimmune disease costs the British economy £13 billion per year [1072]. Meanwhile, the likes of our own Trinity College Dublin Professor of Biochemistry and Immunology, Lukey Kooky co-founded the biopharmaceutical company Sitryx, a company that manufactures immunometabolism drugs to treat autoimmune disease. GlaxoSmithKline (GSK) helped Sitryx raise US$30 million (€26 million) in funding to help advance these immunometabolism drugs toward human testing [1073]. If only the boffins would spend some of their grant money conducting the study comparing vaccinated to unvaccinated, perhaps we wouldn't need immunometabolism drugs.

Vaccine injury compensation programmes: As vaccines carry inherent risk, vaccine injury compensation programmes (VICPs) are no-fault schemes that were established to compensate individuals who experience vaccine injury. VICPs do not require injured parties or their legal representatives to prove negligence or fault by the vaccine provider, the health care system or the manufacturer before compensation. The programmes serve to waive the requirement for accessing compensation through litigation. As the global capacity for vaccine safety surveillance improves and more reporting of AEFI in low- and middle-income countries occur, WHO member states claim to be identifying and documenting reactions with scientific evidence of causal associations [1074]. As discussed in Chapter 12, 'Vaccines aren't Described as Safe and don't Always Work', the Global

Vaccine Safety Summit experts admit to not having adequate post-vaccination surveillance. WHO Chief Boffin Dr Soumya Swaminathan said in 2019,

> *"I think we cannot overemphasise the fact that we really don't have very good safety monitoring systems in many countries and this adds the...the miscommunications and apprehensions because we are not able to give clear cut answers when people ask questions about deaths...this always gets blown up in the media...one should be able to give a very factual account of what has happened and what the cause of the deaths are ..in most cases there's some obfuscation at that level, and therefore there is less and less trust then in the system"* (761).

That gives me so much confidence in vaccines, Heidi.

Scheming: A WHO review of international schemes on no-fault compensation VICPs explains that the schemes reflect a belief that it is fair and reasonable that the community protected by a vaccination programme accepts responsibility for and provides compensation to those injured by it. From a population-level perspective, it is considered that the 'benefits' of widespread immunisation outweighs the 'small risks'. It is deemed ethically acceptable that individuals 'occasionally' bear a significant burden for the benefit provided to the rest of the population. There are currently a total of 19 countries only with vaccine compensation schemes. Germany enacted a vaccine compensation scheme in 1961 after the German Supreme Court had earlier ruled that people affected by vaccine injury through compulsory smallpox vaccination were entitled to compensation. France implemented a vaccine compensation scheme in the 1960s. During the 1970s, concerns over adverse events following diphtheria-tetanus-pertussis (DTP) vaccination led to vaccine compensation schemes being established in Austria, Denmark, Japan, New Zealand, Sweden, Switzerland and the UK. During the 1980s, Taiwan, Finland, the US and Quebec implemented vaccine compensation schemes. During the 1990s, Italy, Norway and the Republic of Korea followed suit. The most recent schemes were implemented in Hungary, Iceland and Slovenia. Even now in 'mandatory vaccine 2021', significant public pressure is being put on Australia, Canada and Ireland to establish similar schemes. Recently, China has shown interest in a no-fault compensation. By 2011, there were still no schemes covering developing countries (1075). Developing countries are now covered for COVID-19 vaccine injury under a world first no-fault compensation scheme discussed shortly [1076]. As will be explained, coverage is vague however.

Vaccine-injured children: The National Vaccine Injury Compensation Programme (VICP) was created after the National Childhood Vaccine Injury Act of 1986. The VICP was created as a no-fault alternative to the traditional tort system (personal injury lawsuits) and began accepting claims in 1988. The VICP provides compensation to people who have been injured by vaccines. Even in cases in which such a finding is not conclusive, claimants (petitioners) may receive compensation settlements. The VICP was established after lawsuits against vaccine manufacturers and healthcare providers threatened to cause vaccine shortages and derail vaccination programmes [1077]. Vaccine injury compensation arose after the historical vaccine scares and withdrawals as described in Chapter 12, 'Vaccines aren't Described as Safe and don't Always Work', particularly the Cutter incident (polio vaccine) and diphtheria-tetanus-pertussis (DTP) vaccine lawsuits. Basically, vaccine manufacturers stopped producing vaccines as they couldn't afford the lawsuits against them. Once our governments agreed to assume liability for vaccine injury, it was full steam ahead to injure.

Vaccines carry inherent risk: Yes, we know the mantra 'vaccines are safe'; 'vaccines save lives'; nevertheless, vaccines carry inherent risk. Reflecting this risk is that, despite authorities doing everything in their power to prevent payouts, US$4 billion in vaccine injury compensations payouts through the VICP have been awarded since 1988 in the US alone. Filing a claim for vaccine injury through the Court of Federal Claims requires a US$250 filing fee, which can be waived for those unable to pay. In 2019, US$46,146,803 in total was paid out in compensation for vaccine injury in the US. The breakdown of the outlays is as follows; 203 injury petitions were filed, 116 compensations were awarded, and 13 payments were made to attorneys. The awards reported in 2019 were, in fact, at the lowest level since 2007. These reductions in payout in the year 2019 are thought to be due to a change in the definition of a vaccine injury known as shoulder injury resulting from vaccine administration (SIRVA).

Removing SIRVA from the Vaccine Injury Table saves money: SIRVA is a preventable injury caused by injecting a vaccine into the shoulder capsule rather than the deltoid muscle resulting in inflammation of the shoulder structures, causing pain, a decreased range of motion and a decreased quality of life. According to an investigational team's reporting, approximately 50% of all the new federal vaccine injury cases alleged a SIRVA, and have little or nothing to do with what was in the vaccine [(1078)]. The Department of Health and Human Service's VICP made a revision to remove SIRVA from the Revisions to the Vaccine Injury Table [(1079)]. The Centres for Disease Control and Prevention (CDC) and the Health Resources and Services Administration (HRSA) now say that most cases of SIRVA are caused by the vaccines being administered too high on the arm and not the actual vaccine. Additionally, the HRSA say, "there is a confidentiality provision in the programme which prohibits the agency from notifying the vaccine administrator of the corresponding SIRVA case". As the person administering the vaccine is protected from liability, the vaccinator is not a party to the lawsuit. Each potential SIRVA victim now has to give written consent that they understand the vaccine injury the vaccinator might cause and how they will not be compensated in such an event [(652)].

COVAX the COVID-19 vaccine liability mechanism: In 1999 the Bill & Melinda Gates Foundation pledged US$750 million to set up Gavi, the Vaccine Alliance (Gavi). Gavi co-leads the COVID-19 Vaccines Global Access (COVAX) Facility. COVAX is one of three pillars of the access COVID-19 Tools (ACT) Accelerator. COVAX is the global risk-sharing mechanism to accelerate development, production, and equitable access to COVID-19 vaccines. Launched by the WHO in April 2020, COVAX is a conglomeration of Gavi, the WHO, UNICEF, Bill & Melinda Gates Foundation, the Coalition for Epidemic Preparedness Innovations (CEPI) and the World Bank [(1076)]. The WHO and G7 leaders have pledged to intensify cooperation on COVID-19 and increase their contribution to the COVAX vaccine-sharing initiative [(1080)].

The breakneck speed at which the COVID-19 vaccine was developed increases the risks of unforeseen events. To support the then vaccine candidates, governments brought in liability waivers that were "focused on the fair distribution, as opposed to turning a profit". They must have overlooked that Pfizer's alone projected earnings are US$33 billion in 2021. Leading the taxpayers who paid for the COVID-19 vaccine to believe that vaccine companies are altruistic is disingenuine. Even 'no-profit pledge' AstraZeneca has raked in US$1.5 billion. COVAX finances COVID-19 vaccine doses for 92 low-income and low-middle income countries. The remaining 97 countries participating in COVAX are self-financing, high-income and upper-middle-income countries. As of December 7th 2020, the US and Russia had thus far opted out of COVAX participation (1081). The 92 low-income and low-middle-income countries in which COVAX is financing COVID-19 vaccines are mainly in Africa and South-East Asia. Essentially, COVAX means that these governments face little or no costs from COVID-19 vaccine injury claims brought by patients. Dozens of middle-income countries, such as South Africa, Lebanon, Gabon, Iran and most Latin American states, are not covered by the COVAX mechanism hence, not protected (1082).

In the past, potential compensation costs have hampered the WHO's efforts to distribute vaccines to low-income countries. The COVAX facilities primary purpose is to allay fears that could hamper a global COVID-19 vaccine rollout. It is also hoped that the COVAX mechanism would avoid a repetition of the delays experienced during the 2009 H1N1 swine influenza pandemic when the H1N1 influenza vaccine (Pandemrix) rollout was hampered in dozens of low-income countries because there was no clear liability. COVAX aims to distribute at least two billion COVID-19 vaccines around the world by the end of 2021 (1083).

As of October 2020, COVAX remained vastly underfunded, having only received about a quarter of the US$16 billion the WHO and Gavi estimated it required by the end of 2021. Under the COVAX scheme, high-income countries assume COVID-19 vaccine liability. A COVAX document says, "Participants will be responsible for deployment and use of approved vaccines within their territories and assuming any liability associated with such use and deployment". These contractual obligations apply to European Union (EU), China and the middle-income countries, including Argentina, Iran, Iraq, South Africa and Mexico. Even though the EU 27 nation bloc pledged money to the COVAX scheme, the potential hidden costs arising from this assumption of liability meant the EU decided not to take delivery of COVID-19 vaccines through COVAX. Instead, the EU separately negotiated with vaccine companies to pay a higher price for the vaccine in return for the firms accepting some liability for potential compensation. Under Donald Trump's presidency, the White House refused to fund COVAX and instead negotiated its own deals with drug companies under which blanket legal immunity was given to COVID-19 vaccine manufacturers [1084].

Good thing Biden got in: As mentioned, Trump's White House opted out of the COVAX scheme in September 2020 [1085]. While President Trump was still in office, founder and executive chairman of the World Economic Forum (WEF) supreme leader Satan Klaus said, *"we've got a bit of a problem because when it comes to COVAX, for example, while the EU was quick to back this, we have players like the US and Russia that are not on board"*. Schwab said that Joe Biden "will boost multilateralism". Multilateralism is an alliance of multiple countries in pursuit of a common goal [1086]. Under Joe Biden's presidency, the White House pledged US$4 billion to the COVAX scheme at the G7 meeting in February 2021 [1087]. Then it was full steam ahead to injure with COVID-19 vaccines.

Liability conditions remain vague: COVID-19 vaccine liability conditions remain a concern as liability terms remain vague. Without clearly stated liability terms, governments of poor countries may still be liable for potential compensation claims. This may put these countries off participating in the COVAX scheme. Whilst Vietnam is covered under the COVAX scheme, Vietnam is eligible for free or cheaper COVAX vaccines and is therefore unlikely to use the COVID-19 vaccines provided by the global facility. A Vietnamese health official described that supply deals it negotiates bilaterally with pharmaceutical companies are more transparent than COVAX's terms. Kenya is also eligible under the COVAX scheme, however Kenya's Chief Administrative Secretary at the Ministry of Health, Rashid Aman, said that Kenya expected the vaccine makers bear some responsibility.

Different horses for different courses: Different vaccine manufacturers are striking different deals with different countries. European governments have agreed to pay claims above an agreed limit against vaccine injury caused by the Oxford-AstraZeneca COVID-19 vaccine. Different terms were agreed with French drugmaker Sanofi, the manufacturer of the Pfizer-BioNTech COVID-19 vaccine. Under this deal, Oxford-AstraZeneca would pay legal costs up to a certain agreed threshold. Exactly how these costs would be shared with individual European governments, or what the cap is, was not elaborated on. In return for the higher price paid for its COVID-19 vaccine, Sanofi, which partners with GlaxoSmithKline, did not get any liability waiver [1088]. The more you pay, the less you pay.

A new and unimproved COVID-19 vaccine injury compensation programme: As mentioned, an important tool for maintaining public trust following the rollout of a new vaccine is to guarantee that victims are rapidly and adequately compensated. Guaranteeing that recipients of COVID-19 vaccines are automatically eligible for compensation that covers healthcare costs and loss of livelihoods helps maintain public vaccine compliance [(1089)]. In the US, the Public Readiness and Emergency Preparedness Act (PREP Act) authorised the Secretary of Health and Human Services (HIH) (the Secretary) to establish the Countermeasures Injury Compensation Programme (CICP) Programme. This CICP programme is designed to benefit the person who sustains serious physical injuries or death as a direct result of administration or use of covered countermeasures identified by the Secretary in declarations issued under the PREP Act [(1090)]. A directive issued by HHS Secretary Alex M. Azar II on March 17th 2020 mandated that individuals who suffer ADRs from COVID-19 vaccines must bring their claims for compensation to the CICP. The CICP was set up specifically to deal with vaccines under Emergency Use Authorisation (EUA) and has replaced the VICP [(1091)].

The C.I.C.P. is C.R.A.P. COVID-19 vaccine-injured face an injury payment 'black hole'. The CICP employs only four people and shares little characteristics of a normal court. Government officials make decisions in secret. There is no route for claimants to appeal to a judge. Payouts for death cases are capped at US$370,376. Cases before the Vaccine Court are heard in the US Court of Federal Claims. George Washington University Law Professor Peter Meyers has studied the CICP for years and calls it a "black hole". Meyers obtained a federal document in the summer of 2020 showing it has awarded fewer than one in ten claims since its inception 15 years ago [(1092)]. Unlike the VICP, the CICP does not allow the programme to payout for either attorneys' or doctor's fees, providing expert reports in support of the petition. Unlike the VICP, the CICP will also not payout for the assistance of counsel or expert testimony required to answer complex medical and legal questions as to whether the COVID-19 vaccine caused the subsequent injury or whether the injury was only temporally (occurred at the same time) associated with the COVID-19 vaccine. In response to a Freedom of Information (FOI) request filed by Meyers, the HHS revealed in June 2020 that the CICP had rejected over 90% of compensation claims filed for ADRs to other new vaccines. Additionally, 100% of compensation claims filed for injuries claimed to have resulted from a new anthrax vaccine were rejected. Over 90% of compensation claims filed for injuries claimed to have resulted from the 2009 H1N1 vaccine were rejected. 72% of compensation claims filed for injuries claimed to have resulted from a new smallpox vaccine were rejected [(1091)]. This doesn't bode well for COVID-19 vaccine-injured Americans. On the bright side, at least the US has a vaccine injury compensation scheme.

Irish vaccine-injured will have no recourse: If you get injured by the COVID vaccine in Ireland, you're on your tod. Calls currently exist for the Irish government to set up a compensation scheme for injuries linked to any vaccines. Calls for a bespoke COVID-19 vaccines compensation scheme are also being urged [(1093)].

Let the tsunami of lawsuits ensue: This are a tiny sample. On April 2nd 2021, it was reported that the family of a woman who died of a blood clot after receiving the Oxford-AstraZeneca coronavirus vaccine had filed a complaint with prosecutors in France. The woman was a social worker and worked at a centre with disabled people and did not have any underlying diseases. Her health rapidly deteriorated shortly after vaccination, and the woman died of a blood clot on the brain (1094). On April 18th 2021, the family of an Italian woman who died from multiple blood clots in her body, including in her brain, weeks after having the Oxford-AstraZeneca COVID-19 vaccine, stated they were taking legal action. The woman, a music teacher, was excited to receive a vaccination and had expressed her joy in a Fascistbook post, writing "fatto", Italian for done. Next post, after she was unable to return to work, the woman posted "Andra tutto bene", Italian for everything will be alright [(1095)]. It wasn't. The vaccine companies have no liability for vaccine deaths. The taxpayer will foot the bill for these payouts, that is if payouts are awarded at all, as the onus is on the vaccine (person receiving the vaccination) to prove injury.

CHAPTER SEVENTEEN

NATURAL IMMUNITY

"My final conclusion after 40 years or more in this business is that the unofficial policy of the World Health Organisation and the unofficial policy of the Save the Children's Fund and almost all those organisations is one of murder and genocide. They want to make it appear as if they are saving these kids, but in actual fact, they don't".

Dr Archie Kalokerinos [1096]

Twenty-twenty (2020) was the year natural immunity ceased to exist. I stand before the altar of western medicine, having taking two grammes of soma (Lord knows I need it), repeating, "there's no immunity like artificial immunity", "natural medicine is quackery". The idea that the human immune system cannot produce a long-lasting immune response to coronavirus disease 2019 (COVID-19) is a criminal notion being peddled by the pharmaceutical owned mainstream media to generate interest in and increase uptake of vaccines. Vaccinating ourselves healthy is an oxymoron. The truth is we don't need vaccines. The human immune system is a finely tuned machine. Public health would do better to promote natural immunity. I studied a Master in Public Health naively thinking there may be a future role for me as a public health policy adviser working to integrate Complementary and Alternative Medicine (CAM) into mainstream healthcare, or a position helping to implement the World Health Organisation's (WHO's) Traditional Medicine Strategy. Then came 2020; the year that sounded the death knell of natural immunity. I advocate natural immunity. As a mother who has raised 7 children, I, like my grandmothers before me, am an expert in the human immune system. I say to my children, your immune systems are practically perfect in every way; don't mess with perfection. Pro-natural immunity is the choice not to use all pharmaceutical drugs, not only vaccines. My family would not benefit from vaccine-induced artificial immunity. I have clients who have taken the COVID-19 vaccine; that is their choice. I protect public health during this outbreak of the novel coronavirus by advising my clients of potential post-vaccination red-flag symptoms that require immediate medical attention.

Mask your own microbiome: Straight from the off, we are covered in germs; more correctly called microbes, which inhabit each and every part of our body. This is positive and is known as our microbiome. Our microbiome includes commensal populations, which are microscopic bacteria, viruses, fungi, archaea and protists. Commensalism is an association whereby microbes benefit from us, and we derive neither benefit nor harm from microbes. In a healthy body, pathogenic and symbiotic microbes coexist in harmony. Our human microbiome regulates immune homeostasis. The sanitising brigade needs to understand that destroying this microbiome weakens our immune system and makes us more susceptible to infections. The only thing we have to fear is fear itself. Biologists estimate there are 380 trillion viruses are living on us and in us. Additionally, an estimated 300,000 different viruses affect mammals (us) [(1097)]. If your immune system hasn't protected you from a novel coronavirus, frankly, you need to boost your immune system.

The daily propaganda only advertises viruses that vaccines exist for. Respiratory syncytial virus (RSV) is a good example of this. RSV is a harmless virus in healthy people and infects almost every child. RSV only negatively affects those with compromised immune systems. Whilst RSV kills 15,000 elderly Americans every year compared with 20,000 to 50,000 influenza deaths per year, we never hear about RSV in the news, or I should say, we don't hear about RSV yet. The biotech company Novavax Inc (CDC sponsor) is closer than any drug developer to a vaccine for RSV. According to Heather Behanna an analyst at Wedbush Securities, an effective vaccine would represent a US$1 billion opportunity in the United States (US) and potentially double that worldwide [(1098)]. With this new mRNA technology and recombinant DNA technology combined with the broad global acceptance of injecting unlicensed, experimental medical products, we will soon have a new vaccine for the 300,000 different viruses affecting mammals.

The human virome is our natural 'vaccine' against all viruses: The human virome is part of the human microbiome. The overprescribing and abuse of antibiotics to treat and prevent bacterial infections led to the antibiotic apocalypse. Knowledge of the human virome is barely a decade old yet we are also taught that viral infections cause disease. Natural selection dictates that the overuse and abuse of pharmaceutical therapeutics towards viruses will lead to an antiviral apocalypse. Not another ruddy apocalypse! Naturopathic medicine is not only aimed toward eradicating pathogenic microbes such as viruses, however also aimed toward promoting symbiotic microbes to keep pathogenic microbes in check. Yet our children are being indoctrinated to destroy their microbiome with advice that really is so last century.

The human immune system: In order to discuss the natural immune response, and indeed to understand the vaccine-induced artificial immune response to coronavirus disease 2019 (COVID-19), it is useful to understand how the human immune system works. We have two types of immune responses; innate and adaptive. The innate response occurs in hours and is non-specific. The adaptive immune response occurs in days and weeks and is a much more sophisticated defence mechanism, specific to the pathogen presented.

Innate (early): The innate immune response is the first line of defence against pathogens. In an attempt to bamboozle us with science jargon, the innate immune response is also called acquired immunity or specific immunity. Innate immunity consists of physical, chemical and cellular defences against pathogens. Physical defences include the cough reflex, enzymes in tears and skin oils. The delicate microbiome that exists on our skin is also part of our innate immune system. Innate immune cells are white blood cells, including basophils, dendritic cells, eosinophils, Langerhans cells, mast cells, monocytes and phagocytic macrophages, neutrophils and natural killer cells (NK cells) [(1099)].

The overuse and abuse of hand sanitiser: Public health advice to overuse and abuse bactericidal and virucidal hand sanitisers weakens our innate immunity. Modern humans are obsessive repulsive about bacteria and viruses. Notwithstanding the environmental impact of hand sanitiser, several lines of evidence exist suggesting that alcohol in hand sanitisers significantly disrupts the microbiome of human skin [(1100)]. The skin provides a passive physical barrier against infection and contains elements of the innate and adaptive immune systems to fight infections. Repetitive exposure to hand sanitising products is well known to be a significant factor in the development of occupational irritant hand dermatitis [(1101)]. Overusing and abusing bactericidal and virucidal products is the last thing we should be doing when a novel virus is circulating. Washing hands with soap and water suffices.

Adaptive (later): The adaptive immune system is also called the acquired immune system. The adaptive immune response is more pathogen-specific and has memory. T cells and B cells are the major cellular defences of the adaptive immune response. Antibodies are produced by B cells to neutralise the virus [(1102)]. Memory T cells are antigen-specific T cells and remain long after an infection is gone. Subsequent re-exposure to that same pathogen, or even a similar pathogen, stimulates the memory T cells to provide a rapid response [(1103)]. This memory is lifelong. Healthy, older people with plenty of exposure to infectious disease throughout their lifetime have robust immune systems. The problem is not that we are ageing; there are plenty of healthy elderly. The problem is that we are increasingly obese, and increasingly unhealthy because we shield ourselves from infectious disease.

The daily propaganda says antibodies decline after natural infection: The daily propaganda would have us believe that natural immunity is far inferior to vaccine-induced artificial immunity. The daily propaganda wilfully withholds or manipulates data intending to indoctrinate us with fear, so we lose faith in our natural immune system and take our shot. But it isn't one shot. It's three shots a year, every year. The next COVID-19 booster will very likely contain an influenza vaccine, and the chip is coming. Our bright future is contemplated in Chapter 20, 'The Future is Vaccines, Vaccines and More Vaccines'.

Human coronavirus-19: Coronaviruses are just a few of the viruses that cause the common cold [(1104)]. The boffins go as far as saying the reason why this coronavirus is so dangerous is because people may think they've only got a cold! COVID-19 is currently an uncommon cold, soon to be just another endemic seasonal common cold-causing coronavirus. Whilst the protective immunity of the seasonal cold caused by coronaviruses is said to be short-lived, reinfection, even of the common cold, has been found to occur most frequently at 12 months post-infection. Whilst COVID-19 vaccines need a booster every six months, true COVID-19 reinfection after natural infection is exceedingly rare [(1014)]. As previously discussed in Chapter 14, 'COVID-19 Vaccines are Effective for Seven Days', there have been five cases only documented in clinical journals; a 25 year old male from the US [(1015, 1016)], a 33 year old male from Hong Kong [(1017)], a 51 year old female, from Belgium [(1018)], a 46 year old male from Ecuador [(1019)] and a 20 year old female from Israel [(1020)]. The rest is hearsay.

Vaccine-induced immunity lasts six months to one year: A study published in the *New England Journal of Medicine* on January 7th 2021, assessed the neutralising antibody count in patients who had received both doses of Moderna's mRNA-1273 vaccine. Whilst only a preliminary analysis, study authors discovered that neutralising antibodies that bind to the virus in a manner that stops infection were not high post-vaccine, therefore the long-term efficacy may be less than hoped for. This study found slight decreases and significant drops in neutralising antibodies 119 days after the first vaccination (90 days or three months after the second vaccination) [(1105)]. The Pfizer-BioNTech COVID-19 vaccine trial data showed the vaccine was effective in reducing symptoms of mild COVID-19 disease seven days after the second shot [(1106)]. Updated initial data from a Pfizer study published in July 2021 recommends a booster shot is needed after six to 12 months to provide the best protection from COVID-19 [(1107)]. Compare this below to cross cell T cell reactivity to past infection with SARS that has been demonstrated to last 17 years and that natural immunological memory to SARS-CoV-2 would likely prevent the vast majority of hospitalisations in people with severe COVID-19 disease for many years, Mother Nature wins hands down.

Preexisting Immunity to SARS-CoV-2 from SARS-CoV-1

Preexisting immunity to SARS-CoV-2 means that you don't need a vaccine. Shh! shut up! Obey! Take your shot! The Centres for Disease Control and Prevention (CDC) acknowledges long-lasting natural immunity to the coronavirus. A study published in the CDC's *Emerging Infectious Disease Journal* in 2007 on the original severe acute respiratory syndrome (SARS) found on average that patients produced SARS specific antibodies and that these remained in the blood for on average two years and up to three years, suggesting that immunity to the SARS virus may remain for up to three years [(1108)]. Bear in mind that the influenza vaccine is annual. SARS-1 protected people from SARS-2, 17 years later. Cross-reactivity is when an antibody our body makes naturally reacts to another antigen, i.e. we get a cold and it protects us from SARS-CoV-2. A study published in *Nature* in July 2020 looked at preexisting memory T cells that could recognise SARS-CoV-2. The study investigated T cell responses in patients who had recovered from COVID-19 and found that robust cross-reactivity occurs. Patients who recovered from the original SARS were found to possess long-lasting memory T cells that were reactive to the N protein of SARS-CoV-2, 17 years after the 2003 SARS outbreak [(1109)]. 17 years ago, I was working in

Chinese hospitals during the SARS outbreak. If I were a person with free will, I would ask if I have cross-reactive immunity and therefore don't need a vaccine.

Before COVID, 57% of people were already immune to COVID-19: People who had never been infected with SARS-CoV-2 were also found to have preexisting natural immunity through cross-reactive T cells from being exposed to the common cold. Preexisting coronavirus-specific memory CD8+ T cells influence immune responses against SARS-CoV-2, thus the immune system is able to see this virus and mount an effective immune response. In July 2020, a preprint study published in *Nature* looked at SARS-CoV-2-reactive T cells in healthy donors and in patients with COVID-19. The paper was the first to measure SARS-CoV-2-reactive T cell responses directly and to determine potential cross-reactive immunity to SARS-CoV-2. The authors demonstrated that preexisting SARS-CoV-2-reactive T cells existed in patients with a history of COVID-19 infection and in a subset of SARS-CoV-2 seronegative healthy donors who had not been previously infected [(598)]. Back in August 2020, the US National Institutes of Health (NIH) said that 57% of people who never had COVID-19 showed preexisting immunity to SARS-CoV-2 due to cross-reactive T cells. Master Mason Fauci's NIH National Institute of Allergy and Infectious Diseases (NIAID) website describes a study where researchers generated T cell lines from the memory cells that recognised SARS-CoV-2 fragments and then tested them for cross-reactivity against other coronaviruses. The CDC found that, of the SARS-CoV-2 'uncommon cold' and 'common cold' coronavirus fragments, there was at least 67% genetic similarity and that 57% of people showed cross-reactivity due to memory T cells [(1110)]. Essentially the NIH was saying back in August 2020, that the science said, 57% of people did not need a COVID-19 vaccine, but that was before the science said 'vaccinate the world'.

Peter Doshi, associate editor of *The BMJ,* noted that by September 2020, there had been at least seven studies reporting T cell cross-reactivity against SARS-CoV-2 in people with no known previous exposure to the virus [(1111)]. In October 2020, *Science* reported that SARS-CoV-2 -reactive CD4+ T cells had been found in unexposed individuals in the US, suggesting preexisting cross-reactive T cell memory to SARS-CoV-2 in 20 to 50% of people [(1112)]. A study published in *Cell* in June 2020 looked at T cell responses to SARS-CoV-2 in humans with COVID-19 disease and in unexposed individuals and detected SARS-CoV-2-specific CD8+ and CD4+ T cells or virus-specific killer T cells in 70%-100% of COVID-19 convalescent patients. Importantly the study found 40%-60% of people were already immune to COVID-19, finding that $CD4^+$ T cells were discovered in 40%-60% of unexposed individuals, suggesting cross-reactive T cell recognition between circulating 'common cold' coronaviruses and SARS-CoV-2 [(1113)]. These studies show that not everyone is susceptible to COVID-19 and we don't need to vaccinate everyone to be safe. These findings are proof the PCR test is dialled up to 'Rockefeller public health is pulling history's most audacious scam to coerce us into taking an experimental vaccine', by literally diagnosing immune people as 'cases' to generate interest in and increase uptake of vaccines.

The common cold-causing rhinovirus offers better protection than a COVID-19 vaccine: It is not only other cold-causing coronaviruses that offer better protection than COVID-19 vaccines against SARS-CoV-2. In June 2021 Yale University's School of Medicine published a study in the *Journal of Experimental Medicine* that demonstrated that another common cold-causing virus, the rhinovirus, is also effective in preventing SARS-CoV-2 infection and reducing serious disease due to COVID-19. The current raft of COVID-19 vaccines are literally so ineffective that an improvement in public health policy would be to simply inoculate people deliberately with rhinovirus as it both prevents SARS-CoV-2 infection and prevents serious COVID-19 disease. Incidentally, the rhinovirus and coronavirus also protect against influenza [(1114)]. Unfortunately, no one at the WEF old boy network would increase their personal wealth using this therapeutic approach.

Post- Infection Immunity to COVID-19

The European Centre for Disease Prevention and Control (ECDC) state most people infected with SARS-CoV-2 display an antibody response between day ten and day 21 post-infection. Detection in mild cases can take a longer time (four weeks or more), and in a small number of cases, antibodies (IgM, IgG) are not detected at all, at least during the study time scale. Studies finding low antibodies post-infection and claiming that natural immunity is inadequate are simply measuring antibodies within too short a period of time.

Iceland found long-lasting immunity to SARS-CoV-2 and a 0.3% mortality rate. As mentioned in Chapter 9, 'Inflated Deaths', Iceland has good data on SARS-CoV-2 immunity. The Reykjavik-based deCODE Genetics study tested 15% of its population, providing a solid base for comparisons. The deCODE Genetics study concluded that antiviral antibodies against SARS-CoV-2 did not decline within four months after diagnosis (the time frame of the study) [(481)].

In November 2020, a preprint study published in *bioRxiv* aimed to fill the knowledge gap as to how long immunity lasts after infection with COVID-19. The study analysed multiple components of circulating immune memory to SARS-CoV-2 in 185 COVID-19 cases. Forty-one of these cases were in people greater than six months post-infection. The study simultaneously measured circulating antibodies, memory B cells, CD8+ T cells, and CD4+ T cells specific for SARS-CoV-2. As SARS-CoV-2 is a new infection, the mechanisms of protective immunity against SARS-CoV-2 have not been defined in humans.

However, it was known that SARS-CoV-2-specific CD4+ T cells and CD8+ T cells are associated with less severe COVID-19 disease and therefore some reasonable interpretations could be made. The study found that spike IgG was relatively stable over six or more months, and spike-specific memory B cells were more abundant at six months than at one month. While SARS-CoV-2-specific CD4+ T cells and CD8+ T cells declined with a half-life of three to five months, that amount of memory cells would likely prevent the vast majority of hospitalisations in people with severe COVID-19 disease for many years [(1115)]. Many years! Shut up! Obey! Take your shot! Then, shut up, obey and take your booster in six months.

Moving into 2021, a study published in *bioRxiv* in January 2021 looked at the evolution of antibody immunity to SARS-CoV-2 and concluded that the memory B cell response to SARS-CoV-2 evolves between 1.3 and 6.2 months after infection [(1116)]. A similar study published in *Science* in February 2021 also looked at multiple aspects of circulating immune memory to SARS-CoV-2, including antibody, memory B cell, $CD4^+$ T cell, and $CD8^+$ T cell memory and concluded that immunological memory existed up to eight months post-infection. The study found that the immunoglobulin G (IgG) antibody to the spike protein was stable over six or more months. Spike-specific memory B cells were more abundant at six months than at one month, and SARS-CoV-2-specific $CD4^+$ T cells and $CD8^+$ T cells declined with a half-life of three to five months [(1117)]. Numerous studies have proved beyond doubt that natural immunity lasts longer than vaccine-induced artificial immunity.

When antibodies (B cells) wane, T cell mediated immunity kicks-in: A study published in the CDC's *Emerging Infectious Diseases* in January 2021 confirmed that low antibodies do not equate to low immunity. The study investigated immune responses against SARS-CoV-2 in convalescent (recovering) German patients who were donating blood to be used as convalescent plasma for the treatment of COVID-19. The study found that whilst 78% of PCR-positive volunteers had undetectable antibodies, they still showed T cell immunity against SARS-CoV-2. In convalescent patients with undetectable SARS-CoV-2 IgG, the authors concluded that immunity may be mediated through T cells (1118).

Professor Lukey Kooky said natural immunity is better than vaccine immunity: They say listen to the 'experts'. On January 11th 2020, appearing on News Talk's, *The Pat Kenny Show*, Professor of Biochemistry in the School of Biochemistry and Immunology at Trinity College Dublin, Luke O'Neill, said that recovered COVID-19 patients have better immunity than artificially induced vaccine immunity. Professor Lukey Kooky referenced an Oxford study published in a preprint in November 2020 that found that COVID-19 infection offers protection from reinfection for at least six months. The study, a major collaboration between the University of Oxford, Oxford University Hospitals (OUH) and the National Health Service (NHS) Foundation Trust, concluded that previous infection with COVID-19 protected individuals for at least six months. The study was conducted in 12,180 healthcare workers (HCWs) working at Oxford University Hospital and covered a 30-week period between April and November 2020. The study was part of a major ongoing staff testing programme supported by the Oxford Biomedical Research Centre and Public Health England (PHE) (1119). Professor Lukey Kooky said,

> *"Nobody in the infected group got infected again, which means it was better than the vaccine. The vaccine would give say 90% protection but, in this case, infection gave 100% protection in that group of people, so it is a really positive sign".*

He also referred to two studies previously mentioned; the study that demonstrating cross cell T cell reactivity to past infection with SARS lasting for 17 years published in Nature, and the study showing immunological memory to SARS-CoV-2 lasting for up to eight months post-infection published in *bioRxiv* [1109, 1117].

Post-infection immunity in Irish hospitals: In October 2020, a Healthcare Worker COVID-19 Antibodies Study conducted at Tallaght University Hospital Dublin found that 20% of frontline HCWs had antibodies to SARS-CoV-2. SARS-CoV-2 antibodies were detected in 18% of participants overall. The rate was 20% for staff with roles involving more direct patient contact [1120]. These same HCWs are currently being harassed and coerced into taking an unlicensed experimental vaccine they do not need and if they don't they are being threatened with redeployment. All HCWs should be offered serological SARS-CoV-2 tests to determine immunity status. All HCWs should stand.

Individual-level serological tests prior to vaccination should be conducted: As the COVID-19 vaccination rollout began, public health experts and scientists were questioning if those with a previous history of COVID-19 infection should defer their vaccination. The scientists and epidemiologists said that herd immunity could be developed faster by vaccinating people who have never been infected therefore don't have protective antibodies [1121]. Commenting on the Oxford study in January 2021, Kingston Mills, Professor of Immunology at Trinity College Dublin, said the COVID-19 vaccine rollout could be expedited if people with a previous history of COVID-19 infection are excluded [1122]. This prioritisation was suggested after a study was done by researchers at the University of Colorado Boulder on COVID-19 vaccine prioritisation strategies by age and serostatus that suggested using individual-level serological tests prior to vaccination to redirect doses of the COVID-19 vaccine to seronegative individuals. Seronegative refers to a person not having antibodies to COVID-19 [1123]. A vaccine is not without risks, and preexisting immunity should be established. However, the CDC recommendations on vaccinating people with a history of infection are that "vaccination should be offered to persons regardless of history of prior symptomatic or asymptomatic infection", and "viral testing to assess for acute SARS-CoV-2 infection or serologic testing to assess for prior infection solely is not recommended" [218].

Skin scratch test for immunity to COVID-19 on the cards: I am a child of the 70s and remember the Heaf test. The Heaf test was a diagnostic skin test that was performed to determine whether or not the child had been exposed to and was therefore naturally immune to tuberculosis infection. Children who exhibited a positive Heaf test did not need the BCG (tuberculosis) vaccination [1124]. Low and behold, the Heaf test was discontinued because the manufacturer deemed it financially unsustainable. A more scientific approach to COVID-19 would be to test people for immunity prior to vaccination. In March 2021 in fact, Tonix Pharmaceuticals announced it had developed a skin scratch test known as TNX-2100 to assess and measure T cell immune responses to SARS-CoV-2. The TNX-2100 skin test measures T cell immunity using delayed-type hypersensitivity (DTH). DTH is the classic measure of antigen-specific T cell protection that has been in use for more than a century. The TNX-2100 skin test consists of three different mixtures of synthetic peptides aimed to discriminate between naïve (never been infected) people, vaccinated people, and people who are COVID-19 convalescent [1125]. What! You want to know if you are immune? You're SELFISH! Doublespeak for 'thinks for one's self'. Shut up! Obey! Take your shot.

Children protect adults from SARS-CoV-2 infection: Irish boffins are currently injecting Irish children over 12 with the vaccine they stopped using in younger age groups as they said the risks outweighed the benefits in this age group. Worse still, far from putting the vulnerable at risk, children protect their parents and grandparents because they are immune and can't get it or spread it! This is called herd immunity or population immunity. It is the responsibility of the healthy in our community to catch and become immune to the virus to protect our vulnerable. A University of Glasgow study of over 300,000 adults living in HCW households looked at households shared with children and found that not only are children at no greater risk from contracting COVID-19, children actually protect the adults they live with. Children have higher levels of exposure to endemic coronaviruses than adults, and, as with adults, evidence exists for B cell and T cell cross-reactivity between SARS-CoV-2 and these endemic coronaviruses. Although a range of potential mechanisms exists, these SARS-CoV-2 responsive T cells provide protection against COVID-19, which is why children are relatively protected from COVID-19 and therefore contact with children also affords adults a degree of protection from COVID-19 [1126]. Vaccinating children is nothing less than criminal. On September 11th 2021, Pfizer-BioNTech announced that it is expected to file its regulatory dossier on vaccinating five to 11 year olds in September and has laid out plans to seek approval in children aged six months to two years later in 2021. Six month old babies being vaccinated for a cold! Asthma and food allergy will go through the roof, and parents will blame their genes then donate to a 'charity' to find a cure.

Newborn babies are not susceptible to SARS-CoV-2 infection! Foetuses receive antibodies from the mother through the placenta. After birth, infants have their naïve immune systems inoculated as they pass through their mother's birth canal. At this time of birth, the infant receives antibodies from the mother to viruses such as measles, RSV, influenza and coronavirus etc. These antibodies are further topped up through breastfeeding. Breastfed babies have fewer infections, allergies and autoimmune diseases. Breast milk also contains numerous protective antibodies against infectious disease [1127]. A child that is delivered by caesarean and not breastfed is more susceptible to infection. The mechanisms of the hygiene hypothesis are that the mode of delivery affects the colonisation of the infant's intestinal human microbiome thereby suppressing the immune system and increasing the likelihood of the development of childhood allergy, asthma and autoimmune disease [1128].

Babies are born with antibodies against SARS-CoV-2 and protected from COVID-19: An article published in *JAMA* in March 2020 reports that six mothers who had experienced mild COVID-19 symptoms all passed down antibodies to their infants. None of the infants had any symptoms of the disease [1129]. Another paper also published in *JAMA Paediatrics* in January 2021 found that out of 83 pregnant, antibody-positive women, 72 gave birth to babies who tested positive for antibodies to SARS-CoV-2. Fifty of these women were completely asymptomatic [1130]. The recommendations remain to vaccinate pregnant women who have had COVID-19 and are naturally immune. Shortly, public health will recommend vaccinating immune babies for a disease they are not susceptible to, to save grandparents they naturally protect!

Being poor and living in squalor protects against COVID-19: Evidence of high levels of natural immunity in poorer communities exists. In September 2020, the results of a seroprevalence study among people who visited public health facilities for antenatal care and routine HIV testing in the Cape Town area found that 40% of respondents had antibodies against SARS-CoV-2. Researchers stressed that the results are preliminary and based on a skewed sample of 2,700 people in South Africa's Western Cape Province who aren't representative of the overall population. A representative seroprevalence study in August 2020 of residents in the Indian capital New Delhi found that 30% had antibodies to SARS-CoV-2. Professor Mary-Ann Davies, Director of the Centre for Infectious Disease Epidemiology and Research at the University of Cape Town, said, "especially in poorer communities, a relatively high proportion of people had been exposed to and infected with COVID-19". The Western Cape Department of Health also said the pressure (due to COVID-19) had eased off considerably, and that hospitals had started reintroducing normal clinical services (1131). It doesn't matter if they are immune; South Africa has been back in lockdown multiple times because of a soon-to-be in December 2021, defunct PCR test.

The hygiene hypothesis and molecular mimicry: This is why the human race is sicker than ever. One need not be an 'expert' or 'authority' to know that children that have multiple siblings and are exposed to animals and outdoor life have more robust immune systems and a lower likelihood of developing asthma, eczema and allergy. The Thought Police, Heidi Larson's Vaccine Confidence Project (VCP) and GSKoogle censor this information and, of late, even worse push industry-sponsored studies showing that children who get colds and flu are at an increased risk of allergy! Enter narrative, 'Children need a flu shot'; No they don't! The Institute of Medicine's (IOM's) Immunisation Review Report (ISR) report entitled *Immunisation Safety Review: Multiple Immunisations and Immune Dysfunction* states that early exposure to infectious disease and environmental microbes educates an immature immune system toward a protective immune response and prevents allergy. The report states that vaccine-induced immune responses differ to immune responses from wild-type infections and summarises that it is not yet clear what the roles of vaccinations have on altering the development of the immune system (7). The precautionary principle says when in doubt, get it out (1132).

Molecular mimicry: The link between vaccination and autoimmune disease was covered in Chapter 12, 'Vaccines aren't Described as Safe and don't Always Work'. Here I explain the mechanisms linking vaccines to the development of autoimmune disease which is known as being caused by molecular mimicry. Molecular mimicry describes a structural similarity between proteins in vaccines (specifically isolated from viral or bacterial pathogens) to proteins in humans. This structural similarity can lead to what is called immune cross-reactivity. This is where the antibodies the immune system makes toward pathogenic antigens attacks the human proteins. This is how autoimmune disease develops [669]. Molecular mimicry is due to a dysregulation of our immune systems caused by living in an overly clean environment and by not being exposed to infectious disease. This is called the hygiene hypothesis. The decreasing incidence of infections in western countries, and more recently in developing countries, correlates with the increasing incidence of both autoimmune and allergic diseases. The rise in autoimmune and allergic disease is due to the overuse and abuse of antibacterials (acceptable), antibiotics (acceptable), antipyretics to suppress fever (acceptable), and vaccines ironically as they work to prevent infection. Now I wear a tinfoil hat, believe that the earth is flat and The King is not dead.

The hygiene hypothesis is based upon epidemiological data, particularly migration studies, which show that people who migrate from a low-income to a high-income country acquire immune disorders with a high incidence at the first generation. Whilst a variety of multiple and complex underlying mechanisms exist, the lack of exposure to infections impedes homeostatic mechanisms that strengthen and educate our immune system; this natural maintenance is termed immunoregulation [1133]. The incidence and prevalence of autoimmune disease has increased significantly over the last 30 years [1134]. Approximately 50 million Americans or 20% of the population have an autoimmune disease [699]. Autoimmune diseases are a leading cause of death among females in the US and UK [1135, 1136]. The hygiene hypothesis remains a hypothesis because the boffins won't disprove the null hypothesis as it would mean comparing the health outcomes of the vaccinated to the unvaccinated.

Interferons are the cure for COVID-19 and every other disease: Interferons are the General of our natural immunity army. Interferons are named for their ability to 'interfere' with viral replication by protecting cells from virus infections and trigger an increase in natural immune response such as natural killer cells, macrophages, phagocytes and other immune cells to eradicate pathogens, not only viruses but also bacteria, fungus, parasites and tumours [1137]. Increasing interferon upregulates antigen (foreign protein) presentation by increasing the expression of major histocompatibility complex (MHC) antigens. This essentially means that inteferon introduces the immune system to the foreign invader and provides a handshake. The importance of MHC proteins is to allow T cells to distinguish foreign proteins from self-proteins. The inability of the body to accomplish this is known as molecular mimicry and is a causative factor in autoimmune disease [1138]. Increasing interferon is thus imperative to decrease the risk of autoimmunity. Enter the other disaster of allopathic medicine; the overuse and abuse of antipyretics to suppress fever.

Fever is not a dirty word: Fever regulates the immune system and increases augmenting interferon-α (IFNα) production in response to infection [1139]. By preventing disease, vaccines prevent childhood exposure to fevers which protect against allergic disease. Fever is a symptom of measles for example, of which exposure to measles has been found to be protective against atopy (allergic disease) [654, 1140]. Although children may develop fevers after vaccination, this reaction is suppressed with antipyretics (medicine to reduce fever) as a matter of course. As a mother and a Complementary and Alternative Medicine (CAM) practitioner, I never suppress a fever unnecessarily. Fever in children is common and caused mainly by benign self-limiting infections, meaning the prognosis is good and will run its own course. Mother's intuition has always known this to be true. Naturopaths teach this. It took DuBois, an American physician remembered for his work on the physiology of fever, a lifetime of study on fever to finally come up with the statement, "Fever is only a symptom, and we are not sure that it is an enemy. Perhaps it is a friend" [1141]. A child or adult running a 'good' fever is a sign that the child or adult is perfectly healthy. However, many parents are overanxious about their children's fevers, even if they are mild, and consult their doctor or Accident and Emergency (A&E). The medical term used to describe this anxiety disorder is called fever phobia [1142]. Taking medicine to suppress the fever is associated with risks including asthma, eczema and increased mortality from many conditions. When it comes to fevers, even from a biomedical perspective there are two basic fields of thought; the fever should be suppressed because its metabolic costs outweigh its potential physiologic benefit, or fever is a protective adaptive response that should be allowed to run its course [1143]. The latter approach, sometimes referred to as the 'let it ride' philosophy, has been supported by several recent randomised control trials (RCTs) [1144]. 'Let it ride' reminds me of 'let it rip', the inflammatory language used by the boffins to turn us off the Greater

Barrington Declaration's 'focused protection'. You don't let a fever ride, you manage a fever.

When fever is a cause for concern: Although infection is the most common cause of fever, fever may be a symptom of a serious underlying cause [1145]. A fever of unknown origin (FUO) is a prolonged fever, with a temperature exceeding 38.3 °C on at least three occasions over a period of at least three weeks, with no diagnosis made despite one week of inpatient investigation. A FUO may have an underlying diagnosis of cancer, infection, or noninfectious inflammatory disease [1146]. The main causes of FUO in paediatric and adult patients are autoinflammatory disease (AID) [1147]. Red flag symptoms require immediate medical attention. Red flag symptoms include, for example, symptoms of meningitis in a seriously ill child that requires immediate referral to A&E. I teach parents Natural Medicine First Aid, which includes how to manage their child's fever and included red flag symptoms warranting immediate medical attention.

What happens during a fever? The febrile response is mediated by endogenous pyrogens (cytokines) in response to invading exogenous pyrogens, originating outside the body, primarily microorganisms such as bacteria and viruses. These endogenous pyrogens act on thermosensitive neurons in the hypothalamus which upgrade the thermostat set point via prostaglandins. Cytokines play a pivotal role in the immune response by the activation of B cells and T lymphocytes. A fever results in simultaneous lymphocyte activation, which demonstrates the clearest and strongest evidence that fever plays a protective role. These protective processes are optimal at high temperatures (around 39.5°C) [1148, 1149]. Fever increases white blood cell macrophages and monocyte phagocytic activity. Antipyretics used to inhibit fever target multiple aspects of the inflammatory response besides temperature regulation and these are postulated to increase associated risks [1150].

Paracetamol risks in adults: Paracetamol is used worldwide for its analgesic (pain-relieving) and antipyretic (fever-reducing/preventing) properties. The exact mechanisms of how paracetamol works remain unknown. The judicious use of antipyretics is unlikely to cause problems, however the overuse and abuse of antipyretics by anxious parents and the general public is widely acknowledged. A large Cochrane study concluded that paracetamol is not only largely ineffective but that paracetamol use is associated with increased mortality from cardiovascular events including heart attack, stroke, or coronary heart disease, adverse gastrointestinal events including ulcers and upper gastrointestinal bleeding, and kidney disease. Patients taking paracetamol for chronic pain are four times more likely to have abnormal liver function tests results and experience twice the rate of acute liver failure [(1151)]. Animal studies found that when inhibiting the fever with acetylsalicylic acid (aspirin), 70% of acetylsalicylic acid-treated animals died as a result of infection, compared with only 16% of animals who did not have their fevers suppressed [(1152)].

Paracetamol risks in children: Several epidemiologic studies suggest that acetaminophen use might be a risk factor for asthma development and asthma exacerbation [(1153, 1154)]. Routine use of prophylactic paracetamol with vaccinations results in lower antibody titres to several vaccine antigens post-vaccination and should not be routinely recommended [(1155)]. Yet paracetamol post-vaccination is always recommended. A Mexican population-based study found exposure to paracetamol significantly increased the risk of rhinitis (colds and allergies) and possibly eczema [(1156)]. A study on paracetamol use in chickenpox found that the chickenpox lesions took longer to crust in the paracetamol group, possibly due to prolonged viral shedding in the absence of fever [(1149)].

What defines a fever? As a mother and qualified CAM practitioner experienced in childhood infectious disease, I don't pay much heed to public health advice, although I am aware of the official rules supplied by public health surrounding fever. Once again, I teach parents Natural Medicine First Aid which includes fever management. Fever management involves learning how to raise the temperature when too low, how to lower the temperature when too high, and how to recognise when your child's temperature is either rising or falling. From a naturopathic perspective, the ability to throw a 'good' fever indicates a person has a strong Vital Force and is a determinant of one's state of health on a physical, mental, emotional and spiritual level.

CHAPTER EIGHTEEN

HERD IMMUNITY

"Those who have the privilege to know, have the duty to act, and in that action are the seeds of new knowledge".

Albert Einstein [1157]

Twenty-twenty (2020) heralded the age of artificial immunity and the worshipping of false idols. Herd immunity is now for exclusive use by Big PhRMA (Pharmaceutical Research and Manufacturers of America). Anyone caught using the term herd immunity in relation to natural immunity is labelled ill-advised, arrogant, reckless, a killer and will be shot (with a vaccine). For the COVID faithful grappling in predicting the course of the coronavirus disease 2019 (COVID-19) pandemonium, one of the important questions they ask is how effective and what length of time immune responses protect the host from reinfection. In order to discuss the herd immunity level (HIT), one must first acknowledge that the human immune system has, since the beginning of time, evolved to be perfectly capable of recognising new antigens (disease) and mounting an immune response. Infection with some viruses provides lifelong immunity, whilst infection with seasonal viruses may be short-lived.

Herd immunity in the old days; it was only the 80s: Herd immunity is also known as community immunity or population immunity. I prefer the term population immunity however I will use herd immunity to highlight what was stolen by Big PhRMA. Herd immunity refers to the protection of susceptible individuals against an infection when a sufficiently large proportion of immune individuals exist in a population.

The chickenpox and indeed the now much-maligned measles party, which I advocate a return of, are examples of mothers encouraging their children to get infected while the child is young, so the child becomes immune before adulthood when the disease is much more severe. To those so abhorred by this idea, mothers didn't send their chronically ill vulnerable children to a measles party or spread the disease willy-nilly. Infected children convalesced at home and mothers knew how to manage the symptoms without the need to go to a doctor or Accident and Emergency (A&E). Measles then did its rounds, herd immunity was reached, the vulnerable were protected, and children remained immune for life. There were undoubtedly far fewer vulnerable children back in the days of measles parties. I stand by the protective effects of contracting measles to decrease the risk of allergic and autoimmune diseases in Chapter 23, 'Measles Shmeezles and the Great Autism Cover-up'. As also described in Chapter 12, 'Vaccines aren't Described as Safe and don't Always Work', 20% of our children have a chronic disease requiring long-term prescription medication. Remember our children were healthier. Remember we were healthier.

Another example of herd immunity is the protection of adults from shingles when adults are exposed to chickenpox in their children [(1158)]. The varicella-zoster virus causes chickenpox. Shingles, also known as herpes zoster, is caused by the varicella-zoster virus's reactivation, which lies dormant in the human peripheral nervous system and spine after the original chickenpox infection. Shingles is a far more serious disease than chickenpox which occurs primarily in the elderly and immunocompromised. The exposure of adults to chickenpox in children stimulates the adult immune system to provide them with protective immunity to shingles. The introduction of the chickenpox vaccine has seen the rate of chickenpox decline and a sharp rise in the rate of shingles [(1159)]. Rather than allowing our children to get chickenpox, an uncomfortable perhaps but completely self-limiting harmless disease, the pharmaceutical companies response is to make a 'safe and effective' shingles vaccine, and public health policy is to add this vaccine to the ever-increasing vaccine schedule [(1160)]. As only mentioned in the previous Chapter 17, 'Natural Immunity', herd immunity has been demonstrated with COVID-19. A University of Glasgow study looked at the risk of COVID-19 in 300,000 adults healthcare workers (HCWs) in households sharing with children found that not only are children at no greater risk from contracting COVID-19, children actually protect the adults they live with [(1126)]. When it comes to vaccinating children, there is no way the benefits outweigh the risks. Children are being placed at unnecessary risk of adverse reactions following vaccination in a completely disproportionate policy response to gain votes.

COVID-19 party anyone? I was calling for a COVID-19 party at the beginning of the pandemonium, but couldn't find anyone with COVID-19 ironically. Fascistbook blocked my invitation. It is the responsibility of the healthy members of the population to catch the virus and gain immunity to protect our vulnerable. In Australia, we say take one for the team. This is herd immunity. You cannot hide from a virus. If a new virus is circulating, I would rather expose myself and my children on the first round and be protected from a potentially more serious mutation or variant of concern (VOC). The Greater Barrington Declaration (GBD) authors support allowing the virus to circulate naturally in the healthy population whilst applying "focused protection" to at-risk groups. The GBD authors are covered in Chapter 24, 'Speaking Truth to Power'. According to GSKoogle, the three public health experts from Harvard, Stanford, and Oxford who authored the GBD are ill-advised, arrogant and reckless. Again, the daily propaganda misreports it as a "let it rip" strategy (1161). This is a lie created to instil fear, to generate interest in and increase uptake of vaccines.

Global health experts are telling porkies about how many people can catch the virus: World Health Organisation (WHO) Director-General Dr scare-the-bejesus-out-of-us is an academic doctor, not a medical doctor. Considering Ghebreyesus has a Master of Science degree in Immunology of Infectious Diseases and a PhD in Community Health, Ghebreyesus doesn't demonstrate a good grasp of the human immune system. In October 2020, Dr scare-the-bejesus-out-of-us, presented this dire warning to promote fear and anxiety, "The vast majority of people in most countries remain susceptible to this virus. Seroprevalence surveys suggest that in most countries, less than 10% of the population have been infected with the COVID-19 virus". Food and Drug Administration (FDA) Deputy Commissioner for Medical and Scientific Affairs and member of the board of Pfizer, Scott Gottlieb, however, said that up to 30% of Americans may be infected with coronavirus by the end of 2020 and that in some states the rate of prior infection will be as high as 50% (473). Listen to the 'expert' they say, unless the 'expert' you're listening to isn't listening to the 'expert' the 'experts' tell them to listen to. Dr scare-the-bejesus continues his fear campaign by applying the public health seven-step recipe; "although older people and those with underlying conditions are most at risk of severe disease and death, they are not the only ones at risk. People of all ages have died" (193). Blow me down with a feather! People of all ages have died 'from any cause within 28 days of a positive test' using a test that has a false positive rate of 97%. The WHO page also states incorrectly that "Never in the history of public health has herd immunity been used as a strategy for responding to an outbreak, let alone a pandemic". Frankly, this statement is an insult to the University of Nottingham where Ghebreyesus got his PhD in Community Health from. Ghebreyesus will have been taught that the term herd immunity had its origins in natural immunity and the concept of herd immunity was commandeered by Big PhRMA to generate interest in and increase uptake of vaccines.

The origins of herd immunity include acquired resistance from natural exposure: An article published in *The Lancet* in 2020 entitled 'A History of Herd Immunity' describes the early origins of the term herd immunity. The phrase 'herd immunity' was originally used in veterinary medicine. Regarding the use of the term herd immunity in humans, researchers never really settled on a clear definition. The term herd immunity was first applied to humans in an article published in *The Lancet* in 1924 by Sheldon Dudley, Professor of Pathology at the Royal Naval Medical School. Dudley focused on what share of a 'herd' had acquired resistance from either natural exposure or through immunisation. Bacteriologist W. W. C. Topley then expanded on the concept. In 1935 Topley explained in the *Journal of the Royal Army Medical Corps* that herd immunity encompassed not just immunity distribution but also encompassed the socioeconomic factors determining the herd's exposure. Topley said that the 'English herd' had herd immunity to plague, malaria, and typhus because of improved living conditions resulting in less contact with the required vectors (fleas and mosquitoes). In the mass vaccination campaigns of the 1950s and 1960s, herd immunity took on fresh importance for public health policy in relation to ascertaining what percentage of a population had to be vaccinated to control or eradicate a disease. The concept of herd immunity resurged after 1990 as public health officials worked to generate interest in and increase uptake of vaccines and achieve 'sufficient' levels of vaccination coverage [(1162)]. So when WHO Director-General Dr scare-the-bejesus-out-of-us says that never in the history of public health has herd immunity been used as a strategy to respond to an outbreak, Ghebreyesus is lying by omission. Modern public health began in the 19th century and mass vaccination campaigns began in the 1950s, so prior to the 1950s, herd immunity was acquired through natural infection and improved living standards only, and achieved every year for every circulating virus.

George Orwell said, "The most effective way to destroy people is to deny and obliterate their own understanding of their history" [1163]. In 2020 the WHO rewrote the English language definition of herd immunity. The WHO acknowledges that herd immunity is the indirect protection from an infectious disease that happens when a population is immune either through vaccination or immunity that develops through prior infection. However, the WHO only supports achieving herd immunity through vaccination, not by, *"allowing a disease to spread through any segment of the population, as this would result in unnecessary cases and deaths"*; doublespeak for 'it would result in that segment of the population not requiring a vaccine and by default, immunometabolism drugs' [1164].

Herd immunity does not exist in healthcare settings: Herd immunity is a coercive control technique used by the daily propaganda to generate interest in and increase uptake of vaccines. As discussed in Chapter 4, 'Vaccine Refusal and the Age of Censorship', the daily propaganda doesn't want you to know that the Holy Grail of vaccine-induced herd immunity does not exist in healthcare settings. HCWs are the most vaccine-hesitant group in society. The WHO says vaccination rates coverage among European HCWs is less than 30% [241, 242]. As the WHO describes vaccine hesitancy as a top ten threat to global health and security, HCWs are one of the top ten threats [285]. Name-calling is a tactic used by the state to divide us in an attempt to increase vaccine compliance.

Herd immunity level: The herd immunity level (HIL) is also called the herd immunity threshold (HIT). The HIL is vitally important as it represents the percentage of people in the population that either need to get the disease naturally or be vaccinated against the disease to achieve herd immunity and protect the vulnerable. It is not surprising that there is no scientific consensus on the HIL for SARS-CoV-2. The HIL depends on the reproduction number (R_0), which is an epidemiologic metric used to describe the contagiousness of a disease. Calculating the R number is complex. The R_0 itself, or transmissibility of a disease, is affected by numerous biological, sociobehavioural and environmental factors and should be estimated, reported, and applied with great caution [1165]. Depending on whether a study accounts for the population heterogeneity (we're all different), both the R number and the HIL will be completely different. We may remember the malarkey about the R number having to be less than 1. Since it has been kept consistently under 1 for six months we no longer hear about it

[1166]. Ireland's Chief Medical Officer (CMO), unapologetic over his CervicalCheck botch job Hooligan just renewed this R number scare tactic in Ireland. In Australia, we would say R for rort.

The pseudoscience of science: Whilst the daily propaganda with their 'experts' and 'authorities' and 'the science' will indoctrinate you to believe that 100% of us are susceptible to COVID-19, even to the point where people who have had COVID-19 are still considered susceptible, this is far from true. In statistics, heterogeneity means that populations are different (diverse in character and genetics), and homogeneity means that populations are the same. Most HIL studies for COVID-19 do not capture the inherent heterogeneity of the population and assume there is no population immunity and that all individuals are equally susceptible and equally infectious [1167]. This is not proper science. We are all different and are thus not all equally susceptible.

Professor Martin COVID-69er Ferguson's notorious modelling at the beginning of the pandemonium unscientifically assumed that there was a cultural homogeneity of our society, resulting in Professor COVID-69er's disastrous, overinflated figures that in part, led to the global shutdowns. Professor Ferguson should look beyond the homogeneity of his gated estate. The UK mad cow disease 'crisis' predicted by Ferguson was a major policy disaster, and the mass carnage predicted by Ferguson did not occur [456]. In a betrayal of trust, Professor COVID-69er quit as a government adviser on coronavirus after admitting an "error of judgement"; doublespeak for, 'I cheated on my wife during lockdown and broke the rules imposed as a result of my own modelling predictions' [1168].

Additionally, regarding heterogeneity, the impact of the lockdown will be very different in the locked-down subset of the population. For example, key workers in the population are more exposed to the virus and thus more likely to have contracted COVID-19 and acquired natural immunity. In all fairness, pandemic forecasting is complex and has a dubious track record. The problem we are faced with is that these modelling and prediction forecasts have become more pronounced with COVID-19, and these predictions are being used to strip us of our freedom; and again, it's not proper science.

Humans can be homogeneously immune or heterogeneously resistant to COVID-19: Whilst the government would love us to be homogenised 'individuals' with homogenised thoughts and be dependent on the state, thankfully, human populations are far from homogeneous. Heterogeneousness is the quality of the human populations not to be equally susceptible and equally contagious. As described, preexisting immunity and post-recovery immunity to COVID-19 means that not everyone is susceptible to COVID-19. A group of scientists published a preprint article in *bioRxiv* refuting the accuracy of current statistical models. The team applied a widely-used inverse binomial method to demonstrate the current risk level of COVID-19 infection and the odds of contracting COVID-19 among heterogeneous (different) populations to provide more accurate estimates. In relation to naturally acquired immunity, study authors acknowledged that the population can in fact be either homogeneously immune or heterogeneously resistant to COVID-19 [1169].

The herd immunity level according to the bought-out 'experts': The number needed to vaccinate to achieve herd immunity is a very different figure to how many they will vaccinate. The media would have us believe that the HIT for COVID-19 is 100%, but it wasn't always the case. Back in October 2020, the UK was seemingly far more level headed. Then UK Chair of Vaccine Taskforce Kate Bingham told the *Financial Times* that less than half the UK population would receive the coronavirus vaccine, adding that vaccinating everyone in the country was, *"not going to happen"*, and that *"we just need to vaccinate everyone at risk"*. Kate said this in an attempt to clear up the public's "misguided perception" of the COVID-19 vaccine programme's aim [1170]. Anthony Fauci is the Director of the National Institute of Allergy and Infectious Diseases (NIAID). Flip-flop Fauci, anti-mask one minute pro-mask the next, also flip-flopped on herd immunity levels. Originally Fauci echoed World Wealth Organisation guidelines that 60%-70% of people needed to be immune to SARS-CoV-2, either through artificially induced vaccine immunity or through natural immunity acquired due to prior infection, for herd immunity to be reached [1171].

By October 2020, Fauci was fear-mongering, *"the nation's top health experts have said a majority of Americans remain susceptible to a coronavirus infection"* [1172]. Then flip-flop Fauci went so far as to say that herd immunity may require nearly 90% of US residents to get coronavirus vaccine [1173]! This U-turning shows that the experts are not 'following the science', they are following their drug lords' demands.

So what is the actual herd immunity level? Even taking into account studies that do not take into account the heterogeneity of the community, the HIL is not that high. The following study published in *JAMA* assumed no population immunity and that all individuals are equally susceptible and equally infectious. Study authors found that the herd immunity threshold for SARS-CoV-2 would be expected to range between 50%-67% in the absence of any interventions [1174]. When mathematicians from the University of Nottingham and University of Stockholm devised a simple model categorising people into groups reflecting age and social activity level, they found that when these differences in age and social activity were incorporated in the model, the herd immunity level reduced from 60% to 43% [859]. Another preprint article published in *medRxiv* found a much lower HIT level for SARS-CoV-2. This study considered that as SARS-CoV-2 spreads, the number of susceptible people declines, causing the rate of new infections occurring to slow and that variations in individual susceptibility or exposure to infection exacerbate this effect. The study concluded the HIL to be around 10-20%, considerably lower than the minimum coverage needed to interrupt transmission by random vaccination, which for R_0 higher than 2.5 is estimated above 60% [860].

Herd immunity is used by Big PhRMA to generate interest in and increase uptake of vaccines. As previously mentioned, former FDA commissioner and Pfizer Board of Director member Scott Gottlieb said that the rate of infection in some US states would be as high as 50% by the end of 2020 [473]. Using another example, it makes no sense whatsoever that Australian Prime Minister ScoMo the clown want a 95% uptake of the COVID-19 vaccine. Whilst, ScoMo made a massive U-turn on his plan to make the coronavirus vaccine mandatory he did however threaten that, "I would expect it to be as mandatory as you can possibly make" [1175]. He meant to say except I'll make it definitely mandatory for truck drivers, constructions workers, healthcare workers, teachers etc. History has shown us that coercion is central to fascist rule. I stand with Melbournians.

Herd immunity was reached long ago: Enough of this already. On March 31st 2021, the Office for National Statistics (ONS) said that 50% of people in Britain already had antibodies to SARS-CoV-2 either through natural exposure or through vaccination [1176]. As previously mentioned in Chapter 13, 'COVID-19 Vaccines are Safe for Two Months', on June 9th 2021, the UK media reported the results of an analysis of a COVID-19 infection survey. Antibody and vaccination data was released showing that eight in ten people in Britain had antibodies to SARS-CoV-2 either through natural infection or vaccination [858]. The HIL has been reached yet we are still masquerading and playing make-believe. The PCR test is literally diagnosing immune people as infective 'cases' and Kary Mullis is having a grand mal seizure in his grave.

The bottom line is, evidence is irrelevant. Shut up! Obey! Take your shot! None of this makes any sense, however it makes absolutely no sense for public health to insist that anyone who has been infected with COVID-19 need to take an experimental vaccine. As previously mentioned in Chapter 17, 'Natural Immunity', individual-level serological tests or a skin scratch test to assess and measure T cell immune responses can be used to determine preexisting immunity to SARS-CoV-2. You want to know if you are naturally immune? You're SELFISH! Doublespeak for thinks for one's self. The science is settled. Shut up! Obey! Take your shot! The objective is universal vaccination; to vaccinate every man, woman, person and child on the planet every year.

CHAPTER NINETEEN

COVID MEDICAL & NATURAL MEDICINE PREVENTION & TREATMENT

"Look deep into nature, and then you will understand everything better".

Albert Einstein (1177)

As a naturopath and an environmentalist, I'm not interested in the medical paradigm of being poisoned and polluted with pharmaceutical drugs when there are natural alternatives. I touch on the medical therapeutics below, as natural medicine is my bag. I do know however, these drugs are being prescribed by (silenced) doctors around the world to treat COVID-19. Scientists should be elated that some drugs have been repurposed and new treatments have been developed as effective therapeutics for COVID-19. Our drug lords however censor the efficacy of these medications as the 'emergency' ends when there is an effective therapeutic. Whilst our drug lords conducted research into vaccines at breakneck speed, the same boffins have not applied the same priority to researching these potential therapeutics. Without an 'emergency', the boffins can't coerce the population into taking an unlicensed experimental vaccine under Emergency Use Authorisation (EUA). These days have seen a return of the Burning Times and once again Complementary and Alternative Medicine (CAM) practitioners are being burned.

The COVID passport used to be called the International Certificate of Vaccination or Prophylaxis (ICVP). The ICVP is a certificate that travellers must carry to enter certain countries which mandate a yellow fever vaccination (217). The P in ICVP stands for prophylaxis. Prophylactic means prevent infection. Theoretically, one should be able to argue from a legal perspective that if one adopts a proven prophylactic procedure, there is no need to take a vaccine when we can take a cheap, safe and effective alternative. We should, except that no one in the World Economic Forum (WEF) old boy network would increase their wealth.

Note: Never self-prescribe prescription medication!

Hydroxychloroquine: Hydroxychloroquine (HCQS) is a disease-modifying anti-rheumatic drug (DMARD). In January 2021, a review published in *The European Journal of Pharmacology* on HCQS found that reports of its efficacy *in vitro* experiments and early observational studies had been mostly positive. However, according to the boffins, those studies had several methodological flaws and were subject to numerous biases and confounders (unlike vaccine studies!).

In the first quarter of 2021, the United States (US) *Clinicaltrials.gov* registry displayed several ongoing studies investigating the role of HCQS in the treatment and prophylaxis of COVID-19. These studies will help identify relevant groups that might receive the most benefit from HCQS use. Until this data emerges from these high-quality clinical studies, the science is not settled. HCQS is currently being administered to COVID-19 patients as per treatment guidelines and strictly under investigational settings, followed by close monitoring of patients [(1178)]. Whilst Trump said it was good, so it must be bad, the Centres for Disease Control and Prevention (CDC) is conducting an RCT Phase IIa study of HCQS, vitamin C, vitamin D, and zinc for the prevention of COVID-19 Infection (HELPCOVID-19) [(1179)]. The CDC must have headhunted Irish Professor Dolores Cahill to run their trials as this is what she recommends, that, and ivermectin.

Ivermectin: The antiparasitic medicine ivermectin is already a Food and Drug Administration (FDA)-approved drug [(1180)]. Whilst the daily propaganda and the fact-wreckers say this is a horse wormer, ivermectin tablets are approved for use in humans for the treatment of some parasitic worms, in particular for the treatment of the neglected tropical disease (NTD) onchocerciasis (or River Blindness), a chronic human filarial disease caused by infection with *Onchocerca volvulus* worms [(1181)]. Countries with routine mass drug administration of what is described as 'prophylactic chemotherapy' against parasitic infections in humans, including the drug ivermectin, have a significantly lower incidence of coronavirus disease 2019 (COVID-19). This correlation is highly significant among both African nations as well as worldwide [(1182)]. Ivermectin has been shown to inhibit the replication of severe acute respiratory syndrome coronavirus 2 (SARS-CoV-2) *in vitro* [(1183)].

Some trials in humans have shown promise, others not so. A Phase II randomised study on chloroquine, hydroxychloroquine or ivermectin in hospitalised patients with severe manifestations of SARS-CoV-2 infection published in *Pathogens and Global Health* in June 2021 found that although CQ, HCQ or ivermectin revealed a favourable safety profile, the tested drugs do not reduce the need for supplemental oxygen, ICU admission, invasive ventilation or death, in patients hospitalised with a severe form of COVID-19 [1184]. The science is not settled, however. The CDC is conducting a double-blind, randomised, double-blind, placebo-controlled (RCT) of ivermectin in adults with severe COVID-19 [1185].

A pilot RCT published in *EClinicalMedicine*, found that in patients with non-severe COVID-19 and no risk factors for serious disease, a single 400 mcg/kg dose of ivermectin within 72 hours of the onset of fever or cough resulted in a marked reduction of self-reported anosmia and cough, and a tendency to lower viral loads and IgG titres. There was no change in the proportion of reverse transcription-polymerase chain reaction (RT-PCR), however. The study concluded these results warrant assessment in larger trials [1186]. An RCT published in the *International Journal of Infectious Diseases* in December 2020 found that a 5-day course of ivermectin was safe and effective in treating mild COVID-19 adult patients [1187].

A meta-analysis of RCTs of ivermectin to treat SARS-CoV-2 infection was published in *Open Forum Infectious Diseases* in July 2021. Researchers investigated ivermectin in 24 RCTs and found ivermectin was associated with reduced inflammatory markers (C-reactive protein, d-dimer and ferritin) and faster viral clearance by PCR. Eleven randomised trials of moderate/severe infection found there was a 56% reduction in mortality with favourable clinical recovery and reduced hospitalisation [1188].

Remdesivir, hydroxychloroquine with or without azithromycin: Remdesivir is an antiviral medication. Azithromycin is an antibiotic. A review on treatment options for COVID-19 published in *Frontiers in Medicine* discussed available antimicrobials that may be very effective in treating COVID-19 and the trials currently underway to detect and confirm the efficacy of these antimicrobial agents. The review concluded that remdesivir and HCQS, with or without azithromycin, were promising treatment options for patients with mild to moderate COVID-19 [1189].

Convalescent plasma therapy: Convalescent plasma therapy has shown promise as a treatment strategy for COVID-19 disease. The therapy has a long history going back more than 100 years and convalescent blood has been used to treat measles, Spanish influenza and many other diseases. The mechanism of protection from SARS-CoV-2 not only comes from the neutralising antibodies in the plasma, immune-boosting antibodies like IgM, IgG and some non-neutralising antibodies have been found to bind to the SARS-CoV-2 virus and may enhance recovery and be prophylactic. Passive antibody therapy is known to be more useful when used for prophylaxis rather than for treatment. Antibodies used for therapy need to be administered soon after the onset of symptoms to maintain their efficacy [(1190)].

Monoclonal antibody treatment: Monoclonal antibodies are man-made proteins that act like human antibodies in the immune system. Neutralising monoclonal antibodies to SARS-CoV-2 have the potential for both therapeutic and prophylactic applications. The main target of SARS-CoV-2 neutralising monoclonal antibodies is the surface spike glycoprotein that mediates viral entry into host cells [(1191)]. In November 2020, the FDA authorised monoclonal antibodies for the treatment of COVID-19 [(1192)]. Yet, the 'emergency' continues...

Vitamin D: Despite the fact that the number of high-quality studies on vitamin D is constantly expanding, scientists and clinicians will tell you controversy and uncertainty exists surrounding the relationship between vitamin D and COVID-19. There is no money to be made from vitamin D. Like influenza, COVID-19 is a respiratory infection. Vitamin D deficiency is described as a European pandemic and deficiency in the Irish is well established [(1193, 1194)]. Influenza-like illness (ILI) is the reason for hospitalisations in influenza. Dr Gerry Schwalfenberg describes how he and a colleague prescribe vitamin D in their practices to both prevent and treat influenza. They have prescribed 100 mol/L for years to most patients and remark that they see very few patients with influenza or ILI. If a patient gets influenza, the doctors treat them with what they describe as a 'vitamin D hammer', a one-off high dose of 50,000 IU ('international unit') vitamin D3 or 10,000 IU 3 times daily for 2 to 3 days. Vitamin D results in treating flu-like symptoms have been described as dramatic [(1195)]. A 2017 systematic review and meta-analysis of over 11,000 participants published in *The BMJ* found that vitamin D protected against acute respiratory tract infection among all participants. Investigators found that in vitamin D deficient individuals, daily or weekly supplementation cuts the risk of respiratory infection in half. Vitamin D was found to protect against ILI among all participants, and that supplementation was safe [1196]. That represents a 100% efficacy.

Additionally, another meta-analysis published in *PLOS ONE* concluded that long-term vitamin D supplementation prevents overall respiratory infection mortality [1197]. A study published in *Nutrients* reported that evidence exists that vitamin D may reduce the risk of influenza and COVID-19 disease and deaths. Investigators found in vitamin D deficient individuals, daily or weekly supplementation cut the risk of ILI in patients with COVID-19 disease in half [1198]. The United Kingdom (UK) National Health Service (NHS) acknowledges that vitamin D can reduce healthcare-associated influenza costs [58]. An analysis of studies on vitamin D and SARS-CoV-2 published in The *International Journal of Clinical Practice* concluded that high-dose vitamin D supplementation, particularly for at-risk groups, could be recommended to achieve and maintain optimal (range 40-60 ng/ml) serum 25-hydroxy vitamin D levels (marker of vitamin D status), both for COVID-19 prevention and treatment [1199]. Yet the 'emergency' continues, let's 'vaccinate the world'.

The UK NHS is recommending vitamin D to prevent and treat COVID-19: Now ex UK Monster-of-Health Matt Hancock was urging people to take vitamin D to protect themselves against COVID-19. In the background of the COVID-19 vaccine rollout, it is worth knowing vulnerable people in the UK were prescribed vitamin D. Prior to the rollout, in November 2020, the UK government gave four months worth of free vitamin D supplements to more than 2.5 million vulnerable and elderly population [1200]. Scotland also rolled out vitamin D to its vulnerable and elderly population. Then health-monster Hancock himself requested guidance from the National Institute for Health and Care Excellence (NICE) and Public Health England (PHE) on the use of vitamin D. A NICE spokesperson, "NICE and PHE received a formal request to produce recommendations on vitamin D for prevention and treatment of COVID from Matt Hancock, on October 29th 2021" [1201]. If the NHS and the CDC recommend taking vitamin D to prevent and treat COVID-19 why are we being coerced into taking a vaccine to prevent and treat COVID-19? Particularly as there is no conclusive evidence that COVID-19 vaccines prevent nasal SARS-CoV-2 infection to block viral transmission and stop the spread of infection [219].

The CDC is running a trial to determine if vitamin D prevents and treats COVID-19: The CDC is currently running an RCT on the efficacy of vitamin D supplementation to prevent the risk of acquiring COVID-19 in healthcare workers (HCWs). Unlike some of the COVID-19 vaccine trials, this trial excluded people with a known history of COVID-19 infection. The estimated study completion date is July 2021. This will prove or disprove if taking vitamin D is prophylactic against COVID-19 [1202]. I looked this up on August 12th 2021 and it still states they are recruiting. I imagine the CDC are busy covering up vaccine injury after their COVID-19 vaccine rollout.

COVIT-TRIAL: In December 2020, the COvid-19 and high-dose VITamin D supplementation TRIAL (COVIT-TRIAL) protocol was published. A trial protocol is written before a trial. The COVIT-TRIAL was to be the first RCT to assess the effect of vitamin D supplementation on the prognosis of COVID-19 in high-risk older patients. The study was to involve 260 participants who were to be followed for 28 days. The primary outcome was to measure all-cause mortality within 14 days of inclusion. Secondary outcomes included scoring changes on the World Health Organisation (WHO) Ordinal Scale for Clinical Improvement (OSCI) scale for COVID-19. The OSCI is a measure of clinical improvement and/or survival, assessed at a pre-specified time post-randomisation [1203].

Vitamin C: This coronavirus is an uncommon cold, soon to be a common cold [1204]. A Cochrane review looking at vitamin C for preventing and treating the common cold reported that, whilst more research is needed, the authors acknowledged that vitamin C reduced the duration and severity of colds when supplemented regularly [1205]. New York hospitals treated coronavirus patients with vitamin C. Dr Andrew G. Weber, a pulmonologist and critical care specialist affiliated with two Northwell Health facilities on Long Island, said his intensive care patients with the COVID-19 immediately received 1,500 milligrams of intravenous vitamin C [1206]. At the time of writing in April 2021, there were a number of RCTs registered globally assessing intravenous vitamin C monotherapy in patients with COVID-19. Since vitamin C deficiency is common in low- to middle-income settings, and many of the risk factors for vitamin C deficiency overlap with COVID-19 risk factors, it is expected that trials carried out in populations with chronic vitamin C deficiency may show greater efficacy [1207]. There are currently other ongoing clinical trials that will provide more definitive evidence on the use of vitamin C as prophylactic for COVID-19 [1208].

Zinc: A systematic review and meta-analysis of RCTs of zinc for the treatment of the common cold found that zinc may shorten the duration of symptoms of the common cold by between two and three days [1209]. A study looking at the potential role of zinc supplementation in prophylaxis and treatment of COVID-19 discussed the medical hypotheses that zinc has been well proven to possess a variety of direct and indirect antiviral properties, therefore the administration of zinc supplements has the potential to enhance antiviral immunity, both the innate and adaptive immune responses, and to restore depleted immune cell function or to improve normal immune cell function in immunocompromised or elderly patients. The authors concluded that it can be hypothesised that zinc supplementation may be of potential benefit for prophylaxis and treatment of COVID-19 [1210].

A review into zinc and COVID-19 based on a current clinical trial published in *Biological Trace Element Research* concluded that due to zinc's direct antiviral properties, it could be assumed that zinc administration is beneficial for most of the population, especially in those patients with suboptimal zinc status. This review integrated the current studies of the antiviral activity of zinc and discussed its potential role in the prevention and treatment of COVID-19 and ongoing COVID-19 clinical studies using zinc [1211]. A study predicting the survival odds in COVID-19 by zinc, age and selenoprotein P (SELENOP) biomarker, was published in *Redox Biology*. Study authors concluded that zinc and biomarker status being within the reference ranges indicated high survival odds in COVID-19 and assumed that correcting a diagnostically proven deficit of selenium and/or zinc through supplementation may support convalescence in COVID-19 disease [1212].

The US Department of Health and Human Services *Clinical.Trials.gov* website shows a phase IV RCT was being conducted in 2021 to evaluate the efficacy of zinc sulphate 220mg for the treatment of COVID-19 in the higher risk COVID-19 positive outpatient setting. The trial end date was February 8th 2021. Results had not been published at the time of writing. The primary outcome measures were the number of participants hospitalised and/or requiring repeat emergency room visits assessed at 21 days. Other outcome measures included the number of participants admitted to the intensive care unit (ICU) assessed at 30 days and, if admitted, the number of days in ICU, the number of patients ventilated, and if so, for how long, assessed at 30 days [1213].

COVID-19 and potential traditional herbal medicines targets: COVID-19 is a coronavirus like severe acute respiratory syndrome coronavirus (SARS-CoV) and the recently identified Middle Eastern respiratory syndrome coronavirus (MERS-CoV) [1214]. Haemagglutinin exists in the structure of the coronavirus and is a target for herbal treatment [1215]. Neuraminidase inhibitors are the cornerstones of the management of patients hospitalised for suspected MERS-CoV infection and the original SARS coronavirus, hence neuraminidase is a potential target for herbal treatment [1216]. Whilst SARS-CoV-2 contains a haemagglutinin-esterase protein, it is said that SARS-CoV and SARS-CoV-2 do not appear to have functions of a haemagglutinin and neuraminidase which is mysterious as most other coronaviruses respond to therapies that target haemagglutinin and neuraminidase [1217, 1218]. Nontheless, these targets warrant investigation.

Antiviral herbal medicines: My allegiances lie with pharmacognosy, the study of herbal medicines in their whole form. COVID-19 is a virus, so antiviral herbs are indicated. Constituents in herbs exhibit a diverse array of antiviral, virostatic, antimicrobial, immune-enhancing and anti-influenza activities [1219]. At the start of the pandemonium, a report of the WHO-China Joint Mission on COVID-19 acknowledged that the Chinese government had initiated a series of major emergency research programmes for many potential therapeutics, but also including traditional Chinese medicines (TCMs). The WHO was also looking to determine the effectiveness of TCMs against COVID-19 [1220]. Many herbal medicines have demonstrated both *in vitro* and *in vivo* antiviral activity.

Antiviral herbal actions required;

- Haemagglutinin inhibition (prevent viral replication)
- Neuraminidase inhibition (prevent viral replication)
- Surface spike protein inhibition (prevent viral entry)
- Increasing interferon (boost natural immunity)
- Inhibit the cytokine storm (prevent the inflammatory cascade)

I write about the human immune system and have an immune tonic geared towards these (and other) pharmacognostical targets. As a result of my natural immunity advocacy, in March 2020, I received an FDA letter that wrongfully accused me of peddling snake oil and GSKoogle posted six pages of warnings regarding the family business we spent 20 years building. According to the FDA, we were one of only seven companies in the world to receive said warning, so we are officially public enemy number one to seven. I don't sell 'cures'. I have an immune tonic that empirical evidence has shown to be effective which is based on my research and geared toward the following herbal actions. This information is from the article I wrote at that time that got their attention. Herbal medicines have demonstrated the following actions *in vitro* (in glass) and *in vivo* (in animals).

Haemagglutinin inhibition: Influenza haemagglutinin (HA) is a glycoprotein found on the influenza virus surface, along with neuraminidase, which assists viral replication (1221). The following herbs have been shown to display HA inhibitory effects;

- Catechins isolated from green tea, like epigallocatechin gallate (EGCG), exhibit a mild anti-influenza effect (1222).
- Elderberry (*Sambucus nigra*) has been traditionally used for treating influenza and colds in western countries. The highly active flavonoids extracted from elderberry inhibit H1N1 swine influenza and is comparable to the anti-influenza drug of Oseltamivir (1223). Flavonoids from elderberry extract block viral entry by binding to H1N1 virions. Elderberry inhibits several strains of influenza virus *in vitro* (1224).
- The polyphenol constituent curcumin in turmeric (*Curcumin longa*) targets HA to inhibit virus entry into cells (1225).
- The constituent andrographolide from andrographis (*Andrographis paniculata*) displays inhibitory activity against avian influenza A (H9N2 and H5N1) and human H1N1 influenza A viruses *in vitro* and *in vivo* (1226). Andrographolide interferes with HA to prevent the virus from binding to cellular receptors (1227).

Neuraminidase inhibition: Viral neuraminidase is found on influenza virus surfaces and enables viral release from host cells (1228). The following herbs have been shown to display NA inhibitory effects;

- The principal active ingredient of the first oral NA inhibitor Oseltamivir is derived from star anise (*Illicium verum*) (1229).

- The constituent rosmaranic acid from rosemary (*Rosmarinus officinalis*) is a potent NA inhibitor [1230].
- Berberine containing herbs such as barberry (*Berberis vulgaris*) are antibacterial, antimicrobial, antifungal and antiviral [1231]. The NA inhibition activity of berberines is comparable with Oseltamivir [1232].
- Ganoderma triterpenoids from reishi (*Ganoderma lucidum*) display NA inhibition against H5N1 and H1N1 [1233].
- Elderberry is also a natural NA inhibitor [1234]. The compound cyanidin-3sambubiocide, an anthocyanin flavonoid, displays potent NA inhibition [1235]. The extract exhibits inhibitory potential on H5N1-type avian influenza A virus [1236].

Surface spike protein inhibitors: Surface spike proteins located on the coronavirus surface are involved in mediating the entry of coronavirus into human host cells. Two small molecules, tetra-O-galloyl-beta-D-glucose (TGG) and luteolin have been identified as displaying anti-SARS-CoV activities in wild-type SARS-CoV infection systems. TGG is isolated from the traditional Chinese medicine Indian gooseberry (*Phyllanthus emblica*) [1237]. More than 200 Chinese medicinal herbal extracts were screened for antiviral activities against SARS-CoV. Four herbal extracts showed moderate anti-SARS-CoV activity.

These herbal medicines were;

- Red spider lily (*Lycoris radiate*)
- Sweet wormwood (*Artemisia annua*)
- Large-lipped rustyhood (*Pterostylis lingua*)
- Japanese evergreen spicebush/ wūyào (*Lindera aggregate*) [1238]

Interferons: As explained in Chapter 17, 'Natural Immunity', Interferons (IFNs) are proteins called cytokines produced by white blood cells. IFN 'interferes' with viral replication to protect cells from virus infections by triggering an increase in natural killer cells, macrophages, phagocytes and other immune cells to eradicate pathogens, not only viruses but also bacteria, fungus, parasites and tumours. IFN up-regulates antigen presentation by increasing the expression of major histocompatibility complex (MHC) antigens which allow T cells to differentiate foreign antigens from self-proteins to avoid autoimmunity [1137].

The following herbs have been shown to increase IFN;

- Elderberry (*Sambuccus nigra*) fruit extract enhances IFN-β response [1239].
- Astragalus (*Astragalus membranaceus*) root extract enhances IFN-β response [1239].
- Astragalus polysaccharides enhance immunity and inhibit H9N2 avian influenza virus *in vitro* and *in vivo* [1240].
- Echinacea's (*Echinacea angustifolia/Echinacea purpurea*) antiviral properties are attributed to its ability to increase IFN [1241-1243]. Echinacea's antiviral properties are comparable with Oseltamivir [1244].
- Curcuma in turmeric (*Curcuma longa*) is immune-stimulant, anti-inflammatory and increases IFN [1245].

Preventing inflammatory cascade (cytokine storm): The cytokine storm is when immune cells and their activating compounds (cytokines) are overproduced. During influenza infection, it is this surge of activated immune cells into the lungs that leads to high mortality rates [1246].

Suppression of the cytokine release correlates with reduced death rates in clinical diseases such as pandemic influenza, where a cytokine storm plays a significant role in high mortality rates [1247].

The following herbs have been shown to inhibit the inflammatory cascade;

- The immune-modulatory activities of echinacea (*Echinacea purpurea*) comprise stimulation of macrophage phagocytic activity and suppression of the proinflammatory cytokines and chemokine responses of epithelial cells to viruses and bacteria [1246].
- The active constituent andrographolide in andrographis (*Andrographis paniculata*) inhibits influenza A virus and reduces inflammatory cytokine expression induced by infection [1248].
- Curcumin (*Curcuma longa*) inhibits key proinflammatory cytokines, interleukin (IL) IL-1, IL-6 and tumour necrosis factor (TNF) TNF-α [1249].

Not following the science protects against COVID-19: I have to acknowledge George Carlin, who is no longer with us, who put his robust immunity in preventing polio down to swimming in raw sewerage in the Hudson. George Carlin in fact said, "Rights aren't rights if someone can take them away. They're privileges" [1250]. Not using hand sanitiser, not social distancing and not wearing masks protects against COVID-19 [1251]. Being taught to fear bacteria and viruses is completely irrational and not scientifically based. Our microbiome, which was covered in Chapter 17, 'Natural Immunity', has become all the rage yet is still not fully understood. The microbiome consists of trillions of microbes, including bacteria, viruses, fungi and archaea that live inside us and help in digestion, protect against pathogenic causing microbes, regulate the immune system and produce vitamins. Whilst the bacterial microbiota has been studied extensively, the functional role of and interaction with each other or with the host immune system of these non-bacterial microorganisms has not been as widely explored [1252]. Not to matter, the 'science is settled'; kill viruses and bacteria. The microbiome is irrelevant, drugs 'cure' disease.

Next season in Europe, due to our overly sanitised lifestyle, Eurosurveillance expect influenza deaths to rival COVID-19 deaths as there is no population immunity (herd immunity) from naturally acquired influenza infection [1253]. The boffins will tell us that this is because we are not taking enough vaccines, however this will be a lie created to generate interest in and increase uptake of vaccines. Influenza vaccine efficacy studies are exaggerated due to healthy vaccinee bias that is introduced by not testing vaccines in the elderly or frail [611]. The truth is the number of influenza cases fell so dramatically because the number of samples submitted for testing for influenza dropped by 61% during the COVID-19 pandemonium [542]. Enter more lockdowns to 'cure the flu' if we allow it.

Indian researchers studied the potential of the microbiome to explain the disparity in COVID-19 deaths between high and low-income countries. The article, published in *Medical Hypotheses*, suggested that low hygiene, lack of clean drinking water, and unsanitary conditions may have actually saved many lives from severe COVID-19 disease. The study authors, Kumar and Chander from Dr Rajendra Prasad Government Medical College, examined data from 122 countries, including 80 high and upper-middle-income countries and found that COVID-19 deaths are lower in countries that have a higher population exposed to a diverse range of microbes, particularly Gram-negative bacteria. These bacteria are typically responsible for severe pneumonia, blood and urinary tract and skin infections. Gram-negative bacteria however are also believed to produce interferon, the antiviral cytokine molecule, which protects cells against SARS-CoV-2 [1254].

Another study assessing COVID-19 mortality in different countries in relation to the demographic character of these countries and the prevalence of autoimmunity published in *medRxiv* found a positive correlation between improved hygiene and a higher incidence of autoimmune disorders with COVID-19 deaths. The study used a multivariate linear regression model to assess countries' demographic statuses, such as the prevalence of communicable and non-communicable diseases, BCG (tetanus) vaccination status, sanitation levels etc. The study found a negative correlation between the incidence of communicable diseases and COVID-19 mortality, i.e. the more infectious diseases you have; the less likely you are to die from COVID-19. In contrast, the study found a positive correlation between a countries' Gross Domestic Product (GDP), hygiene levels and the prevalence autoimmune disorders, i.e. the richer and cleaner a country is, the more COVID-19 deaths. India, for example, has one-sixth of the world's population and equally one-sixth of the world's cases yet accounts for only 10% of the world's deaths. The case fatality rate (CFR) in India is among the lowest in the world at less than 2% [1255]. The daily propaganda didn't share this fact in their fearmongering about India and the dreaded Delta.

CHAPTER TWENTY

THE FUTURE IS VACCINES, VACCINES ..& MORE VACCINES

"If we define an American fascist as one who in case of conflict puts money and power ahead of human beings, then there are undoubtedly several million fascists in the United States".

Henry A. Wallace (1256)

The latest and greatest COVID mantra being pumped out on the daily propaganda is 'nobody will be safe until everybody is safe' (474). Safe from who exactly? Safe from Pfizer? Ireland, with a population of 4.9 million, will be receiving 4.9 million Pfizer COVID-19 vaccines in 2022 and another 4.9 million in 2023 (1257). I'll altruistically donate mine to someone who has enjoyed living in a cage for the past 18 months.

The ruling class say life will never return to normal: In this video between 20-42 seconds, you can hear our supreme leader, Klaus Schwab, in full maniacal persona saying:

> *"I sink vun lesson vich ve take out of zis crisis is ze notion of mutual interdependence, because even as individuals ve have to take care not to infect somevun else and not to be infected. It's ze same ve have to apply now on a global level. As long as not everybody is vaxzinated, nobody vill be safe"* (1258).

Not this body, vill be vaccinated! On April 9th 2020, Bill Gates spoke to the *Financial Times* on the COVID-19 vaccine. When questioned on the financial outcomes of the pandemic at 44 seconds, Mr Smirk says, "You don't have a choice. People act like they have a choice (about taking the vaccine)...people don't feel like going to a stadium if they might get infected". At 1 minute 29 seconds, Gates tells us, *"Normalcy only returns when we largely vaccinated the entire global population and so"* (1259). The Coalition for Epidemic Preparedness Innovations (CEPI) estimates global COVID-19 vaccine manufacturing capacity at between two and four billion doses annually and that it will be 2023-2024 before enough vaccines can be manufactured (1260). Then we all need that booster shot for that variant of concern (VOC) and emerging disease with pandemic potential. It's a slippery slope. Damn straight we have a choice! CEPI of course was founded in Davos by the Norwegian and Indian governments, the Bill & Melinda Gates Foundation, Gate's Wellcome Trust and Satan Klaus' World Economic Forum (WEF). Enter 'Ze Grrreat Rrreset'.

In a video Irish Grinch ex-Taoiseach Leo-the-Liar Varadkar now Tánaiste (second in command) says:

> *"Maybe it will be the case that International travel is not possible this summer (2021) and not possible this Christmas (2021)...I certainly don't want to close off that possibility, but maybe we have to. If you're serious about elimination and if you're serious about COVID being zero, surely it would go on for a couple of years or maybe indefinitely...a lot of hypothetical here...that you have vaccinated 70-80% of your population that 70-80% is enough to confer herd immunity. Would you then take the risk around Christmas (2021) of allowing at that point huge numbers of people? I think you probably wouldn't...let's say we did get to levels of mass vaccination...I don't think you would say everyone come home for Christmas now. I really don't"* (1261).

Indefinitely? Zero COVID? We didn't vote for that. Varadkar took the risk in September 2021 and flew to a festival in the UK because there are none he could attend in Ireland.

Dr Clare Wenham, Assistant Professor of Global Health Policy at the London School of Economics, reminded us that life in the UK will not return to normal until 2024 or until the global population is vaccinated (1262). If we obey and take our shot, will we not be free! We have relinquished control and we will never get it back without a struggle. We won't be free until 'ze vorld iz vaxzinated'. Oui Oui bourgeoisie. I'll take my shot for the common good.

Perpetual project fear: Our ruling class are already stoking the fear factor toward the next wave of infectious diseases for which we will need new vaccines. Ten of the world's most infectious diseases currently not being catered for by pharmaceutical companies have been identified by the World Wealth Organisation. GlaxoSmithKline (GSK) CEO says GSK is committed to improving research, access and development of new medicines and vaccines for global health diseases for future pandemics. Pandemics are a very lucrative business. The global COVID-19 vaccine market will be worth US$25 billion a year by 2024 [1263]. Access to Medicine Foundation, a not for profit for us but profit for our mates, is preparing us psychologically for the new wave of emerging viruses. The Access to Medicine Foundation is funded by the UK and Dutch governments, the Bill & Melinda Gates Foundation, the Wellcome Trust and Axa Investment Managers. The next viruses lined up for our indoctrination of fear are Nipah, Chikungunya, Marburg, Zika, Ebola, Rift Valley fever, Lassa Fever, Crimean-Congo haemorrhagic fever, enteroviruses and other coronaviral diseases including COVID-19 [20,21][1264]. These in addition to the other greatest global threats, the three diseases that the World Wealth Organisation has created extensive drug resistance in; HIV, TB and malaria [1265]. That's the list for the next onslaught of 'safe and effective' vaccines.

Combination of adult measles vaccines and COVID-19 vaccine: Immunity to measles from measles vaccination is not lifelong. Waning immunity to measles in teenagers and young adults is a dominant issue in populations who are highly vaccinated at a rate greater than the WHO recommended uptake of 95%. Yet, the daily propaganda continues to blame vaccine failure on failure to vaccinate. Measles-mumps-rubella (MMR) vaccine failure is discussed in greater detail in Chapter 23, 'Measles Shmeezles and the Great Autism Cover-up'. The boffins are working on enhancing pre-travel vaccination with an aim to increase uptake of an adult measles vaccine [1266]. COVID-19 is being seen as an opportunity to kill two birds with one stone. In July 2020, a study by researchers from the Paul Ehrlich Institute in Germany describes a measles-virus based COVID-19 vaccine. The measles virus-based vaccine expresses the severe acute respiratory syndrome coronavirus 2 (SARS-CoV-2) spike glycoprotein. Researchers say that this vaccine has the advantage of eliciting both an antibody response and cellular immunity to the SARS-CoV-2 virus and the measles virus. In December 2020, this measles-virus based platform was being used by CEPI to launch anti-SARS-CoV-2 vaccine development [1267].

DNA and RNA-based gene vaccines are the future of vaccines: Jedi mind trick; the COVID-19 DNA and RNA-based vaccines are not genetically modifying vaccines. Genetic vaccines in fact consist only of deoxyribonucleic acid (DNA) as plasmids, or ribonucleic acid (RNA) as messenger RNA (mRNA) which is taken up by cells and translated into protein [1268]. Once the vaccine delivers the genetic material into cells, the cells follow the genetic instructions to churn out the viral spike protein [963].

In 1999, DNA and RNA-based vaccines were called 'gene vaccines'. Gene vaccines were described as a new approach to immunisation whereby, rather than a live or inactivated organism being delivered, one or more genes that encode proteins of the pathogen are delivered [(1269)]. CRISPR is the tool used for genome editing [(1270)]. CRISPR is used in the development of mRNA vaccines [(1271)]. Scientists used CRISPER to design the mRNA instructions for cells to build the unique spike protein into the mRNA vaccine [(967)]. CRISPR technology is also used in viral vector vaccines. 'Viral vector vaccines' were previously known as 'DNA vaccines' [(1272)]. That was before they realised we know that the DNA is in the nucleus of the cell which contains our genetic material, so it would be exceedingly difficult to say that a DNA vaccine doesn't modify our DNA.

mRNA vaccines enter the cell's cytoplasm: The Pfizer and Moderna COVID-19 vaccines are both mRNA vaccines. The CDC say "that mRNA never enters the nucleus of the cell, which is where our DNA (genetic material) is" [(1273)]. The mRNA vaccines enter the ribosomes, the sites of protein synthesis, in the cell's cytoplasm [(1274)].

DNA vaccines enter the cell's nucleus: In our civil rights conversations, there is a lot of talk about mRNA vaccines and none on DNA vaccines. There are currently three DNA vaccines being rolled out which are even more concerning, AstraZeneca, Johnson & Johnson (J&J) and Sputnik V are COVID-19 vaccines [(1275)]. Oxford-AstraZeneca's COVID-19 vaccine is a recombinant DNA vaccine that uses double-stranded DNA inserted in a chimpanzee adenovirus. Once inside, the adenovirus escapes from the lipid-based bubble and travels to the nucleus, the chamber where the cell's DNA is stored [(1276)]. The CDC refer to the COVID-19 DNA vaccines as 'Viral Vector COVID-19 Vaccines' and reassure us that "The genetic material delivered by the viral vector does not integrate into a person's DNA". The CDC website wilfully omits that the vaccine ingredients enter the cell's nucleus [(1274)]. J&J (Janssen) COVID-19 vaccine also uses DNA inside a chimpanzee adenovirus. J&J is a single dose recombinant vector vaccine using live replicating viruses that are (genetically) engineered to carry extra genes originating from the pathogen, which produce proteins against which we want to create immunity [(1277)]. Gavi, the Vaccine Alliance (Gavi) says that viral vector vaccines/DNA vaccines, once injected into the body, the vaccine viruses begin infecting our cells and inserting their genetic material, including the gene for the antigen, into the cells' nuclei. Human cells then manufacture the antigen as if it were one of their own proteins and this is presented on their surface alongside many other proteins. When the immune cells detect the foreign antigen, they mount an immune response against it and make antibodies [(1278)]. Sputnik V is also a viral vector vaccine based on chimpanzee adenovirus DNA [(1275)]. There are no two ways about it. This is gene therapy using genetically modified ingredients, which is also called genome manipulation and modifies a person's genes [(1279)]. There is a problem with this technology. A preprint paper by a team of German scientists at Goethe University in Frankfurt said they believed they had worked out why vector-based vaccines like Oxford-AstraZeneca and J&J's cause the vaccine-induced thrombocytopenia that results in the blood clots experienced in a growing number of people. Rolf Marschalek said, "The viral piece of DNA, deriving from an RNA virus, is not optimised to be transcribed inside of the nucleus". After arriving in the cell's cytosol (the liquid found in cells), the mRNA is again translated into the spike protein. "These unintended splice events are destroying the reading frame, resulting then in aberrant (abnormal) proteins being made in the cytosol". Scientists say the vaccines can be improved so as not to cause this aberrant reaction [(1280, 1281)]. 'Not optimised to be transcribed inside of the nucleus'? 'Aberrant proteins'? That gives me so much confidence in vaccines, Heidi.

Big Tech bosses aren't on the same page: Mr Smirk likes DNA and RNA-based vaccines. In the video entitled 'The race for a COVID-19 vaccine, explained' at 1 minute 40 seconds Bill Gates says, "One final way that is new and it's promising, is called the RNA vaccine. With RNA and DNA instead of putting that shape in you put instructions in the code to make that shape" [(1282)]. As mentioned in Chapter 13, 'COVID-19 Vaccines are Safe for Two Months', Zuckerberg doesn't like DNA and RNA-based vaccines. Zuckerberg says (in reference to the COVID-19 vaccines),

> *"but I do just want to make sure that I share some caution on this because we just don't know the long-term side effects of basically modifying people's DNA and RNA"* [(345)].

Zuckerberg is a conspi-racist!

The good news just doesn't stop: Moving away from recombinant DNA vaccines and mRNA vaccines and hark back to a good old fashioned inactivated whole virus vaccine with a twist; a novel adjuvant. On January

29th 2020, our ruling class promised us yet another weapon of mass salvation. Scotland began manufacturing the COVID-19 vaccine Valneva from a French Biotech Company [1283]. Valneva announced in June 2021 that it had completed recruitment for the phase III trial of its inactivated, adjuvant COVID-19 vaccine candidate known as VLA2001. This vaccine falls into a category of vaccines known as inactivated whole virus vaccines. This vaccine contains two adjuvants, alum and Cytosine phosphoguanine (CpG) 1018 [1284]. CpG is a synthetic form of DNA that mimics bacterial and viral genetic material [1285]. Aluminium-containing adjuvants have been used since the 1930s.

Variants of concern? No worries: Moderna made an announcement at a J.P. Morgan healthcare conference that the immunity from Moderna's COVID-19 vaccine should last a year. Whilst this may disappoint the masses, the company was quite upbeat, optimistically adding that it was confident that the mRNA technology could be rapidly utilised to make a new vaccine based on this new emerging VOC [1286]. John Bell, Regius Professor of Medicine at Oxford University, said that it might take a month or six weeks to get a new vaccine [997]. Pfizer says their vaccine-induced artificial immunity wanes (decreases) after six months and now recommends a COVID booster shot, although the FDA and CDC currently say wait; until the next U-turn [995]. The COVID-19 VOCs from Alpha to Lambda (and now Mu), were covered in Chapter 14, 'COVID-19 Vaccines are Effective for Seven Days'.

Next-generation 'Wave 2' vaccines: Populations that receive the first round of COVID-19 vaccines will have waning immunity and require boosting using improved second-generation COVID-19 vaccines [1287]. It is expected that vaccine-induced artificial immunity will be short-lived, thus a proportion of the population will need to be vaccinated every year with a COVID-19 vaccine [1288]. Billionaire 'philanthropist' Mr Smirk has already offered his tainted donations to develop the next onslaught of vaccines. In December 2020, before the current COVID-19 vaccine rollout, CEPI announced a collaboration with South Korea-based SK bioscience to develop a next-generation or 'Wave 2'vaccines against SARS-CoV-2 [1289]. There's the CEPTIC tank again. 'Next-generation' is doublespeak for 'covid generation'. More vaccines than you can shake a stick at. How lucky are we!

CHAPTER TWENTY-ONE

CHIPS, DOTS AND BOTS

"Conformity is the jailer of freedom and the enemy of growth".

John F. Kennedy [1290]

As explained in Chapter 1, 'The New Normal / World Order', Bill Gates and Rockefeller play an increasingly active role in global health and security agenda-setting and funding priorities of governments and international organisations, which undermines the UN bodies. Bill Gates is a philanthrocapitalist and makes money for investors under the guise of 'social return' on investment (SROI). Bill Gates is not a prophetic visionary who called the pandemic. The powers that be were expecting the next global pandemic, and the powers that be knew the world was woefully unprepared [1291, 1292]. The powers that be also knew how they could turn a profit on a pandemic. The Global Health Security Agenda (GHSA) includes not only more vaccines than you can shake a stick at, but also chips, dots and bots. Their agenda is total control via radio-frequency biometric identification and on-person vaccine records.

The end goal is transhumanism: God is so last century. Who needs God when our new saviour is vaccines? Nowadays, we don't have to age, disease or die (and they say I wear a tinfoil hat). Transhumanism promises us freedom from our own inherent biological limitations. Transhumanism aims to enhance physical, emotional and cognitive capacities, thus opening up new possibilities and horizons of experience [1293]. Transhumanist technologies utilise genetic, robotic, computer and information, and nanotechnologies to enhance the mind and body [1294]. Eugenicist and founder of transhumanism in the mid-1950s, Julian Huxley obviously hadn't experienced psilocybin mushrooms [1295]. How serendipitous that mass vaccination campaigns also started in the mid-1950s. Whilst I embrace the power of herbal medicine to prevent ageing and disease, I have no problem accepting my human limitations and acknowledge that death is a part of life. Before Covid (BC), I applied to do a PhD in biomedicine at a research centre focusing on stem cell research to answer the question, which Chinese herbal medicines are effective in promoting neural stem cell proliferation and differentiation to induce neuroprotective and neurodegenerative benefits. We don't need Klaus' 'Ze Fourth Industrrrial Rrrevolution' to enhance the mind and body.

Bill Gates of Microsoft is involved in microchips in medicine: If we have or want children now, we are eco-terrorists! If I may briefly highlight that half the world is obese and half the world's food is thrown away. Common sense says if we only ate what we needed and industry was more frugal with food there would be no impending food shortages. Jedi mind trick; Bill Gates has nothing to do with depopulation. Bill Gates has a depopulation agenda. Bill Gates says in a Ted Talk entitled 'Innovating to Zero',

> *"Now, if we do a really great job on new vaccines, healthcare, reproductive health services, we could lower that (the population) by, perhaps, 10 or 15%* [(60)].

Bill Gates wants to snuff out the lives of over one billion people. Jedi mind trick; Bill Gates has nothing to do with microchips in medicine. Bill Gate's and his peanut gallery of fact-checkers deny that Bill Gates has anything to do with microchips in medicine [(1296)]. It should come as no surprise however that Bill Gates of Microsoft is involved in microchips in medicine. Microchips in medicine are a new technology capable of releasing various drugs on-demand over a prolonged period of time. The first microchip drug delivery devices were developed back in 1998. Women are soon going to be offered a microchip birth control that can be operated by remote control. Microchips Biotech has developed a microchip-based implant female contraceptive device. Microchips Biotech was co-founded by Massachusetts Institute of Technology (MIT) researchers Robert Langer and Michael J. Cima, and is funded by healthcare and technology vulture investors Polaris Partners, Medtronic, InterSouth, Flybridge Capital and InterWest [(1059)].

Human microchip implants use the same technology as microelectronic integrated circuits and microelectromechanical systems. This thumbprint sized microchip contains a microreservoir of drugs. A voltage is applied between the thin, metallic, (copper, gold, platinum, titanium) anode membrane and a cathode to electrochemically dissolve the drugs microreservoir cover. The electrical potential can be activated wirelessly by remote control, or result from metabolic changes in the host [(1297)]. Who shall hold the remote control? How far is the range on the remote control? What metabolic changes in my body activate drug release?

Bill Gates investment and patent for microchips in medicine: In January 2014, the Bill & Melinda Gates Foundation gave a grant of US$20,470,038 to Microchips Biotech for the 'Purpose: to develop a personal system that enables women to regulate their fertility' [1058]. In the current market, a San Diego-based biopharma company called Daré Bioscience aims to advance these new forms of birth control. Daré Bioscience has developed a pipeline for experimental devices and treatments specifically for women's 'health'. In November 2019, the company announced that it secured an agreement to acquire another contraceptive to add to its product base, the Gates-funded Microchips Biotech microchip-based implant [1298].

In addition to Gates investment in Microchips Biotech, Gates also holds a patent for microprocessor-based systems and cryptocurrency. The patent has UK 'charity' Full Fact working overtime to censor this information, so chances are it has some truth to it. Take the Full Fact webpage regarding Bill Gates and Microsoft patent numbered 060606 (666!) for technology allowing people's activity to be monitored in exchange for cryptocurrency (return to slavery chip). The Full Fact peanut gallery attempt to refute by saying, "Patent application 060606 doesn't reference 'injectable microchips'. It is true that Microsoft has a patent application with the numbers 060606 in it, but it's for a system which rewards physical activity with cryptocurrency" [1299]. The truth is Bill Gates and Microsoft patent is numbered WO2020060606 and entitled 'Cryptocurrency System Using Body Activity Data'. The patent description further states, "may include any device capable of processing and storing data/information and communicating over communication network...For example, user device may include personal computers, servers, cell phones, tablets, laptops, smart devices". Gate's patent is looking to include *"microprocessor-based systems"* [1300]. The word microchip is short for microprocessor chip [1301]. The global agenda is monitoring work. The WEF old boy network just got us used to counting steps.

Poor demented Gates denies it. Here's what Bill Gates of Microsoft has to say about those COVID-19 'conspiracy theories'. *"I've never been involved in any microchip type thing"*, Gates says. *"It's almost hard to deny this stuff because it's so stupid or strange that even to repeat it gives it credibility"*, Gates says. Gates describes it as "bizarre". I would have to agree with him. It is bizarre, and denial is not a river in Egypt. Gates has the fact-wreckers working overtime to suppress the connections between Gates and

Microchips Biotech Inc [1296]. If one needs further convincing that Mr Smirk wants to implant microchips in us, Google Wickedpedia 'Microchip implant (human)' [1302]. The most conspiratorial aspect is that Wickedpedia doesn't mention the Gates Foundation's US$20,470,038 donation in January 2014 to Microchips Biotech [1058]. Bill Gates 'you have been weighed, you have been measured, you have been found wanting'.

Other Dubious Patents

Rothschild patent for a COVID-19 test: Rothschild patented a test for COVID-19 on May 17th 2020. The patent is numbered US20200279585A1. The applicant and inventor named is Richard A. Rothschild, London, UK. The provisional application No. 62 / 240,783 was filed on October 13th 2015. These provisional and subsequent applications were for a method for acquiring and transmitting biometric data (vital signs) of a user and be analysed to determine whether the user is afflicted with a viral infection. The method includes using a pulse oximeter to obtain pulse and blood oxygen saturation percentage, which is then wirelessly transmitted to a smartphone. The smartphone accelerometer measures movement of the smartphone and/or the user to ensure that the data is accurate. Accurate data then uploads to the cloud (or host), where data is used alone (or with other vital signs) to determine whether the user is afflicted with (or likely to be afflicted with) a viral infection. The application may not necessarily be COVID-19 specific, however the patent for a system that analyses biometric data to determine whether the user is suffering from COVID-19 was applied for on May 17th 2020 [1303]. Monitoring vital signs to see if we are infected, or likely to be infective, or rebellious perhaps? Send in the drones to give us that mind-body experience.

The CDC took out a patent on SARS coronavirus in 2007: Dr David Martin is Associate International Director of the Royal College of Physicians. Dr Martin provides insight into the COVID-19 pandemic in America. Martin gives a deposition to Reiner Fuellmich on a *BitChute* video entitled 'Spike Protein Depopulation Patents Since 2002!' Martin describes how he has combed thousands of patents since the early 2000s for the SARS-CoV spike protein injections. Martin names all of the companies, universities and major players involved, including the Defence Advanced Research Projects Agency (DARPA). Martin describes the coronavirus and vaccines, and the interest of DARPA in creating a biological weapon out of this as a tool for population control. Martin says "we are not having a vaccine for a virus, we are injecting a computer simulation of a sequence which has been known and patented for years". Martin says (I have extracted the main points), "This is an opportunity marketing campaign". Martin reads a statement made in 2015 by Dr Peter Daszak, President of EcoHealth Alliance (who funds the Wuhan Institute of Virology), published in *National Academies Press* on February 12th 2016. Daszak said,

> *"We need to increase public understanding of the need for medical countermeasures such as of pan coronavirus vaccine, a key driver is the media and the economics will follow the hype. We need to use that hype to our advantage to get to the real issues; investors will respond if they see profit at the end"*.

As Public Enemy says "Don't believe the hype".

Dr Martin reviewed 400 patents issued around SARS coronavirus and says there are 120 patented pieces of evidence to suggest that the declaration of the novel coronavirus is entirely a fallacy. There are countless variations of sequences of viruses that have been uploaded to GISAID (Global initiative on sharing all influenza data). Martin explains that up until 1999, patents of coronavirus applied to veterinary sciences. Martin explains;

> *"The first patent for coronavirus vaccine was sought by Pfizer. The application for the first vaccine for coronavirus was filed on January 28th 2000; 21 years ago...US patent 6372224 which was the spike protein virus vaccine for the canine coronavirus. Fauci and the NIAID (National Institute of Allergy and Infectious Diseases) found the malleable coronavirus to be a potential candidate for HIV vaccines. ...SARS is...not a natural progression of a zoonotic modification of a coronavirus...In 1999 Fauci funded research at the University of North Carolina... specifically to create a... filed on April 19th 2002 ...where the National Institute of Allergy and Infectious Diseases built an infectious replication-defective coronavirus specifically targeted for human lung epithelium ... in other words we made SARS, and we patented it on April 19th 2002 before any alleged SARS outbreak in Asia...The patent issued as number 7279327 clearly laid out in gene sequencing the fact that we knew the ACE 2 binding domains and spike protein and other elements... was not only engineered but could be synthetically modified in the laboratory using nothing more than gene sequencing technologies using*

nothing more than a computer code. Harness coronavirus as a vector to distribute HIV vaccines...".

"We started monitoring...National Institutes of Health (NIH), NIAID, US AMRIID (Army Medical Research Institute of Infectious Diseases)...our concern was coronavirus was being seen as a potentially manipulable agent as a vaccine vector but...also...being considered as a biological weapon candidate. In April 2003 filing by US CDC...in addition to filing the entire gene sequence which became SARS coronavirus... you cannot patent a naturally occurring substance...patent No 7220852...also had series derivative patents associated with it, these include US patent 46592703P & US patent 776521 which not only covered gene sequences of SARS but also covered the means of detecting it using RT-PCR."

Martin continues, *"If you...own a patent on the gene itself and you own a patent on its detection, you have a cunning advantage of being able to control 100% of the providence of the virus itself and its detection; you have the entire scientific and message control. The patent office rejected the patent on the gene sequence as it was unpatentable as the gene sequence was already in the public domain".*

Martin affirms the CDC got the patent on SARS coronavirus in 2007 [(1304)].

The COVID-19 smart vaccine: In a world first development, researchers are currently creating a COVID-19 smart vaccine patch that will deliver the vaccine, as well as measure vaccine efficacy. The COVID-19 smart vaccine is being developed in collaboration with Imperial College London and Swansea University Institute for Innovative Materials, Processing and Numerical Technologies (IMPACT). The COVID-19 smart vaccine patch uses microneedles that break the skin barrier to deliver the vaccine and also "measure inflammatory responses to the vaccination by monitoring biomarkers in the skin". It is said the COVID-19 smart vaccine design allows for both lower doses of the vaccine and offers a personalised approach to vaccination. Researchers are looking to conduct human clinical studies on transdermal delivery [(1305)]. The daily propaganda does not tell us that biosensors are required to measure biomarkers in the skin. Microfluidic chips equipped with biosensors are called biosensors-on-chip or chips [(1306)]. The chips are coming, and they're not frites. Microneedles are used to insert quantum dots, discussed next.

Quantum dots: The following is difficult for me to grasp fully, but this information is important for us to understand the future agenda of transhumanist medicine. Quantum dots (QDs) are being seen as promising agents to combat COVID-19. QDs are multifunctional nanoparticles that can act as biosensors and can potentially act as targeting agents for viruses and cancer cells. A possible role of QDs in attenuating (lessening the effect of) SARS-CoV-2 is now being explored [(1307)]. QDs are invisible to the naked eye yet become detectable when exposed to near-infrared spectroscopy (NIR) light. QDs contain a copper indium selenide core and aluminium-doped zinc sulphide shell. QDs can be tuned to emit in the NIR spectrum by controlling stoichiometry (the elements) and shelling time [(1308)]. The human implantable QD microneedle vaccination delivery system will deliver the vaccine and invisibly encode vaccination records in the skin [(1309)].

QDs are nanomedicine. Nanomedicine uses nanoparticles. A single nanoparticle is a multifunctional nanocarrier or vector, with the potential to accommodate drugs, affinity ligands (related to antibodies), and imaging moieties (fluorescent visualisers) to enable targeted and traceable drug delivery [(1310)]. Researchers at MIT, the institute that collaborates with Microchips Biotech, developed a novel way to record a patient's vaccination records by storing the data in a pattern of dye that is invisible to the naked eye but that can is delivered under the skin at the same time as the vaccine. The dye consists of QDs nanocrystals that can remain under the skin for at least five years. Under the skin, the QD dye can emit near-infrared light that a specially equipped smartphone can detect. These on-person medical records being developed are copper-based quantum dots. The dots are approximately four nanometres in diameter but are encapsulated in microparticles spheres measuring about 20 microns in diameter. The red nanoparticle dye is designed to be delivered by a microneedle patch as opposed to a syringe and needle, such as the COVID-19 smart vaccine patch currently in development. The microneedles are made from a mixture of dissolvable sugar and a polymer called PVA, as well as the QD dye and the vaccine ingredient. After applying the patch to the skin, the microneedles, which are 1.5 millimetres, partially dissolve and release all the microparticle ingredients within approximately two minutes. The researchers say the advantage of this technology is that it will *"enable the rapid and anonymous detection of patient vaccination history to ensure that every child is vaccinated"* [(1308)]. Child is doublespeak for 'everyone'.

Microchips in COVID-19 diagnostics: Microchips are currently being developed in COVID-19 diagnostics. Biosensor-based diagnostics (biosensors on-chip or chips) are described as the frontiers in rapid detection of COVID-19. Novel biosensor-based diagnostics currently used to detect RNA-viruses include CRISPR-Cas9 based paper strip, nucleic-acid based, aptamer-based, antigen-Au/Ag nanoparticles-based electrochemical biosensor, optical biosensor and surface plasmon resonance (SPR). These tools allow rapid, portable and more accurate diagnosis [(1311)].

Microchips in COVID-19 therapeutics: Again, DARPA is a research and development agency of the US Department of Defence, responsible for developing emerging technologies for military use. DARPA funded microchip technology is currently being used to optimise convalescent plasma (blood of recovered patients) therapy for COVID-19 patients. The DARPA microchip technology was initially developed to study the contagiousness of influenza and common cold infections, including common coronavirus infections. DARPA-funded microchip technology is being used to comprehensively measure SARS-CoV-2 specific antibodies to allow physicians to choose the most effective donors for convalescent plasma therapy. The research was conducted to develop platform technology for new therapeutics to address the current coronavirus pandemic and emerging pathogens with pandemic potential. Pandemic 2; *"You'll pay attention next time"*, said Gates while he rubbed his hands together gleefully. The research was funded in part by the NIH and the Defence Threat Reduction Agency [(1312)]. Sounds like biological warfare on us, to me.

Forgot your wallet? No problem: Microchips are being used to store medical records and our cryptocurrency. In 2004 the Food and Drug Administration (FDA) approved Verichip, an implantable radiofrequency identification device (microchip) that would allow doctors to access patient medical records [(1313)]. A Danish firm called BiChip released a microchip implant with wireless connectivity in 2018. The company's intentions for its microchip implant are to link into the Ripple cryptocurrency and allow payments to be made via the implanted microchip [(1314)].

Millibots and microrobots: Microchips are being used to store medical records and our cryptocurrency 3D fabrication technologies can now manufacture wirelessly controlled millibots and microrobots with integrated sensors. Millibots and microrobots are said to be revolutionising micromanipulation-based medical interventions and enabling doctors to perform minimally invasive procedures not previously possible. Micromanipulation refers to the microscopic manipulation of cellular organelles using specific tools capable of moving an object with high precision. Encouraging results using these novel technologies have been achieved in cancer and gastrointestinal, neurological, cardiovascular and ocular disease, along with oral vaccine delivery. Whilst this technology may be valuable in certain surgical procedures, the application of this technology in vaccines has more sinister connotations. Such microrobotic systems could be used for local targeted delivery of imaging contrast agents, medications, genes and mRNA [(1315)]. That bodes well for, as Gates says, "*this great new mRNA vaccine technology*".

What happens when animals are chipped? Researchers conclude that microchips in animals are associated with microchip-associated tumours or malignant sarcomas. Microchip-associated tumours have been reported in rodents and dogs and are observed around or adjacent to the microchips implants. Carcinogenic fibrosarcomas are also microchip-associated tumours in animals [(1316, 1317)].

Our dystopian future is chips in all drugs: Pharmaceutical firms are currently exploring a new technology known as microphysiological systems (MPS), also known as 'organ-on-a-chip', 'body-on-a-chip', or 'human-on-a-chip'. The aim is to reach the point where these chips are adopted as a standard component in drug development [(1318)]. This technology is being described as being useful in the quality control of live viral vaccines and is being considered to analyse mutations in the oral poliovirus vaccine (OPV). Mutations in the OPV can be analysed using microchips which can be used to deduce the original complementary DNA (cDNA), and results can be registered and quantified by a computer-linked charge-coupled device (CCD) camera [(1319)].

In 2015, a propositional review on synthetic biology devices and circuits for RNA-based smart vaccines was conducted. The review found that DNA or RNA based vaccinations would programme these nucleic acids and allow immunologists the power to control the production of antigens and adjuvants through the administration of small molecule drugs as chemical triggers. Modified RNA gene delivery methods will allow mammalian synthetic biologists (synthetic biology) to create genetic circuits encoded exclusively on RNA [1320]. Microchips to monitor mutations in viruses! Immunologists using microchips to control the production of antigens and adjuvants! That gives me so much confidence in vaccines, Heidi.

Synthetic biology and smart dust, that other conspiracy: Synthetic biology involves redesigning organisms for more useful purposes by engineering them to have new capabilities. Synthetic biology aims to control gene regulation and can lead to increased production of chemicals and pharmaceuticals. DNA nanotechnology is one aspect of synthetic biology. Nanoparticles have the ability to self-assemble into complex, organised superstructures on patterned surfaces through fluid-mediated interactions. 'Smart dust' is a term that originally referred to cubic-millimetre wireless semiconductor devices manufactured using fabrication techniques derived from the microelectronics industry. Smart dust are nanostructured devices with optical, chemical, and mechanical properties that can be utilised to perform sensing, signal processing, communication and motive functions [1321]. Later, smart dust came to include functional micron-sized porous silicon particles used to monitor smaller environments. An article published in *Nature Nanotechnology* in 2009 explained that biosensors (such as the ones used in the 'smart COVID-19 vaccine') can be miniaturised by injecting smaller volumes into micro-and nanofluidic devices or submerging increasingly sophisticated particles known as smart dust into the sample. The smart dust miniature wireless semiconducting sensor devices can invisibly monitor the environment in buildings and public spaces. The report described a hybrid microdevice that is powered by adenosine triphosphate (ATP) (the energy of living things) and relies on antibody-functionalised microtubules and kinesin motors (used to control actuation and transport in nanoscale dimensions). The authors envisaged that large numbers of such smart dust biosensors could be inserted into organisms or distributed into the environment for remote sensing [1322]. I wonder how the ruling class would distribute such biosensors into our environment. No matter; the 'smart' dust is coming in the 'smart' vaccines.

Scientists want to control our brain with their big remote control: Welcome to the new age of magnetogenetics. In 2016 geneticists from Rockefeller University published an article in *Nature* explaining that neuroscientists had successfully genetically engineered neurons to become responsive to magnetic fields so that the scientists could remotely control the activity of particular neurons in the brain and even control the animal's behaviour. Interestingly, the study used a chimpanzee adenovirus; the same virus vector being used in the Johnson & Johnson, Oxford-AstraZeneca and Sputnik V vaccines [1323]. Magnetic strategies allowing scientists to control neuronal activity in the brain have been successfully used in zebrafish and mice [1324].

We don't need synthetic biologists manipulating our bodies for more useful purposes by engineering them to have new capabilities. That is playing God. We have an immune system and it is practically perfect. The era of microchip implants in medicine to embed our medical records, synthetic biology devices and circuits in DNA and RNA-based vaccination, and genetically engineered neurons to control our brain is on us. These are highly unethical and do not adhere to European General Data Protection Regulation (GDPR). Confidential health records could potentially be accessed and used by unauthorised persons [1325]. The ethics of microchips in medicine should be debated, not dismissed and labelled a conspiracy.

CHAPTER TWENTY-TWO

VACCINES ARE NOT GREEN

"Tread softly! All the earth is holy ground. It may be, could we look with seeing eyes, this spot we stand on is a Paradise".

Christina Rossetti [1326]

Environmentalists wake-up! Once an environmentalist always an environmentalist! Vaccines incentivise global shark culls, the wanton destruction of river and lake beds and drive CO2 emissions. The whole so-called green push from the Greta Reset is hypocrisy in its true form. The Greta Reset stays silent about the detrimental effects of the pharmaceutical industry and of non-renewable fossil fuel-derived plastic personal protective equipment that is incinerated. The Greta Reset stops the proletariat from going on holidays whilst the bourgeoisie pretend to take their ungreen vaccine and enjoy the return of the jet set days, then take their wealthy cronies to inner space.

Not enough trees on the planet: There is simply no justification for the environmental impact of the coronavirus disease 2019 (COVID-19) vaccine rollout. The Greta Reset makes us feel guilty to drive a car, to go on holiday or to eat a burger, while those dependent on pharmacological drugs remain unaware that these drugs drive climate change. An article published in the *Journal of Cleaner Production* stated the pharmaceutical industry global carbon emissions are 55% higher than the automotive industry, with total global emissions of the pharmaceutical industry being 52 megatonnes of CO2e in 2015 [1327]. Vaccines are hugely detrimental to our planet. The production, distribution, transport and storage of vaccines has a huge environmental impact. This is particularly true of the requirements for refrigeration gases and insulation foaming agents [1328]. When I was 14 years old I stood against chlorofluorocarbons (CFCs) to protect our ozone layer.

There is a push to 'green' the pharmaceutical industry, but it's a smokescreen. One of these is to use electric vehicles (EVs) to deliver vaccines and medicines and solar energy linked to the electricity grid to meet all energy needs for storage, cooling and transportation of vaccines and medications. This is still estimated to take between seven and ten years to implement [1329]. EVs and solar power require batteries that require minerals. The minerals needed to make batteries for EVs, electrical cables etc. are manganese, nickel, copper and cobalt which lie at the bottom of our oceans in polymetallic nodules. The region of greatest interest to the mining companies is called the Clarion-Clipperton Zone (CCZ), where these minerals are abundant. Deep-sea mining is as environmentally unfriendly as land mining. Deep-sea mining involves scraping and vacuuming nodules from the seafloor. Deep-sea mining destroys habitats and releases plumes of sediment that blanket or choke seafloor filter-feeding species, reefs and fish swimming in the water column [1330]. Sediment input is one of the great killers of coral reefs [1331]. We are being sold a lemon. The Greta Reset push for a 'cleantech revolution', and 'green' electric vehicles will destroy habitat, fish, the reef and contribute to global warming. I stood against the dredging of Cairns Bay to protect the Great Barrier Reef. I went to the Great Barrier Reef in 2015. One need not be a marine biologist to realise that what you see is coral bleaching. So what do the boffins do to mitigate the detrimental effects of the pharmaceutical industry on our environment? Why; develop a vaccine that makes methane blocking antibodies to mitigate greenhouse gas emissions in agriculture [1332].

The pharmaceutical industry will benefit from global warming: Climate change is an opportunity for Big Pharmaceutical Research and Manufacturers of America (PhRMA) to make even greater profits and further increase their power. A warming planet and rising temperatures are expected to accelerate the spread of vector-borne diseases and result in an increased demand for vaccines [1333]. Where's Greta? Where's Extinction Rebellion? Where's Green Peace? Where's the World Wildlife Fund? Where's the Australian Conservation Foundation? Where are the green anarchists? All lining up for their shot.

Not enough horseshoe crabs in the sea: The pharmaceutical industry plunders and pillages natural medicine resources while discrediting natural medicine and painting herbalists as quacks. There is a reason for this. Almost two-thirds of all small molecules approved by the Food and Drug Administration (FDA) between 1981 and 2014 were derived from natural products including animals and plants. The COVID-19 vaccine has been developed using the blue blood of a living fossil known as the horseshoe crab which has existed for 450 million years. The horseshoe crab is an endangered species. The horseshoe crab's declining population is attributed to pollution, deteriorating coastlines, sea level rise, overfishing, and blood harvesting for pharmaceutical products, in particular for vaccine development [1334]. Anyone injecting a COVID-19 vaccine is directly responsible for the decimation of this ancient species. I stand for the horseshoe crabs.

Not enough sharks in the sea: Many animal oil emulsions are used in vaccine production, where they are described as vaccine oils. Animal sources of vaccine oils are fish oils, including shark and orange roughy, and mink oil [1335]. The triterpene oil squalene is an essential component of nanoemulsion vaccine adjuvants [1336]. Before the vaccine rollout, it was announced that 19 of the 193 candidate COVID-19 vaccines in clinical or preclinical evaluation stages use adjuvants, and 5 use the adjuvant shark-based squalene [773]. There are not enough sharks in the sea to fulfil The Global Health Security Agenda's (GHSA) wet dream for universal vaccination. Shark Allies, a global nonprofit organisation whose goals are to restore and conserve shark populations by improving conservation policies, have estimated that 536,412 sharks globally will be killed to fulfil the current global vaccine rollout. To determine this figure, Shark Allies calculated the mass of squalene in one dose of the adjuvant/vaccine based on quantities that are used in current vaccines [1337]. This figure is for the current global vaccine rollout and does not include yearly booster shots, which are the case. How coincidental that another source of squalene for vaccine use is mink liver and that Denmark found mink-specific mutations of severe acute respiratory syndrome coronavirus 2 (SARS-CoV-2) in humans then culled 17 million minks under a belief that these mutations could negatively impact the effect of COVID-19 vaccine candidates [1338]. I stand for all the animals used in vaccine oils.

Not enough sand in the rivers and lakes: Glass vial manufacturing is big business and getting bigger. In 2019 the pharmaceutical glass tubing industry was worth US$12.35 billion, and this figure is projected to reach US$20.75 billion by 2025 [1339]. There is currently a shortage of glass vials needed to deliver the COVID-19 vaccines, which may have contributed to the slow vaccine rollout seen in certain places in the beginning. The immediate shortage was due to manufacturing issues combined with a surge in demand. Other supply challenges are long-term. The glass vial production industry is a heavily capital-intensive business. Additionally, the equipment used to manufacture the glass vials is energy-intensive, with the furnaces needing to be run at 2000°C even when no vials are being produced. As a result of the intricacy of the procedures in glass vial manufacturing and the additional cost required, there are only a handful of large medical glass vial manufacturers globally. Schott, Corning and Nipro Pharma Corporation, Gerresheimer in Germany, SGD Pharma in France and Stevanato Group in Italy control the market. A lack of the key ingredient, sand, is driving the global glass vial shortage. The type of sand suitable for making glass vials for vaccines is called borosilicate glass. Borosilicate glass contains large amounts of silicon dioxide, resulting in the glass being chemically inert. Most silica sand is found in river beds and lakes. Sand is already the second most consumed resource, only after water [(1340)]. I stand for the rivers and lakes.

Vaccines are neither vegan, cruelty-free, human tissue free Kosher or Halal: In pharmacology, gelatin derived from pork is called porcine, and gelatin derived from beef is called bovine. Bovine and porcine gelatin has numerous uses throughout the pharmaceutical industry as components in drug capsules and stabilisers in vaccines, including measles-mumps-rubella (MMR), varicella, yellow fever, rabies and some influenza vaccines. Children in receipt of these animal-derived vaccine stabilisers have been shown to have an increased risk of allergy to gelatin containing foods, vaccines or other medical products due to the presence of IgE anti-gelatin post-vaccination [(1341)]. Vaccine companies have worked for years to develop pork-free vaccines. The Swiss pharmaceutical company Novartis produced a pork-free meningitis vaccine, and the Saudi and Malaysia based AJ Pharma is said to be working on one. Spokespeople for Pfizer, Moderna and AstraZeneca have purported that pork products are not part of their COVID-19 vaccines, however Secretary General of the British Islamic Medical Association, Dr Salman Waqar, said that demand, existing supply chains, and the cost and shorter shelf life of porcine gelatin-free vaccines means porcine gelatin is likely to be used in the majority of vaccines for years to come. Currently, limited supply and preexisting deals with other companies mean that the vaccines received by countries with large Muslim populations, such as Indonesia, will not be certified gelatin-free [(1342)]. Pork products are forbidden in Islam and Judaism, and Hindus question the inclusion of cow blood in vaccines. Don't worry about your religious or ethical dilemmas; Orthodox Jews, Muslims, Hindus and Vegans, your ethical and religious beliefs are selfish! Shut up! Obey! Take your shot! I stand with the Orthodox Jews, Muslims, Hindus and Vegans.

The pope has told us Catholics that we will be guaranteed our place in Heaven if we inject vaccines that contain human tissue [(1343)]. I do not support injecting human tissue-derived substances such as growth hormone from human cadavers or immortalised cells from an aborted foetus back in 1969. I stand against cannibalism. Vaccines need to be studied in animals where the physiology and disease process is similar to that in humans. Nonhuman primates (NHPs) have been used for vaccine testing for a number of viral, bacterial and parasitic diseases. NHPs used in medical research are mainly macaques monkeys [(1344)]. As mentioned on numerous occasions, the DNA vaccine protection against SARS-CoV-2 of the COVID-19 vaccine was demonstrated in rhesus macaque monkeys [(1345)]. I stand against animal testing.

Not enough CO2: The Pfizer-BioNTech COVID-19 vaccines require ultra-cold storage and special distribution and administration requirements. A shortage of dry ice and strict regulations about its transportation was slowing down the distribution at the beginning of the COVID-19 vaccine rollout [(1346)]. As dry ice melts, it turns into carbon dioxide (CO2). Transporting large quantities of carbon dioxide emitting dry ice poses a danger on aeroplanes. A 2009 memo circulated by the Federal Aviation Administration (FAA) stated, "There have been very few reported incidents of carbon dioxide hazards aboard aircraft resulting from sublimation of dry ice". The statement continued, "The FAA is working with manufacturers, air carriers, and airport authorities to provide guidance on implementing current regulatory requirements for safely transporting large quantities of dry ice in air cargo". The FAA responded by allowing United Airlines to carry 15,000 pounds of dry ice per flight, which is five times more than normally permitted [(1347)]. I thought we are sequestering CO2.

Drugs and vaccines contain an array of inexplicable health-damaging contaminants: A pharmaceutical product analysis published in *The Microscope* used polarised light microscopy, Fourier transform infrared spectroscopy, Raman microscopy, and several types of electron microscopy with energy dispersive spectrometers (EDS) and wavelength dispersive spectrometers (WDS) detectors to identify contaminants in pharmaceutical drugs. Common contaminants found in pharmaceuticals drugs included natural and synthetic fibres, silicon, plastics or polymers, rubber, metal particles and corrosion products, glass particles and glass delamination flakes, skin flakes, char particles, detergents, lubricant oils, Teflon and graphite [(1348)]. As previously mentioned in Chapter 13, 'COVID-19 Vaccines are Safe for Two Months', the contents of vaccines baffle scientists. Scientists examined 44 vaccine samples from Italy and France and found that vaccines were contaminated with lead, stainless steel, iron particles and other inorganic material. The authors said, *"The quantity of foreign bodies detected and, in some cases, their unusual chemical compositions baffled us"*. The findings surprised the authors so much so that they admit the undue presence of the inorganic material is "for the time being inexplicable" [(823)]. I stand against the pharmaceutical industry as it destroys our planet.

Vaccines contain heavy metals: Injectable products such as vaccines contain heavy metals. 85 samples of injectable biological products regulated by the Centre for Biologics Evaluation and Research (CBER) of the FDA surveyed vaccines such as measles virus, typhoid and tetanus toxoid vaccines for the presence of aluminium, arsenic, barium, cadmium, chromium, lead, mercury, selenium, thallium and zinc. The metal concentrations found in the majority of these products were described as low or undetectable [(1349)]. Aluminium offers promise as a key adjuvant for COVID-19 vaccines as it helps achieve high levels of neutralising antibodies. The SARS vaccine, known as COV-RBD219N1, developed by Bottazzi and colleague, Dr Peter Hotez, is aluminium containing [(1350)]. PiCoVacc is one of China's COVID-19 vaccine candidates and contains aluminium [(1351)].

As previously described, today's vaccine schedules include 30-40 injections, with up to five injections being simultaneously administered in one sitting. Vaccines that contain aluminium compound adjuvants may predispose a person to allergy. Many researchers have called for a reevaluation of aluminium adjuvants and for the simultaneous administration of multiple vaccines to be stopped to avoid the combined negative effects of multiple food proteins and adjuvants [(1352)]. The narrative that carcinogens, mutagens, teratogens and neurotoxins are 'safe in small amounts' is a ludicrous notion peddled by pharmaceutical companies, which are chemical companies that benefit from us being sick. A number of persistent organic pollutants (POPs) such as pesticides, polychlorinated biphenyls (PCBs) and dioxins, and heavy metals are detected at high concentrations in blood samples of the United States (US) population, with more than one-tenth of the US population having ≥10 POPs each at concentrations in the 10% [782]. As explained in Chapter 12, 'Vaccines aren't Described as Safe and don't Always Work', pollutants in humans prevent the immune system from mounting an antibody response post-vaccination. When in doubt, get it out. If you are an earth-loving greenie and take your shot, it is said that conscience keeps more people awake than cocaine.

CHAPTER TWENTY-THREE

MEASLES SHMEEZLES & THE GREAT AUTISM COVER-UP

"Love is like the measles; we all have to go through it. Also like the measles, we take it only once. One never need be afraid of catching it a second time".

Jerome K. Jerome [1353]

Measles has very low morbidity/death rate. The ruling class trained us on measles, a completely harmless disease in children. Before COVID (BC) all we heard was measles, measles, measles. Measles shmeezles! Imagine turning a childhood disease such as a common cold into an issue of national security. Sound familiar? Imagine actually falling for it! As a little experiment as to how effective public health indoctrination is, ask any person on the street how many children died from measles in your country last year. The responses I receive indicate that the general public believes 20 kids die from measles a year in Ireland. These beliefs are completely irrational. Putting things in perspective, in 2017, about 85% of the world's children received one dose of measles vaccine by their first birthday and there were 110,000 measles deaths globally. The majority of these deaths were in children under five. According to the World Wealth Organisation, measles vaccination resulted in an 80% drop in measles deaths between 2000 and 2017 worldwide [708]. According to the WHO also, more than 95% of measles deaths occur in countries with low per capita incomes and weak health infrastructures [1354]. Additionally, the WHO state that severe measles is likely among poorly nourished young children, especially those with vitamin A deficiency or whose immune systems have been weakened by HIV/AIDS or other diseases [1355].

In high-income England and Wales, by comparison, there have been 12 deaths from the measles virus since 2000 [1356]. Twelve deaths in 20 years yet BC, measles was rammed down our throats every second day on the daily propaganda. One person dies every six seconds from diabetes, but the same propaganda machine pushes junk food. By comparison also, the common childhood illness slapped-cheek syndrome, also called fifth disease or parvovirus B19, has killed four children since 2006 [1357]. No official death notification website exists for parvovirus. No media attention is paid to parvovirus deaths. No vaccination exists for parvovirus (yet). My children have had parvovirus and are immune to parvovirus. In July 2015, the United States (US) reported their first confirmed measles death in more than a decade [(1358)]. Centres for Disease Control and Prevention (CDC) data shows there have been ten deaths in which measles has been put as a cause of death on the death certificate since 2000 [(1359)]. 10 deaths in 20 years! Yet the media greatly exaggerates the morbidity of measles to generate interest in and increase uptake of vaccines. Measles is practically a nothing disease in children. Asthma on the contrary is life-limiting, life-threatening and lifelong. As explained in Chapter 12, 'Vaccines aren't Described as Safe and don't Always Work', and again reiterated here, measles infection protects against asthma.

Measles outbreaks are due to both failure to vaccinate and vaccine failure: Primary and secondary vaccine failure was discussed in Chapter 12, 'Vaccines aren't Described as Safe and don't Always Work'. Primary vaccine failure occurs when a person does not mount immune response after vaccination and secondary vaccine failure refers to waning of vaccine-induced immunity. Whilst natural infection to measles is lifelong [(763)], despite sustained high vaccine coverage, the reemergence of 'vaccine-preventable diseases' (VPDs), including mumps and measles is linked to waning vaccine immunity [(763(764)]. It is a great business model the vaccine companies have whereby they blame failure to vaccinate and not vaccine failure due to waning immunity. BC, all we heard on the daily propaganda was measles, however the daily propaganda wilfully omitted that these measles outbreaks were be enlarge occurring in highly vaccinated populations and due to primary vaccine failure. Blaming failure to vaccinate is public health's agenda; however this ignores the greater picture. Public health's job is to survey. Public health experts and other stakeholders, including policymakers, immunisation programmes managers, paediatricians, family physicians, and other experts and individuals involved in delivering immunisations, must broaden their knowledge and understanding of vaccine epidemiology [(765)].

Just as near-total vaccinated Seychelles, Guam, Israel, and Iceland experienced high Delta-driven pandemic surges in the double-jabbed, the following measles outbreaks have all occurred in areas that have near-total measles vaccination coverage of between 95-99%. Just as in Seychelles,

Guam, Israel, and Iceland also, the daily propaganda uses these outbreaks in the vaccinated as an opportunity to generate interest in and increase uptake of measles vaccines, by blaming the 'pandemic of unvaccinated'. Examples of measles outbreaks in near-total measles vaccination coverage include the 1991 Quebec outbreak, which had 99% vaccination coverage (1360). South Iran had 95% vaccination coverage (1361, 1362). New Zealand had 95% vaccination coverage (1363, 1364). Australia had 95% vaccination coverage (1365). The WHO confirmed the vaccine coverage was above the 95% target in the Romanian measles outbreak (1366). Primary vaccine failure was observed in a measles outbreak in São Paulo (1367). All measles outbreaks in these countries are due to primary vaccine failure, due to waning immunity. My children and I have had measles. Unlike the general population, which now includes adults susceptible to measles and requiring a measles-mumps-rubella (MMR) booster vaccine, my children and I have lifelong immunity and will never be at risk, or pose a risk, to our vulnerable (1368).

Breakthrough infection, as we are hearing with the 'safe and effective' COVID-19 vaccines is not unusual and is often attributed to waning immunity over time. Where their definition of herd immunity has been achieved, as has been achieved in these areas of high vaccine coverage, outbreaks can indicate virus evolution, where the virus takes on genetic mutations. This phenomenon is known as antigenic drift and results in vaccine-induced escape mutants (VEMs) (1369). VEMs were discussed in Chapter 12, 'Vaccines aren't Described as Safe and don't Always Work'. Public health should survey evidence of measles VEMs by comparing nasopharyngeal samples of the vaccinated and unvaccinated. There is no possibility of robust vaccine science however when the overwhelming majority of the population is vaccinated, thus there is no control, and public health wrongfully blames measles outbreaks on the unvaccinated.

A study published in *Epidemiology and Infection*, the first time of its kind in measles epidemiology, used avidity testing to separate primary from secondary vaccine failures. Low-avidity (LA) and high-avidity (HA) virus-specific IgG antibodies indicated primary and secondary failure, respectively. The study concluded that secondary measles vaccine failures are more common than previously thought, particularly among individuals vaccinated early in life and among re-vaccinees (1370). Measles vaccine failure also occurs due to secondary vaccine failure due to cold chain management failure. An adult measles outbreak in the Federated States of Micronesia in 2014 was attributed to vaccine cold chain management failures that caused the vaccine to spoil [784].

Measles Mary: The contraction of measles by fully vaccinated individuals and the spread of measles to fully vaccinated individuals in populations is acknowledged [1371]. Her name was also Mary, just like poor Typhoid Mary, whose life public health destroyed. Typhoid Mary suffered extreme punishment for something she had no control over, spent 26 years in forced quarantine on North Brother Island and then died alone [1372]. Public health could have retrained Mary in a new role where she wouldn't pose a threat. On the contrary, modern-day Measles Mary is a hero, with the daily propaganda blaming failure to vaccinate, and the vaccinated going on to catch measles and drive infection. Vaccine refusers will be sent to 'the island' (FEMA camps); unless we stand.

Global deaths asthma: Back in the days when I was at primary school, we had a token child with asthma. Oh how times have changed. Up to one in five children now have asthma [1373]. Putting things into perspective, asthma is a common chronic allergic disease affecting 300 million children and adults worldwide [709]. The WHO estimated there were 383,000 deaths due to asthma in 2015 [653]. This number of deaths is nearly four times the number of deaths from measles. The CDC state one in 13 people in the US has asthma [711]. That equates to 8.4% of people in the US having asthma compared with 4.3% of the population worldwide [710].

Measles may protect children against allergies and asthma: As previously discussed in Chapter 12, 'Vaccines aren't Described as Safe and don't Always Work, the study entitled 'Prevention of Allergy-Risk Factors for Sensitisation in Children Related to Farming and Anthroposophic Lifestyle (PARSIFAL)' was conducted in 14,893 children in Austria, Germany, the Netherlands, Sweden, and Switzerland. 73% of children were vaccinated against measles, 20% had been infected with measles (including 11% of vaccinated children), and 14% had been neither vaccinated nor naturally infected. The study found that children that had a measles infection had a reduced risk of atopic disease including, atopic eczema, hay fever, allergic asthma and atopic keratoconjunctivitis. Among the children who never had measles infection, vaccinated children were more likely to have hay fever. Further analysis showed that allergies were less likely in children who had measles than those vaccinated against measles [654]. Another investigation into whether measles infection protects against the development of atopy in children was conducted in Guinea-Bissau, West Africa. The study's authors concluded that measles infection was associated with a large reduction in the risk of atopy [1140]. I don't need any study to know my unvaccinated children who have had measles don't suffer from atopic (allergic) disease.

Measles vaccine is associated with increased female child mortality: A *Lancet* reanalysis of West African studies acknowledged that high-titre measles vaccine and associated subsequent diphtheria-tetanus-pertussis (DTP) and inactivated poliovirus vaccination was found to be associated with excess mortality in female children in West Africa. The study authors concluded that a change in the sequence of vaccinations, rather than the high-titre measles vaccine, may have been the cause of increased female mortality in these trials [1374].

Mumps reemergence: After decades of declining mumps incidence amid widespread MMR vaccination campaigns, the US and other developed countries have experienced a resurgence in mumps cases over the last decade. As with measles, outbreaks have affected vaccinated people and communities with high vaccine coverage. A study published in *Science Translational Medicine* attributed these outbreaks due to waning immunity [1375]. A population-based surveillance study published in *The Lancet Infectious Diseases* described a protracted mumps outbreak that occurred in Western Australian aboriginal children despite high vaccine coverage as being due to waning immunity and recommended decreasing the interval between booster shots [1376]. A study examining recent mumps outbreaks in vaccinated populations published in the *Journal of Virology* argued against immune escape [1377]. Public health's motto is 'when the drugs don't work, give them more'. Mumps is literally a nothing disease in healthy children.

The Great Autism Cover-up

"Charity is suppose (sic) *to cover up for a multitude of sins", Bob Dylan.* [1378]

Wakefield is a smokescreen. When *The Sunday Times* 'investigative journalist' posing as a concerned parent of a newborn kept pressing me on Wakefield, I said, "all I know about Wakefield is he was a respected gastroenterologist that set out to study something else and found a correlation he didn't expect which he reported on, and, as a result, he was denigrated and vilified and struck off". The question is not does the measles vaccine cause autism, the question is, do vaccines cause autism? To answer that question is simple. We must compare the health of completely unvaccinated children to completely vaccinated children according to the CDC schedule. We parents of unvaccinated children would enrol our children in this study, and we wouldn't need to be financially coerced.

The documentary we aren't allowed to watch: Brian Hooker and Andrew Wakefield released the documentary *Vaxxed: From Cover-Up to Catastrophe* in 2016. The documentary was produced by Tobias Tommey and directed by Andrew Wakefield. The documentary included a video of recorded phone conversations with Dr William Thompson, a senior scientist at the CDC, about publishing a reworking of data from a controversial study published in 2004. The documentary highlighted that for over a decade this study had been cited to deny compensation to parents of MMR vaccine-injured children (1379). Andrew, Yes, Andrew, the supposed 'origins of the anti-vax conspiracy theory'. Yes, Wakefield, who falsified data and was found guilty of deliberate fraud, picked and chose data that suited his case; not unlike the CDC finagling statistics. Wakefield, and indeed MMR, is a smokescreen for the study that has not been done nor will ever be done unless we demand it.

Boy-girl, black-white and autism: The rate of autism diagnoses has increased alarmingly in the US and is about 25% higher in black children. Boys are far more likely than girls to receive this diagnosis. A CDC surveillance study published in 'The Morbidity and Mortality Weekly Report (MMWR) Surveillance Summaries' noted that males are four times more likely than females to be identified with autism spectrum disorder (ASD). Previous reports from the Autism and Developmental Disabilities Monitoring (ADDM) Network estimated ASD prevalence among white children to exceed that among black children by approximately 30% (1380).

This science behind 'Vaxxed': A National Immunisation Programme (NIP) CDC population-based study by DeStefano et al. entitled 'Age at first measles-mumps-rubella vaccination in children with autism and school-matched control subjects: a population-based study in metropolitan

Atlanta' was published in *Paediatrics* in 2004. The study explored the connection between the MMR vaccine, sex, race, and autism diagnosis. The study looked at the age at first MMR vaccination in children with autism and school-matched control subjects in metropolitan Atlanta. The study involved the CDC Metropolitan Atlanta Developmental Disabilities Surveillance Programme (MADDSP). The MADDSP estimates the number of children in metropolitan Atlanta that have selected developmental disabilities. The study aims were to compare ages at first MMR vaccination between children with autism and children without autism in the total population and in selected subgroups, including children with developmental regression. DeStefano et al. concluded that the overall distribution of ages at MMR vaccination among children with autism was similar to that of matched control children. CDC employee William W. Thompson, also an author of this study, later blew the whistle on how the statistics were massaged so as not to show a link between vaccination timing and the onset of autism in black males [(1381)].

A reanalysis of CDC data surrounding MMR vaccination timing and autism among young African American boys entitled 'Measles-mumps-rubella vaccination timing and autism among young African American boys: a reanalysis of CDC data' was published in *Neurodegeneration* on August 27th 2014. This article was retracted on October 3rd, 2014. The study reanalysed the data set obtained from the US CDC, used by DeStefano et al. 2004, in relation to the timing of the first MMR vaccine and autism diagnoses. Brian S. Hooker, from Simpson University, Redding, California, evaluated the same data to ascertain whether a relationship existed between a child's age at administration of first MMR in cases diagnosed with autism and controls born between 1986 through 1993 among school children in metropolitan Atlanta. Hooker's results showed that there was a statistically significant increase in autism cases, specifically among African American males who received the first MMR prior to 36 months of age [(1382)].

A further reanalysis of CDC data pertaining to the relationship of autism incidence and the age at which children got their first MMR vaccine by Brian S. Hooker was published in the *Journal of American Physicians and Surgeons* in 2018. This study also noted statistically significant relationships observed when African American males who received the MMR vaccine before the age of two or three years were more likely to receive an autism diagnosis. Hooker's reanalysis also found increased risks of earlier vaccination were observed for African American males and among cases of autism without MMR (potentially pointing to other vaccines), and that both phenomena warrant additional investigation. Hooker noted the flaws in the trials included that the CDC officials had observed similar relationships by November 2001 but failed to report them in their final publication. The original 2004 paper had reported on a relationship that was seen when specifically considering children diagnosed with autism without mental retardation, but that this relationship was not discussed, nor was any follow-up study conducted. Hooker also noted that preliminary results suggested a possible link between thimerosal (mercury-based preservative) exposure and MMR timing increasing the risk of autism. Hooker's discussion noted that the analysis of the MADDSP data used by DeStefano et al. did not consider gender separately and only considered race in the smaller 41% 'birth-certificate sample'. This obscured the statistically significant observation of the effect of vaccine timing on the incidence of autism in black males. Hooker explained their methodology departed substantially from the original study protocol, which indicated that race information was to be abstracted from school records for all individuals in the sample in the analysis. The DeStefano et al. earlier analysis included the entire sample for the race analysis and showed a statistically significant effect for blacks, yet no such effect for whites and others. Hooker concluded that these results warranted further investigation [(1383)].

A press release by the unknowing 'whistleblower' William Thompson was released on August 27th, 2014. The Statement of William Thompson regarding the 2004 article examining the possibility of a relationship between the MMR vaccine and autism that Thomson coauthored stated:

> *"My name is William Thompson. I am a Senior Scientist with the CDC where I have worked since 1998. I regret that my coauthors and I omitted statistically significant information in our 2004 article published in the journal Pediatrics. The omitted data suggested that African American males who received the MMR vaccine before age 36 months were at increased risk for autism. Decisions were made regarding which findings to report after the data were collected, and I believe that the final study protocol was not followed. I want to be absolutely clear that I believe vaccines have saved and continue to save countless lives. I would never suggest that any parent avoid vaccinating children of any race.*

Vaccines prevent serious diseases, and the risks associated with their administration are vastly outweighed by their individual and societal benefits. My concern has been the decision to omit relevant findings in a particular study for a particular sub-group for a particular vaccine. There have always been recognised risks for vaccination, and I believe it is the responsibility of the CDC to properly convey the risks associated with receipt of those vaccines. I have had many discussions with Dr Brian Hooker over the last ten months regarding studies the CDC has carried out regarding vaccines and neurodevelopmental outcomes, including autism spectrum disorders. I share his belief that CDC decision-making and analyses should be transparent. I was not, however, aware that he was recording any of our conversations, nor was I given any choice regarding whether my name would be made public or my voice would be put on the Internet...I am providing information to Congressman William Posey, and of course, will continue to cooperate with Congress. I have also offered to assist with reanalysis of the study data or development of further studies...I will do everything I can to assist any unbiased and objective scientists inside or outside the CDC to analyse data collected by the CDC or other public organisations for the purpose of understanding whether vaccines are associated with an increased risk of autism. There are still more questions than answers" [(1384)].

Still more questions than answers!? That gives me so much confidence in vaccines, Heidi. I'll take my children down to the vaccinator now.

Previous whistleblowers say Merck overstated their MMR vaccine effectiveness: An article published in *Forbes* magazine on June 27th 2012, entitled 'Whistleblower Suit A Boon to Vaccine Foes Even As It Stresses Importance of Vaccines' described a whistleblower lawsuit against Merck filed in 2010 by two former employees who accused Merck of overstating the effectiveness of its MMR vaccine. Merck was accused of misleading both regulators and consumers about its MMR vaccine. The suit alleged that Merck defrauded the US government by causing it to purchase approximately four million doses of mislabelled and misbranded MMR vaccine every year for at least a decade. The scientists said the allegedly ineffective MMR vaccine helped ignite two recent mumps outbreaks, referring to a 2006 mumps outbreak in the Midwest that recorded 6,500 among a highly vaccinated population and a 2009 mumps outbreak that recorded 5,000 cases, also in a highly vaccinated population.

Rather than reformulate the vaccine whose waning efficacy Merck itself acknowledged, Merck reportedly endeavoured on a complicated scheme to adjust its testing technique so that it would yield the desired potency results. The virologists said they witnessed the fraud firsthand and were asked to directly participate in the dishonest testing, dubbed "Protocol 007", outlined in great detail in the complaint. The article was updated on June 28th, 2012 to include a statement from a Merck spokesman that said the lawsuit is without merit and the company intends to vigorously defend itself in court (1385).

'The Civil Action NO. 10-4374 CIVIL ACTION NO. 12-3555 Stephen A. Krahling and Joan A. Wlochowski, Relators v. MERCK & CO., INC., Defendant' is available to view online. The case confirms the Relators (private person making the application) were employed as virologists in the Merck laboratory and allegedly witnessed firsthand the allegedly fraudulent efficacy testing. Relators alleged the Defendant (Merck) first tested their vaccine with a Mumps Plaque Reduction Neutralisation assay comparing pre and post-vaccinated blood to test whether the vaccine neutralised the virus. Relators note that rather than using the 'gold standard' approach and testing the vaccine against a 'wild-type mumps virus' the Defendant tested it against the attenuated virus strain that had been used when creating the vaccine in the 1960s. Relators alleged that comparing a vaccine to its originator virus strain would likely overstate the vaccine's effectiveness.

In addition, the Defendant added animal antibodies to pre and post-vaccinated blood samples. Relators claim that the use of animal antibodies created a high number of pre-vaccinated positive results, which the Defendant systemically destroyed or falsified in order to legitimise the use of animal antibodies. Relators also alleged that senior management was aware, complicit, and in charge of this testing. Relators were barred from participating in the mumps vaccine testing. Relators assert that Defendant continued to make false representations of its inflated 95% efficacy rate to the government while deliberately covering up the results of the tests showing a diminished efficacy. Plaintiffs alleged that Defendant falsified, abandoned, and manipulated testing data that should have been shared with the government in order to fraudulently mislead the government into purchasing the mumps vaccine (1386).

Why people do not believe that pharmaceutical companies manufacturing the 'saviour' COVID-19 vaccines are not falsifying, abandoning and manipulating test data now is beyond reason.

Even the revered Cochrane has been bought out: The Cochrane Collaboration describes itself as;

> *"The reliable source of evidence in health care"* and *"an international nonprofit and independent organisation, dedicated to making up-to-date, accurate information about the effects of healthcare readily available worldwide".*

The Cochrane Database of Systematic Reviews describes itself as, *"the definitive resource for evidence-based health care"*. Since its establishment in 1993, Cochrane has gained an internationally respected reputation around the world. Unfortunately, it is no longer the case that Cochrane is independent. Cochrane's ability to appear above commercial conflicts of interests is dependent on UK governmental funding in particular. In 2004, UK governmental 'core funding' was reduced considerably. This reduction in income led to a decrease in productivity and staff redundancies, forcing Cochrane to consider commercial sources for the first time. Cochrane essentially went up for sale to the highest bidder, and Cochrane is now dependent on both government and commercial funding.

Questions on the independence and reliability of Cochrane Reviews in relation to the MMR vaccine exist. In 2005, Cochrane published a vaccine safety and effectiveness review of the MMR vaccine against a background of litigation in the UK over vaccine damage claims. The conclusions of the Cochrane MMR review were not supported by and contradicted the evidence presented in the review, and Cochrane continued to support the British government's recommendations on the MMR vaccine. The review's conclusion that the millions of doses of MMR vaccine administered worldwide are safe was not science-based. The review itself found that studies into the extent of the adverse events following MMR vaccination are too limited to say. The review admitted it could not evaluate MMR vaccine safety and effectiveness against other measures, such as single vaccines, placebo, no vaccine, or modern treatment options. The review's conclusion was literally based on the circular theory that without cited evidence of vaccine safety, that the MMR vaccine is safe simply because millions of doses are administered.

The Cochrane review duplicates an almost identical paper published in 2003 by members of the same team yet contains no reference to the earlier paper, thereby breaking its own rules on authors attempting to conceal the existence of duplicated publication. The Cochrane review provided no evidence to refute the Wakefield hypothesis of an association between MMR vaccine, regressive autism, and a novel form of inflammatory bowel disease. As the taxpayer and not vaccine companies foot the bill for vaccine injury, the UK government has substantial financial interests in vaccine injury compensation claims failing. The UK government is directly involved in media and political campaigns that discredit the expert medical evidence underlying vaccine injury claims [(1387)].

Additional studies: Moving away from the smokescreen that is the MMR vaccine, let's discuss the full schedule of vaccines. A regression analysis between 2001 and 2007 using data from the US National Centres for Health Statistics (NCHS) was published in the *Journal of Toxicology and Environmental Health* in 2011. The study authors investigated the prevalence of autism or speech or language delays and the relationship between the number of children who had received the CDC recommended vaccines by their second birthday. The study found a positive and statistically significant association between the prevalence of autism and childhood vaccination uptake across the US population. The authors concluded that the higher the proportion of children receiving recommended vaccinations, the higher the prevalence of autism or speech and language delays [(1388)].

Just answer the ruddy question! We can continue to go back and forth and search and research to answers the question do vaccines (not MMR) cause autism. The childhood vaccination schedule has between 1 and 69 antigens, and a child receiving the recommended vaccines is exposed to up to 320 antigens by the time they are two years old [(645)]. The science is not out. This censored debate around vaccine safety could be put to bed once and for all by conducting a cohort study comparing the health outcomes (neurodevelopmental disorders, inflammatory disease and autoimmune disease) of completely unvaccinated to completely vaccinated children. It could be randomised, restricted, matched and adjusted for confounders. But instead, Heidi Larson's Vaccine Confidence Project trolls the internet flagging and censoring vaccine safety concerns to increase our confidence in vaccines.

CHAPTER TWENTY-FOUR

SPEAKING TRUTH TO POWER

"The revolution is not an apple that falls when ripe.
You have to make it fall".

Che Guevara [1389]

I don't get my information from social media. That's an insult pushed by the daily propaganda to tarnish the reputations of people with vaccine safety concerns. With three health science degrees in Complementary and Alternative Medicine (CAM) and a Masters in Public Health, I conduct my own research and draw my own conclusions. We can all conduct our own research. I don't follow anyone *per se* however, I like to keep abreast of those who are risking their careers and reputations to take a stand and speak truth to power. I personally wanted to know if there was anyone I could vote for, and to let you know who deserves our support. The list is by no means exhaustive, if you do not appear in these pages, you are not unappreciated.

Professors, scientists and Nobel Laureates: The Greater Barrington Declaration (GBD) acknowledges the damaging physical and mental health impacts of the current COVID-19 lockdown policies and calls for lifting of all COVID-19 restrictions in healthy people. The GBD recommends "focused protection", that is to protect the vulnerable while letting the disease run its course naturally in the healthy population. The three original authors of the GBD are infectious disease epidemiologists and public health scientists including, Harvard Medical School Professor, Dr Martin Kulldorff, Oxford University Epidemiology Professor, Dr Sunetra Gupta, and Stanford Epidemiology Professor, Dr Jayanta Bhattacharya. As of February 20th 2021, the signature count of concerned citizens was 749,895, medical and public health scientists was 13,618 and medical practitioners was 41,244 [375]. According to GSKoogle, the three public health experts from Harvard, Stanford, and Oxford who authored the GBD are ill-advised, arrogant and reckless. The daily propaganda misreport it as a "let it rip" strategy [1161].

In a rather lacklustre response to the GBD, the ruling class and supporters of public health police powers to mandate masks, mandate social distancing, mandate travel restrictions, mandate quarantine, mandate vaccines, and mandate vaccine passports responded with the John Snow Memorandum (JSM). The JSM calls to maintain the status quo to crush humanity under the guise of 'public health'. This has great support from those in the pocket of the pharmaceutical giants who want to lock us up until we take our shot. In February 2021, this memorandum had a mere 6000 signatures, according to the website, but only showed 4,200 (376). Take one gramme of soma and repeat, 'some scientists are more equal than others', until you shut up, obey and take your shot.

On September 24th 2020, hundreds of healthcare workers (HCWs), medical specialists, lawyers and economists signed two separate open letters posted on *The American Institute of Stress* website. The letters were addressed to all Belgian authorities and all Belgian media. The first letter had 40 signatories and called into question the use and legitimacy of Belgium's coronavirus policy and the experts and policymakers behind them. *De Tijd* and *L'Echo*, two business newspapers in Belgium, reported that the authors were asking for a thorough evaluation of the effectiveness of the current measures to contain the coronavirus. The authors wrote that "the errors of the past can no longer be reproduced" and that "the future management of the crisis must be scientifically sound, rational and proportionate". The authors asserted that "citizens have the right to objective and honest information" and that "the current climate of coviphobia is completely unjustified and generates harmful anxiety for a large part of the population" (1390).

On February 28th 2021, a group of scientists and doctors issued an open letter calling on the European Medicines Agency (EMA) to answer urgent safety questions regarding COVID-19 vaccines or withdraw the vaccines' authorisation. The letter noted that a range of adverse events were being reported following COVID-19 vaccination in previously healthy younger individuals and the numerous global media reports of care homes being struck by COVID-19 within days of the vaccine rollout. The letter stated that, in the absence of post-mortems examinations, there is inadequate scrutiny of the possible causes of illness or death. The letter described serious potential consequences of COVID-19 vaccine technology, warning of possible autoimmune reactions, blood clotting abnormalities, stroke and internal bleeding, "including in the brain, spinal cord and heart" (1391).

John Ioannidis, a renowned Stanford University Professor of Medicine and Epidemiology and Population Health, created uproar when he contradicted public health officials by questioning if lockdowns were causing more harm than good. It goes without saying that the esteemed Professor was unfairly denigrated and his professional opinion was dismissed as lunacy [(1392)]. Nobel Laureate Michael Levitt, Biophysicist and Professor of Structural Biology at Stanford University, said he believed that eventually, COVID-19 will be another mild circulating coronavirus and that lockdowns "may not have been needed". In 2020 Noble Laureate and HIV discoverer Dr Luc Montagnier said he believed the coronavirus was created in a Chinese virology laboratory [(1393)].

Geert Vanden Bossche PhD is an independent virologist and vaccine expert. Dr Bossche previously worked for the Bill & Melinda Gates Foundation and Gavi, the Vaccine Alliance as Senior Ebola Programme Manager. In this video posted on You-will-obey-Tube, Dr Bossche discusses COVID-19 vaccine immune escape and the calls to stop the global COVID-19 vaccine rollout. At 3 minutes 24 seconds, Bossche discusses the general principles of vaccinology and microbiology.

> *"If you put living organism such a bacteria or viruses under life-threatening pressure, and you do it in a way that you still allow the microorganism to replicate...If you cannot really kill them all, prevent completely the infection, and there is still some microorganism that can replicate they will start to select mutations that enable them to survive...COVID 19 has a high capacity for mutation, and they are not under pressure...The pressure (in the case of vaccines) arises from antibodies that you develop from natural infection or immunisation. The viruses then choose among a multitude of mutations that will enable them to survive. This is in its own right is not a recipe for disaster...viruses can only replicate in living cells...So if these guys are released from the cell and if they don't find another living cell"*.

Simply put, Dr Bossche describes when the antibodies made against the vaccine-induced spike protein strain do not match against the variant spike protein strain, thus rendering the current COVID-19 vaccines ineffective [(1394)].

Michael Yeadon was Vice President and Chief Scientist for Allergy and Respiratory at drugs giant Pfizer where he spent 16 years as an allergy and respiratory researcher. Michael later co-founded a biotech company that Novartis, a Swiss drugmaker, bought for US$325 million. Michael co-authored a petition to the EMA demanding that the COVID-19 vaccine clinical trials be immediately halted. The petitioners speculated that the vaccines could cause infertility in women. Michael Yeadon appears in a podcast on Dellingpod Podcast, from approximately 37 minutes he says;

> *"...it 99.7% identical...I assure you that the human immune system is much cleverer than that...There is no chance...it's, it's impossible for a variant that differs by 0.3% ... there's no chance that that will evade human immunity...the stuff that you hear that about not quite sure the vaccine will work against this new variant...Bullshit!...The government advisers are trying to get you to believe...They've shut the international borders to stop you bringing home something that's pretty identical to what you've already got. Why are they doing that? It makes no sense. The grounds they have are just not true... they're not viable, they're not plausible...I started to get a really frightened feeling you can't trust the government or the government advisers because whatever they're doing or whatever they're telling you is not matching up with the immunology".*
>
> *"The really terrifying part is they're telling you, don't worry we can tweak these vaccines ...change mRNA sequence...update production line, and there's a jab for you to update your immunity...Well, the variants are nowhere near different enough to convict or require any kind of different immunity...Your immune system would easily recognise it as a brother or a cousin...I still vote for the human immune system every time...You don't need a new vaccine. The people who had* severe acute respiratory syndrome *(SARS) in 2003, 17 yrs ago, if they survive that infection...they recognise severe acute respiratory syndrome coronavirus 2 (SARS-CoV-2), and they are 20% different. Empirical evidence, I've got theory on my side, sorry you've been misled by government and its advisors".*
>
> *"I've got two terrifying other bits of information for your listeners... I've heard some of the pharmaceutical companies are already manufacturing top-up vaccines for ya... you'll be called up for your top-up vaccination, which I'm telling you, you don't need...The last terrifying bit of information...if you can't put this together, I really can't help*

you...The global medicines regulators, the Medicines and Healthcare products Regulatory Agency (MHRA), EMA, the Food and Drug Administration (FDA) got their heads together months ago said...the top-up vaccines being so similar to the originals they don't require the producers to do clinical safety studies. So there's a conspiracy here...I know...six other immunologists who agree...the variants are so nowhere near different enough to possibly need another vaccine yet you are told that they're needed, and the countries shut borders...They're gonna go from the whiteboard or the computer screen of drug companies into 100s of millions of arms without passing go or any regulator".

"In brief, why would they possibly want to do that? Why did they pick this method... a dead pathogen would take a lot of time...The other reason, gene vaccines, is that you can put whatever gene you like in the...theoretically, you could give someone to express a gene that would have some benefit...You certainly could give them a gene that would give them some harm, that harm may be short-term or long-term...I cannot think of a benign explanation for the claim that you need top-up vaccines, which I'm sure you don't...to say that they are so similar to the original vaccines and don't need safety trials is an insult to your listeners...right now the regulators are wrestling with how safe the parent vaccines are... there's not a benign explanation. If you wanted, say, to depopulate a significant proportion of the world and to do it in a way that wouldn't require the destruction of the environment with nuclear weapons...and you wanted plausible deniability...I actually don't think you could come up with a better plan of work that seems to be in front of me" [1395].

Doctors: Peter C. Gøtzsche is a Danish physician, medical researcher, and former leader of the Nordic Cochrane Centre at Rigshospitalet in Copenhagen, Denmark. He is a co-founder of the Cochrane Collaboration. Currently, Professor Gøtzsche is Director of the Institute for Scientific Freedom, Copenhagen. Gotzshce authored a book entitled *Deadly Medicines and Organised Crime* about how Big Pharma has corrupted healthcare. In a letter dated November 2020, addressed to the *British Medical Journal* at the end of November 2020, Gøtzsche challenged a coronavirus disease 2019 (COVID-19) fatality risk analysis in Spain. Gotzshce claimed that the infection fatality rate was comparable to a median of "about 1% for laboratory-confirmed influenza during the mild influenza pandemic in 2009" and that the draconian pandemic responses have forced a further 100 million people into extreme poverty [1396].

German Doctor Dr Heiko Schöning was arrested by the Met Police at Speakers' Corner at Hyde Park, where Karl Marx, Vladimir Lenin and George Orwell demonstrated free speech [1397]. Dr Schöning is in the World Doctors Alliance (WDA). The WDA is a collaboration of medical professionals from around the world that aims to address issues surrounding the handling of the COVID-19 pandemonium. The WDA was formed by Dr Mohammad Adil, Consultant General Surgeon Global Nishtarian Organisation (GNO) (All Pakistan Medical Association (APMA) United Kingdom (UK) and WDA chair. Dr Adil had his licence suspended by UK's General Medical Council (GMC) for speaking the truth to power [1398]. The WDA's independent nonprofit is an alliance of HCWs worldwide that united in the aftermath of the COVID-19 response, intending to end all lockdowns and associated damaging measures to humanity's psychological and physical wellbeing. The WDA includes Irishwoman Professor Dolores Cahill and You-will-obey-Tube sensation, 'Old Man in a Chair' also known as Dr Vernon Coleman, who does not suffer fools gladly [1399].

County Kildare doctor, Dr Gerard Waters calls himself, "a conscientious objector" to the vaccine. Dr Waters said he will refuse to give the COVID-19 vaccine to his patients and instead send them elsewhere [1400]. Dr Marcus De Brun, Department of Surgery, Our Lady of Lourdes Hospital, Drogheda, and former member of the Irish Medical Council (IMC), has been an outspoken critic of COVID-19 restrictions and holds 'anti-lockdown' and 'anti-mask' views, which is doublespeak for 'civil rights activist'. The IMC threatened to suspend Marcus, who then decided to close his surgery [1401].

County Limerick Dr Pat Morrissey declined to administer COVID-19 vaccines to his patients, saying he is prepared to go to court to fight any potential moves by the Health Service Executive (HSE) to remove him as a general practitioner. Dr Morrissey said he does not support the government's lockdown measures or the national vaccination programme against COVID-19, because, he argued, the vaccines that are currently available are "untested, unlicensed and experimental". Dr Morrissey said he will not take the COVID-19 vaccine or administer the vaccine to patients until there is strong evidence that it poses no long-term health risks. Dr Morrissey's patients are still able to receive the vaccine at his clinic by someone else. Dr Morrissey said, "I'm not refusing vaccinations to anyone, but I'm going to make sure that they are fully consented and that they are aware of the true status of these therapies that are being provided" (1402). Dr Morrissey spoke at organised rallies to protest National Public Health Emergency Team's (NPHET's) advice on the pandemic organised by Health Freedom Ireland.

America's Frontline Doctors (AFD), founded by Dr Simone Gold, aims to deliver unbiased and uncensored medical information to help people make an informed decision about their healthcare. AFD opposes medical cancel culture and censorship. AFD unveiled a 'Vaccine Bill of Rights' to protect oneself from unconstitutional experimental vaccine mandates. AFD doctors promote a book on their website entitled *I Do Not Consent: My Fight Against Medical Cancel Culture*, and have a 'Say No To Forced Experimental Vaccines' petition. AFD opposes lockdowns and social distancing mandates and cites what the daily propaganda describe as 'alleged' and 'unapproved' treatments for COVID-19 that these doctors are experienced in prescribing (1403). A video on *BitChute* posted on a *Health Impact News* website entitled 'Doctors Around the World Issue Dire Warning: Do Not Get the Covid Vaccine' shows numerous doctors and allied health professionals warning not to get the experimental COVID-19 vaccine and expressing their views on how the pandemic is non-existent (1404).

Front Line COVID-19 Critical Care Alliance (FLCCC), a group of scientists and physicians from the United States (US), UK, European Union (EU), South America and Israel, is calling for an end to the COVID-19 pandemic restrictions by immediately adopting policies that allow for the use of ivermectin in the prevention and treatment of COVID-19. FLCCC doctor, intensive care specialist Dr Pierre Kory, believes that ivermectin is the drug that can end the pandemic and that it is absurd that global health agencies refuse to approve its use in COVID-19 (1405).

Christchurch-based doctor, Dr Samantha Bailey, who appeared on Television New Zealand's (TVNZ's) medical show, *The Check Up*, appeared in a video on You-will-obey-Tube, entitled 'COVID-19: Behind the PCR Curtain'. The video, posted in early September 2020, contradicted New Zealand's Ministry of Health, saying the polymerase chain reaction (PCR) test was unreliable (1406).

Natural Medicine Organisations: The UK based Alliance for Natural Health (ANH) International is a nonprofit organisation with a mission to safeguard and promote natural and sustainable approaches to regenerating and managing human health globally. Founder, Executive and Scientific Director Dr Robert Verkerk and Executive Coordinator Meleni Aldridge openly challenge the COVID narrative, provide information to help people make informed decisions about their health and encourage us to stand against medical tyranny. The Washington based Institute for Functional Medicine (IFM), whilst not so openly blatant in challenging the COVID narrative, do offer advice about functional medicine approaches to prevent and treat COVID-19 including nutrition and lifestyle advice to strengthen host defence. IFM also offer information on COVID-19 vaccines, variants, and breakthrough infections.

Judges and Lawyers: The Coronavirus Act 2020 was passed in March 2020. British Supreme Court justices don't think there is justice in the coronavirus emergency laws. In October 2020, retired British Supreme Court justice, Lord Jonathan Sumption criticised, "a loss of effective parliamentary scrutiny of emergency COVID powers" and lambasted the "cavalier use of coercive powers" and "loss of freedom". Lord Sumption condemned the way "the British state exercised coercive powers over its citizens on a scale never previously attempted". In his address at the Cambridge Freshfields annual law lecture, Sumption said the emergency measures were "the most significant interference with personal freedom in the history of our country". He stated;

> *"I do not doubt the seriousness of the epidemic, but I believe that history will look back on the measures taken to contain it as a monument of collective hysteria and governmental folly".*

Lord Sumption, like we who see, was simply flabbergasted, exclaiming, *"The ease with which people could be terrorised into surrendering basic freedoms which are fundamental to our existence...came as a shock to me in March 2020"* [(1407)]. Lady Hale, former president of, and the first woman to lead the Supreme Court in 2017, said that parliament had resumed much of its traditional role, *"but it did surrender control to the government at a crucial time"* and made a plea to *"get back to a properly functioning constitution as soon as we possibly can"* [(1408)].

Tracey O'Mahony is an Irish barrister registered with the Legal Services Regulatory Authority. Tracey opposes the introduction of Ireland's Emergency Measures in the Public Interest (COVID-19) Bill 2020, including the wearing of facemasks, and posts information for citizens on how to protect their rights. Tracey started a Go Fund Me fundraising drive to help pay for a COVID-19 Legal Challenge. In January 2021, it was reported that the COVID-19 Legal Challenge fund had raised €100,000. Tracey since increased her fundraising target to €250,000 [(1409)]. A late addition, Lawyers for Justice Ireland is a group of collaborating Irish pro bono lawyers and associated professionals committed to achieving justice and equality for all Irish people. The setting up of The Peoples Tribunal of Ireland in July 2020 in response to the documented 'inadequacy' of the Irish Courts and government to maintain and preserve the Rule of Law is another promising initiative that could provide a template for other countries to follow.

Lawsuits: Reiner Fuellmich is a consumer protection trial lawyer specialising in the prosecution of fraudulent corporations globally. Dr Fuellmich is one of four members of the German Corona Investigative Committee. Fuellmich plans on issuing a class-action suit in the US against Director-General of the WHO Dr Tedros Ghebreyesus, the head of virology at Berlin's Charité Hospital, Dr Christan Drosten, and the head of Robert Koch Institute (RKI), the German counterpart of the Centres for Disease Control and Prevention (CDC), Dr Lothar Wieler, for knowingly misleading governments across the world. The main concerns of the group of lawyers who plan to sue the WHO are that control measures have damaged people's livelihoods and caused huge economic damage, and to ascertain the correct mortality estimate and PCR test accuracy in relation to whether it shows if someone is infective [(1410)]. On a webpage entitled 'Stop World Control', Fuellmich describes the pandemic as the "worst crime against humanity ever committed" [(1411)].

Michael O'Bernicia is a comedian and filmmaker and self-described anarcho-missionary. Michael worked from 2009-2018 as coproducer /writer/director/editor on *The Great British Mortgage Swindle,* a documentary about institutionalised mortgage fraud and eviction by court order. On September 30th 2020, Michael announced that he was bringing private prosecutions against all of Britain's MPs for voting through the Coronavirus Act 2020. Michael is also taking his Four Horsemen of the

UK COVID-19 Apocalypse to court; Chris Whitty, Patrick Vallance, Martin Ferguson and Matt Hancock [1412].

Del Bigtree is the founder of Informed Consent Action Network (ICAN), a nonprofit organisation focused on the scientific integrity of vaccines and the pharmaceutical industry. ICAN asserts that we have the authority over our health choices and those of our children. ICAN's goal is to empower people with evidence-based health research to enable one to make an informed consent that is not medically coerced [1413]. ICAN has also submitted numerous Freedom of Information (FOI) requests for information regarding vaccine safety. ICAN and Del Bigtree are currently taking *Facebook* and *YouTube* to court in a Bivens action, which is a lawsuit for damages. Prior to the COVID-19 pandemonium, ICAN shared their information on a *Facebook* page and *YouTube* channel which were subsequently terminated without prior warnings [1414].

American Oversight is an activist and litigation organisation that focuses on filing open records requests that target Republican interests. American Oversight tracks the latest developments in federal and state government response to the COVID-19. American Oversight has submitted multiple FOI requests to the CDC for records of urgent importance related to the pandemic, but the CDC has engaged in a practice of improperly claiming that reasonably described requests are "overly broad". The lawsuit asked the court to order the CDC to comply with the law and highlighted the significant issues they experienced in attempting to get the CDC to process requests and issues that have led to unnecessary and inappropriate delays. Austin Evers, Executive Director of American Oversight said, "At a time when public disclosures are especially critical, the CDC has systematically obstructed the public's right to information about the coronavirus pandemic. The CDC must abandon the obstacles it has erected against transparency and lean into its responsibility to honest, timely disclosures" [1415].

In Ireland, Data Analytica, run by David Egan, has a webpage entitled 'Evidence for Criminal case against NPHET', Minister for Health, Tony Holohan, Micheál Martin and RTE'. The *Data Analytica* website includes details of a first criminal charge and a statement made to police at Kevin Street Garda Station, Dublin city, on May 7th 2021. Also included is the book of evidence, a scientific report compiled by top scientists and medical doctors in pdf format, and 15 other criminal charges to be brought in the summer of 2021 [1416]. Egan works closely with Dr Stephen Manning, author, publisher and public speaker, who is currently the administrator of Integrity Ireland, an association seeking to bring justice, transparency and accountability to Irish State institutions, particularly in the legal profession, law enforcement and the Courts. Manning is currently fighting to protect Irish school children from the threat of mandatory COVID-19 vaccination under Ireland's Emergency Measures in the Public Interest (Covid-19) Act 2020 [1417] and has recently published a book on what he names 'The Covid-19 Phenomenon' from a perspective that incorporates the concepts of Universal Law vs historical, systematic and institutionalised evil in social, govermental and corporate formats. The book is entitled, *"CRISIS, CULL or COUP? What, How & Who? Facts & Truths to Make You Think!"* Watch these spaces.

Cardinals and Bishops: On December 13th 2020, Cardinal Raymond Leo Burke spoke truth to power when he delivered a powerful homily for Saturday's celebration of the Solemnity of Our Lady of Guadalupe at the Shrine of Our Lady of Guadalupe. From 30 seconds, Cardinal Burke says, *"Our nation is going through a crisis which threatens its very future as free and democratic"*. Cardinal Burke continues,

> *"The worldwide spread of Marxist materialism...now seems to seize the governing power over our nation...To attain economic gains, we as a nation have permitted ourselves to become dependent of the Chinese Communist Party and the ideology totally opposed to the Christian foundation"*.
>
> From 1 minute 42 seconds, *"then there is the mysterious Wuhan virus about whose nature and prevention the mass media daily give us conflicting information ...what is clear however, is that it has been used by certain forces inimical to families and to the freedom of nations to advance their evil agenda, these forces tell us that we are now the subject of the so-called great reset, the new normal, which is dictated to us by their manipulation of citizens and nations through ignorance and fear"*.
>
> Cardinal Burke continues, *"Now we are supposed to find in a disease the way to understand and direct our lives rather than in God and in His plan for our salvation. The response of many bishops and priests and of*

many faithful has manifested a woeful lack of sound catechesis, so many in the church seem to have no understanding how Christ continues his saving work in times of plague and other disasters. At a time that we need to be close to one another in Christian love, worldly forces would isolate and have us believe that we are alone and dependent upon secular forces that would make us slaves to their Godless and murderous agenda" [1418].

Archbishop Viganò is an archbishop of the Catholic Church. Archbishop Viganò is a strong voice for true Catholics. He believes the church has been hijacked and that COVID is a scam, and he's not afraid to call a spade a spade [1419]. A traditional Catholic client of mine told me about two other Bishops that speak truth to power; Bishop Strickland of Tyler, US, and Bishop Athanasius Schneider of Kazakhstan. The head of my church is to host the Devil incarnate at the Vatican in a conference in 2021 called Exploring the Mind, Body and Soul.

The pope will join vaccine promoter Anthony Fauci, birth control advocate Chelsea Clinton, population control advocate Jane Goodall and others, including the propaganda machine's usual big heads, religious leaders, leading physicians, scientists, policymakers, and 'philanthropists'. Exploring the Mind, Body and Soul will discuss the latest breakthroughs in medicine (transhumanism) and how to make healthcare affordable; doublespeak for 'let's increase the price of medicines!' [1420]

Human rights organisations: A report commissioned by The Irish Human Rights and Equality Commission (IHREC) and authored by the COVID-19 Law and Human Rights Observatory in Trinity College Dublin, found that the use of emergency COVID powers has sidelined human rights and equality scrutiny and that the Irish government is blurring the lines on these powers [1421]. Where's Amnesty? Lining up for their shot.

Journalists: In June 2020, Australian former politician, David Leyonhjelm shared his opinion in *The Australian Financial Review* that Australia's response to the coronavirus outbreak was a massive overreaction. Leyonhjelm went on to say that keeping the infections surge below the health system capacity could have been achieved with moderate social distancing and personal hygiene and that the forced closure shut down of the economy was unnecessary. Leyonhjelm wrote that the pattern of infection would have been different, with more infections occurring early in the piece. Leyonhjelm continued to say that the endpoint of herd immunity can be deferred but not avoided and that herd immunity would be achieved through a combination of infection and vaccination. Finally, he said the lockdown will not have saved additional lives [1422].

In August 2020, Greg Ip of *The Wall Street Journal* said that blanket business shutdowns had led to a deep recession. 400 million jobs worldwide and 13 million in the US had already been lost, and according to the International Monetary Fund (IMF), global output was set to fall 5% in 2020. Ip went on to say economists and health experts say there could be a better way and called for new thinking on COVID-19 lockdowns. Ip described lockdowns as an "overly blunt and economically costly tool". Ip urged policymakers to pursue an approach of targeted restrictions and interventions [1423].

Irish columnist and author John Waters and journalist Gemma O'Doherty have spoken out. Wickedpedia calls them 'conspiracy theorists'. In relation to Ireland's Emergency Measures in the Public Interest (COVID-19) Bill 2020, Waters and O'Doherty were seeking to challenge the constitutionality of these laws and have these various legislative measures declared unconstitutional. Waters and O'Doherty lost their appeal over COVID-19 restrictions. The three-judge Court of Appeal (COA), comprising the COA President Mr Justice George Birmingham, Ms Justice John Edwards and Ms Justice Caroline Costello dismissed all grounds of their appeal saying it was, *"misconceived and entirely without merit"* [1424].

Irish journalist and television presenter Aisling O'Loughlin, speaks out against mandatory experimental unlicensed vaccines and against the emergency COVID laws, which she describes as equating to a tyrannical dictatorship [1425]. In June 2021, Twaddle blocked her account, which is great news for Aisling, as it means she's doing her job to hold our government to account. Aisling is a mother like myself, speaking out for our children, and shared a video of one of my speeches.

Robert Pierzynski is a Galway based photojournalist and Managing Director of RPV media. He runs Hello Irlandia and Action-Covid-1984 Ireland. Pierzynski and his family are constants at the Irish protests [1426]. *The Irish Sentinel* offers online alternative news and speaks out on how to protect our right to informed choice. The *Irish Light Paper* is a people funded paper who to holds power to account and exposes corruption that Irish mainstream media does not.

Politicians: Former Fianna Fáil Minister, GP and ex-Donegal Teachta Dála [(TD) /members of parliament] Jim McDaid is among a group of 15 Irish doctors that called on the government to change its pandemic strategy to co-exist with COVID-19. The letter to the Irish Taoiseach, Tánaiste, and Minister for Health stated that lockdown measures have little impact on the disease and proposed a "proportionate de-escalation of the current exclusive focus on COVID-19 to the exclusion of all other health and wellbeing needs of our Irish society". The frontline doctors in the group said that as the pandemic has played out, they felt more confident in managing the disease. Other signatories included surgeon Martin Feeley, who resigned as Clinical Director of the Dublin Midlands Hospital Group in September 2020 after criticising NPHET's approach to tackling the virus, and Dr Andrew Rynne who spoke at a pro-freedom protest in Dublin in October 2020 with Derry former Aontú councillor and retired GP, Dr Anne McCloskey [(1427)].

On March 1st 2021, Daragh O'Flaherty who ran in Galway West, and David Irish Chariot O'Reilly who ran for Galway East, spoke outside the Galway District Court in Ireland. The two were arrested for reporting from the Galway hospital during the COVID-19 'crisis'. The 'crisis' during which the hospital undertook massive road works which blocked half the car park. The pair said that the government was creating false information about the case numbers and called on HCWs with a conscience to come forward anonymously on alternative media to break the silence, restore the truth and break lockdown. In the video, O'Flaherty asks why the Irish people haven't been informed about COVID-19 prophylactics such as vitamin D and highlights the essentially meaningless PCR test. O'Flaherty says, "silence is consent" [(1428)]. On May 24th 2021, three Irish TDs (members of parliament) voted against the extension of COVID emergency laws in Ireland; Sharon Keogan, Michael McDowell and Rona Mullen [(1429)]. Catherine Connolly, Michael McNamara, Mattie McGrath and Michael Healy-Rae have since joined this list. In early November 2021 – and just as this book was going to print – a discussion was held in the Irish Parliament about the extension of Covid-19 restrictions, with the Labour Party siding with the government to continue restrictions until February 2022.

Interestingly, several more TD's opposed the motion including: Róisín Shortall, Social Democrats; Verona Murphy, Independent; Michael Collins, Independent; Michael McNamara, Independent, and Catherine Connolly, Independent. Meanwhile, while sitting in Dail chambers, Minister for Health Stephen Donnolly tweeted that those opposing the extensions were 'reckless'.

In a video someone sent me entitled 'Vaccines', Ben Gilroy, Irish political and anti-eviction activist standing in Dublin, and founder and former leader of Direct Democracy Ireland describes Article 41.1.1° of the Irish Constitution. Gilroy says;

> *"The State recognises the Family as the natural primary and fundamental unit group of Society, and as a moral institution possessing inalienable* (rights that cannot be surrendered) *and imprescriptible rights* (rights that cannot be lost because they have not been exercised over time), *antecedent* (previous or preexisting) *and superior to all positive law",* and guarantees its protection by the state [1430, 1431].

Positive laws are human-made laws set down by a central authority that oblige or specify an action. Common law is based on our current standards or customs of the people. Common law acts in concordance with natural law principles, to make free men and women living in the fellowship of a free community [1432]. As Gilroy says, *"There's always an excuse for corporations to come and take away your rights. The only way they can do it is by positive law".* He then goes on to say that Article 41.1. 1° is superior to all positive law, be it for the common good or not [1433]. Gilroy also took aim at state corruption and unlawful evictions in a Fascistbook video entitled 'Ben Gilroy Debunks 5 KM' [1434].

Boris backstabber Michael Gove demanded fellow Conservative MP Desmond Swayne apologise and issue a retraction of statements he made about the coronavirus pandemic that were described as 'dangerous misinformation'. During the interview, Desmond Swayne said, "It seems to be a manageable risk, particularly as figures have been manipulated. We're told there is a deathly, deadly pandemic proceeding at the moment. That is difficult to reconcile with intensive care units (ICUs) actually operating at typical occupation levels for the time of year and us bouncing around at the typical level of deaths for the time of year". The daily propaganda responded by saying that the Office for National (fiddling) Statistics showed deaths were 14% above the five year average at the time the comments were made. A person with free will may consider if the 14% increase in deaths were caused by lockdown [1435].

This Australian politician is ace. Reignite Democracy Australia (RDA) was founded by Monica Smit in response to the Victorian government's handling of the COVID-19 pandemic. RDA aims to provide an alternative to the mainstream media to empower people with honest, timely and truthful information and to represent those who are unrepresented. RDA members and other fringe groups arrange pro-freedom rallies [1436]. Take a teaspoon of concrete, Australia, it's a cold! And ferals don't take vaccines!

I love this Italian politician; she speaks to me. On May 14th 2020 Sara Cunial, an independent member of the Italian Chamber of Deputies (part of the Italian parliament) and formerly a member of the 5 Star Movement party, appeared in a video on You-will-obey-Tube strongly criticising the decree and the Italian government's position towards the pharmaceutical industry. Sara Cunial says it as she sees it;

> *"You go on anaesthetising the minds with corrupted mass media with disinfectant and NLP, with words like regime to allow to permit...We understood that people don't die for the virus alone...it will be allowed to die and suffer thanks to you and your laws for misery and poverty, and as in the best regimes, the blame will be dropped only upon the citizens. You take away our freedom, saying that it is our fault. Divide and rule, our children will lose more. Raped souls...the right to school will be granted only with a bracelet, to get them used to probation, slavery and to virtual lager in exchange for a skateboard and tablet.*
>
> *All this to satisfy the appetite of a financial capitalism, whose driving force is the conflict of interest, well represented by the WHO, whose main financier is the well-known philanthropist and saviour of the world, Bill Gates. The real goal of all of this is total control, absolute domination on human beings transformed into guinea pigs and slavery violating sovereignty and free will...While you rip up the Nuremberg code with force fines and deportation, facial recognition and intimidation... endorsed by dogmatic scientism...We outside, the people will multiply the fires of resistance in a way that you won't be able to oppress all of us"*.

Cunial continues, *"Gates does business with several corporations that own 5G facilities in the United States. So with all of this is the entire Italian Deep state Sanofi, together with Glaxo friends of Ranieri Guerra, Assistant Director-General for Strategic Initiatives (polio eradication, polio transition, antimicrobial resistance and migrant health). Previously, Ricciardi (Director-General for Preventive Health of the Italian Ministry of Health and Chief Medical Officer of Italy), as the well-known virologist that we pay €2000 every ten minutes for the presentation on the television. He signed agreements with medical societies to indoctrinate future doctors making fun of their own judgement and their oath"* [(1437)].

Non-political: The non-political movement Yellow Vest Ireland ran a full-page advertisement funded by Moorezey's Holdings, a Dublin finance company owned by entrepreneur John Moore. The full-page advertisement was addressed to "our leaders" and called for an alternative approach to the current COVID-19 restrictions. The advertisement suggested that the restrictions will cause "further damage to our country" and asked if there was, *"another way to take care of the few who are vulnerable while letting our economy and future survive"* [(1438)].

Health Freedom Ireland is a group aligned to empower Irish people to make informed medical decisions for themselves and their families. Health Freedom Ireland provides a resource for impartial information. The group supports medical freedom in relation to vaccination [(1439)]. A letter regarding excessive deaths in Irish nursing homes was signed by M.B. Murran on behalf of Health Freedom Ireland. The letter, addressed to the Dáil Deputy, discussed concerns surrounding a sudden unexplained rise in nursing home deaths and, whilst these may be due to a number of factors, that these excess deaths occurred directly after the COVID-19 vaccination rollout and may indicate a serious adverse event following immunisation [(1440)].

Brandy Vaughan was an activist who founded Learn the Risk in 2015, a US-based nonprofit aimed to educate people worldwide on the dangers of pharmaceutical products, including vaccines. Learn the Risk ran a billboard campaign stating vaccines are responsible for a large number of children's deaths. In December 2019, Vaughan posted a message on Fascistbook saying that she never had any suicidal thoughts and went on to say that she was not on anti-depressants or taking any daily pharmaceuticals.

"If something were to happen to me, it's foul play, and you know exactly who and why given my work and mission in this life".

Vaughan previously worked for the pharmaceutical industry selling Pfizer's painkiller Vioxx, which was withdrawn as it doubled the risk of heart attack and stroke. "From that experience, I realised that just because something is on the market doesn't mean it's safe" Brandy said. "Much of what we are told by the healthcare industry just simply isn't the truth". Vaughan's nine year old son discovered his dead mother [(1441)]. Ar dheis Dé go raibh a anam dílis.

Andy Heasman is an Irishman who stands against wearing masks and stands for our freedom. Heasman was recently sentenced to two months in jail for not wearing a mask [(1442)]. Heasman is doing exactly what we need to do; flood the courts. Heasman has his own website called Andy Heasy Life where he asks people to join him in his fight against tyranny. Hugo Talks covers a broad range of subjects on his channels and has been kept particularly busy keeping people up to date with COVID propaganda and vaccine dangers [(1443)]. Also, from the UK, author and social critic Carl Vernon has a You-will-obey-Tube channel that discusses the anxiety and mental health challenges brought on by the lockdowns and uses comedy to warn us about our dystopian future.

CHAPTER TWENTY-FOUR – PART II

CELEBRITIES & SPORTS PERSONALITIES

Tucker Carlson questions vaccine safety and effectiveness. Referring to the pausing of the Johnsons & Johnson's COVID-19 vaccine in the US and the complete cessation of the rollout of the Oxford-AstraZeneca COVID-19 vaccine in Norway and Denmark, and other limitations to over 60s in the EU, Carlson says, "Don't dismiss those questions from anti-vaxxers". Carlson says people have a right to be concerned about blood clotting. "Shh. Don't ask questions. Just take the shot", he says. I like this man. Carlson also discusses if the vaccine works to prevent the spread of infection, why the need to still wear a mask? "Maybe (the COVID-19 vaccine) doesn't work, and they're simply not telling you that" [1444].

Robert F. Kennedy Junior is a well-known vaccine safety activist. Kennedy is the chairman of Children's Health Defence which aims to end the pandemic of poor health affecting our children. RFK Jr joined Alec Baldwin for an Insta-gramme-of-soma live discussion on August 6th 2020, where the pair discussed the COVID-19 pandemic and the attempt to find a vaccine against the virus. In the video, Kennedy explains that the COVID-19 lockdown is claiming more lives than the virus [1445].

Australian celebrity chef Pete Evans was censored after what the daily propaganda described as repeatedly sharing misinformation about the coronavirus. Evans had 1.5 million Fascistbook followers. Fascistbook said it removed Pete Evan's page for repeatedly violating its policies. The company said, "We don't allow anyone to share misinformation about COVID-19 that could lead to imminent physical harm or (about) COVID-19 vaccines that have been debunked by public health experts" [1446]. We've all heard that old chestnut.

Novak Djokovic's anti-vaccination stance may stop his return to tennis. "Personally I am opposed to vaccination" said Djokovic [1447]. The best thing about being the world number one is you will still get a sponsor when you speak the truth. Djokovic must have enjoyed the 'Vic Vax Boo' during the Australian Open in Melbourne when the Board President of Tennis Australia, Jayne Hrdlicka, had to pause her speech and looked quite taken aback as the crowd booed the introduction of the new saviour vaccine [1448].

Comedian and actor Russell Brand takes the mickey out of the COVID-19 pandemonium and has reportedly flouted the 'Rule of Six' at his comedy show entitled *Brand-emic*. I call it 'the rule of sux'. Brand has a You-will-obey-Tube channel where he provides information in a straight-talking, witty, taking-a-poke-manner, that encourages people to put two and two together [1449].

Jessica Biel opposed SB277, the California bill removing personal belief as a reason for an exemption from the vaccination. Existing law prohibits the governing authority of a school or other institution from admitting for attendance any pupil who fails to obtain required immunisations within the time limits prescribed by the State Department of Public Health. Existing law allowed for exemption from parents in the form of a written statement by a licensed physician stating that immunisation is not considered safe for that child and indicating the specific nature and probable duration of their medical condition or circumstances [1450]. When I first filled out a conscientious objection to vaccination form in Australia back in 1993, I was one of only 5,000 conscientious objectors. I understand that this figure went up to 35,000, hence the tightening of exemption laws. Rather than use this valuable data to conduct a trial comparing the health outcomes (in relation to autoimmune, inflammatory, allergic and neurological disease) of these completely unvaccinated children to completely vaccinated children, what public health does is tell us is, 'the science is settled'. Shut up! Obey! Get your kids shot!

Jim Carey has spoken out against mandatory vaccination. Alicia Silverstone has been highly critical of vaccination, saying there are no proper safety studies. Jenny McCarthy said her son's autism was caused by vaccines. Bill Maher gave Robert F Kennedy Jr a voice on this talk show to discuss vaccine safety concerns. Robert Schneider has made numerous public statements lobbying against mandatory vaccination. Lisa Bonet expressed concern about vaccine ingredients. Toni Braxton said her son's autism was caused by vaccines. Selma Blair lobbied against SB277, the California bill to remove personal belief exemptions. Jenna Elfman, Juliette Lewis and Daniel Peter Masterson are all vocal opponents of SB277. Kristin Cavallari doesn't vaccinate her son. Mayim Bialik doesn't vaccinate her children.

Robert De Niro co-funded the 2016 documentary film *Vaxxed: from Cover-Up to Catastrophe* about the CDC cover-up. Charlie Sheen didn't want to vaccinate his children, but the mother of the children did, and it went to court. American rapper Kevin Gates said his children were advanced in school because they had not been vaccinated [(1451)]. Trump famously spoke out about vaccine safety until his Operation Warp Speed (OWS) and then went on to receive a 'vaccine' in secret after declaring he was immune [(1452)]. What a spineless wonder.

Musicians: Van the man I loved you before, now I love you more. Van has written four protest songs. 'Born to be free' says it all;

> *"Give them an inch, they take a mile. The new normal is not normal, it's no kind of normal at all"* (and) *"The birds in the trees know something we can't see, Cos they know, we were born, to be free".*

'No More Lockdown' says;

> *"No more taking of our freedom, and our God-given rights, pretending it's for our safety, when it's really to enslave".*

'As I Walked Out' says;

> *"As I walked out all the streets were empty. The government said everyone should stay home, and they spread fear and loathing and no hope for the future, not many did question this very strange move"* [(1453)].

No Van, not many did question. Eric Clapton joined him on the fourth song, 'Stand and Deliver', and shared his negative experiences after taking the COVID-19 vaccine. Clapton described how the COVID-19 vaccine aggravated his peripheral neuropathy symptoms and left him unable to play. *The Rolling Stone* described these songs as, *"the four worst songs of 2020"*. Mr Morrison, fancy a 'Freedom Concert' in Phoenix Park? When you stand with us the world will pay attention.

Jim Corr a member of the Irish family pop group The Corrs is described by the daily propaganda as a COVID-denying, anti-vaccination, COVID conspiracy theorist. Goodman yourself! Jim has been criticised for contributing to conspiracy theories on his Twaddle account. Jim is taking legal action against Twaddle after his account was suspended, with the social media giant claiming Jim had breached its policy on 'COVID-19 misleading information' [(1454)].

Noel Gallagher refused to wear a face mask saying, *"There's too many fucking liberties being taken away from us now".* Noel applied his common sense by observing how remarkable it is that a person is impervious to the virus when they take off their mask to eat. Ian Brown from the Stone Roses can also see through the propaganda and has the cojones to speak out [1455].

Morrissey this charming man! In a new interview conducted by his nephew posted on Twaddle in July 2021, Morrissey describes the pandemic as "Con-vid" and likens government restrictions to "slavery". Morrissey also says he can't be cancelled. *"You can't cancel someone who has always been cancelled...I unintentionally invented the condition of being cancelled"* [1456].

Mick Jagger who sings we are free to do what we want any old time, doesn't like freedom. Lyrics from his new song with Dave Grolh, 'Eazy Sleazy' mocks everyone I have mentioned in this chapter, *"Shooting the vaccine, Bill Gates is in my bloodstream; it's mind control..."* [1457]. Co-conspirator Dave Grolh, is doing some pro-vaxxer concert to 'reunite the world', doublespeak for 'increase the socioeconomic divide even further'. The concert aims to raise US$27 billion to vaccinate 27 million HCWs [1458]. These pop tarts should know that 14 million of these HCWs have refused the COVID-19 vaccine.

The people's resistance in the courts: In January 2021, what started out as a seemingly inconsequential case of a German man who took his case to court after being fined for violating strict German lockdown rules in Thuringia turned out to be so significant that the German media described it as "politically explosive". The German court acquitted the defendant and wiped the €200 fine. The court said that at the time, according to the German Robert Koch Institute, the COVID-19 reproduction number was below 1, and the health system was at no risk of collapsing. The judge stated that the government lacked sufficient legal grounds to impose the restrictions as there was no, *"epidemic situation of national importance".* The German court described the Thuringia lockdown as;

> *"The most comprehensive and far-reaching restrictions on fundamental rights in the history of the Federal Republic.."*

..and described the lockdown measures as, *'an attack on the "foundations of our society that was "disproportionate".'* The court said that Thuringia's spring lockdown was, *"a catastrophically wrong political decision with dramatic consequences for almost all areas of people's lives"* [1459].

UK families sued the UK government over *"little or no education"* for their children. The families' lawyers stated that the Department for Education failed to ensure access to online learning by providing laptops and access to the internet. London School of Economics researchers described school closures as opening a chasm of education between the children of low-income and working-poor families and those from well-off families [1460]. A test case was to go to the Irish High Court, with nearly 200 Irish parents of children with special needs threatening to sue the Department of Education and Teachers Unions over the failure to re-open special schools. A leading human rights solicitors' firm reiterated what Education Minister Norma Foley's stated, that remote teaching is not suitable for children with special needs [1461]. More than 100 American parents of students with disabilities filed a nationwide Individuals with Disabilities Education Act (IDEA) class action lawsuit in the US District Court for the Southern District of New York against COVID-19 school closures [1462].

The people's resistance on the streets: The revolution is gathering pace, albeit, the revolution will not be televised; Gil Scott-Heron. The following is a small example of what has been a constant global battle for civil rights. In January 2021, protests occurred in the Netherlands after a curfew was introduced to further increase lockdown measures. Protesters set fires in the Dutch city of Eindhoven, Amsterdam and in a fishing village in Urk where protesters burned a coronavirus testing facility to the ground and pelted police with rocks at the banned demonstration against COVID-19 lockdowns. These pro-freedom protesters were described as, *"white supremacists"* or *"supporters of the anti-immigrant group PEGIDA"* [1463]. In early 2021, pro-freedom protests continued in France, Spain and Denmark [1464]. Other revolutions not being televised; the pro-freedom protests in Brussels, Budapest and Vienna, Belgium, Austria and Slovenia [1465, 1466]. London, Berlin, Stuttgart, Warsaw, Melbourne, Sydney etc. A person of free will may ask why the revolution is not televised.

In August 2020, Irish Gardaí in County Kilkenny investigated an incident in which the €30,000 COVID-19 testing unit was destroyed in a large fire in the Wetlands area of Kilkenny city [1467]. In October 2020, protesters in Berlin attacked the offices of Germany's health authority, the Robert Koch Institute, with Molotov cocktails during demonstrations against COVID-19 restrictions [1468]. In April 2020, Ivorian protestors in Africa set fire to a COVID-19 testing centre then literally tore the centre apart with their bare hands [1469].

I have been speaking at a protest in Galway on the west coast of Ireland since April 2021. Riseup Eireann, and the Galway offshoot Riseup Galway, and concerned citizens have been keeping the candle of resistance lit on the Wild Atlantic Way to Freedom. For speaking out and standing up against public health police powers and tyrannical rule, I have been called anti-islamophobic, racist, new-wave fascist, a holocaust denier etc. We have our little counter-protesters every weekend, the ones who like to live as salves, enjoy masking and stand for freedom from responsibility. At the beginning of the pandemonium, people said to me, *"I don't know what to think"* or even worse, *"I don't' know how to think"*. I said, *"It's easy, just put one brain cell next to the other and rub them together and think"*.

I know what I think and feel. I think discrimination is wrong! I feel civil disobedience is my moral duty. I call on everyone to stand together to challenge inequality and discrimination and to protect our right to informed consent.

Aristotle said, *"The whole is greater than the sum of its parts"* [1470]. Thank you everyone with the strength to speak out. Let's finish this!

EPILOGUE

"That men do not learn very much from the lessons of history is the most important of all the lessons of history".

Aldous Huxley [1471]

OPEN DEBATE: There's a fine line between opinion and bias. I don't care what anyone's opinion is as long as they have formed it themselves through life experience and questioning. No one questions anymore. We all need to relearn how to cross over into the mindset of the person with the opposite opinion and have a discussion. In this cancel culture age, there are very few healthy discussions. I am the first to admit I am guilty of many biases. My biases exist because I am a woman [1472]. I am less committed to the organisation called globalisation, so have greater perceived risks [1473]. I don't believe in taking pharmaceutical drugs so I am guilty of errors of omission. Aware of the extent of drug resistance, I am guilty of availability bias. Aware of iatrogenesis (deaths caused by medical activity) statistics, I am guilty of anchoring bias. I am guilty of confirmation bias by selectively referencing this book. I also understand that when high vaccine coverage is achieved, and that vaccine is 'effective', that my concern regarding vaccine-related morbidity is greater than for the prevented disease. An unbiased person in science does not exist however, bias in science must be eliminated. Public health is supposed to critically analyse both the evidence and policy to ensure maximum effect whilst minimising harm. The evidence of vaccine effectiveness (VE) and of adverse events following immunisation (AEFI) is conflicting and bias exists. Frankly, I believe it is this bias that contributes to falling rates of confidence in vaccines. To eliminate bias, it is essential to assess vaccine effectiveness and safety with a nonindustry-funded cohort study comparing the health outcomes (neurodevelopmental disorders, inflammatory disease, autoimmune disease) of completely unvaccinated to completely vaccinated children. It could be randomised, restricted, matched and adjusted for confounders.

Get healthy and don't vaccinate: With half the globe immunocompromised, for the most part, due to obesity and the overuse and abuse of allopathic medicine, which suppresses natural immunity, those of us who barely use public health are threatened with lockdowns as the hospitals 'can't handle the strain'. Public health doesn't care about our health! If they did they would tell us not to vaccinate. We must stop being so reliant on allopathic medicine. We must get healthy and control our own destiny. If you are not healthy, get healthy (or as healthy as you can). Go and see a Complementary and Alternative Medicine (CAM) practitioner. I train parents in natural medicine first aid. Train yourself. Ask what your grandmother would have said. Stop reading self-help books and listen to you. Never do what you're told! Use your intuition. To really help society we need to help ourselves and our family first. My children and I have robust immune systems and I make no apologies for it. I educated myself on how to raise my family without drugs. Public health are terrified of parents like myself whose unvaccinated children are not dependent on drugs and not dependent on services; no antibiotics, no steroids, no inhalers, no speech or other therapist, no isms and no schisms. My unvaccinated children do not suffer from allergic or inflammatory disease, neurological disease or impairment, or chronic degenerative illness requiring lifelong medication, yet society describes parents like myself as irresponsible. Enough is enough! Society must accept that some of us out rightly reject western medicine and this is our informed choice. Answer the ruddy question boffins; do vaccines cause autoimmune disease, allergic disease and neurological disease?

Boost natural immunity; get dirty: Essentially, every piece of public health advice, bar washing your hands with soap and water, weakens our immune system and makes us more susceptible to diseases, including COVID-19. Public health should be encouraging us to eat a balanced diet, get out in the garden and dirty our hands, and take vitamins and herbal medicine that boosts our immune system. Public health should have advised healthy people to live their lives as normal and told them that if they caught the virus, they would be naturally immune and act as a barrier to the spread of disease to protect the vulnerable. My children had COVID-19 and got over it in a day. They have natural immunity and pose no risk to the elderly and vulnerable.

Stop believing the hype that public health saves lives: Let's face it. Antibiotic resistance is frankly the biggest threat to global health and we are heading for a post-antibiotic era that will make COVID look like a walk through a meadow. If we want to prevent infectious drug-resistant disease we need strong natural immunity and the only way to achieve this is to expose ourselves, not shield ourselves from infectious disease. I am not suggesting that vaccines don't work to prevent infectious disease. I am saying that it is because vaccines work to prevent infectious disease that they cause autoinflammatory (immune system) disease, resulting in deaths from these non-communicable illnesses which are a far more pressing global health concern. The new era of public health is supposed to depend on good science, but it does not (452). Public health is damaging global health by overprescribing drugs and by excluding traditional medicine. Traditional medicine is the answer to many of the major global health threats however traditional medicine is denigrated and vilified. Public health should acknowledge their mistakes regarding antibiotics and learn not to repeat this mistake by overusing drugs or vaccines. The WHO says extensive drug resistance in human immunodeficiency virus (HIV), malaria and tuberculosis (TB) are the greatest threats to global health (1474). Multi, extensive and totally drug-resistant TB exists yet the vaccine faithful still believe that TB is a vaccine-preventable disease (121, 125). There is no effective TB vaccine! The Bacillle Calmette-Guerin (BCG)/TB vaccine is ineffective in preventing pulmonary TB in adults (1475). Homeless people in many of the world's super cities have a tenfold increase in the incidence of TB (1476). Adults have been hoodwinked. TB disappeared when our living standards improved. The antibiotic apocalypse and the obesity pandemic are caused by public health. The solution is, where you can, avoid doctors and public health nurses.

What public health should be doing: The new era of public health is 'vaccinate the world'. Shut up! Obey! Take your shot! It wasn't always this way. As described previously, when I was a child I remember the TB skin scratch test (TST) also known as the Mantoux test or Heaf test. The Heaf test was to both detect for active TB and also to detect if a person had been exposed to TB and was therefore naturally immune and didn't need a TB vaccine. The idea at the time was to prevent complications due to preexisting immunity to mycobacterial antigens and unnecessary adverse reactions following immunisation (1477). We don't need any vaccines. However, regarding this novel coronavirus, individual-level SARS-CoV-2 serological tests should be utilised to prioritise COVID-19 vaccine strategies. A seronegative person does not have antibodies or T cells to COVID-19 as they have not been previously infected (1123). A seropositive person does not need a vaccine. In my opinion, from a public health perspective, the best policy would be to merely inoculate people deliberately with rhinovirus, a common cold-causing virus, as rhinovirus both prevents SARS-CoV-2 infection and prevents serious COVID-19 disease, and unlike a vaccine, there are less serious side effects (1114). Public health should lower the cycle threshold of the PCR test so that only infective cases are diagnosed. Public health should integrate natural medicine into mainstream healthcare.

Set a new precedent: I'm not a lawyer, but I know how to defend myself and prosecute someone using evidence. Today's public health police power to mandate masks, mandate quarantine, mandate vaccines, etc., are still based on our great, great grandfather's law known as Jacobson v. Massachusetts. Jacobson v. Massachusetts was the United States (US) Supreme Court case argued back on December 6th 1904, in which the court upheld the authority of states to enforce compulsory vaccination laws, arguing the view that individual liberty is not absolute and is subject to the police power of the state. Jacobson v. Massachusetts is still the only law that is used today by our ruling class when instigating public health police powers that strip our fundamental freedoms under the guise of 'public health'. For the greater good. For the common good. For money, power and control. In order for us to be free, this is the law that needs to be overturned. How do we do it?

In affirming Massachusetts' compulsory vaccination law, the court established a floor of constitutional protections that consists of four standards: necessity, reasonable means, proportionality, and harm avoidance. Under Jacobson v. Massachusetts, the courts are to support public health matters insofar as these standards are respected (1478). We can prove that emergency COVID-19 measures are unnecessary, unreasonable, disproportionate, and cause harm. Jacobson the defendant, lost the case as he did not prove that he was not fit for vaccination or that the vaccination could impair his health or be a probable cause of death. If the boffins conducted the study that definitively answered the question do vaccines cause autoimmune disease, allergic disease and neurological disease, the court could never mandate vaccines. We need to argue in court, that the court must order a prospective control trial comparing the health outcomes of unvaccinated to vaccinated is conducted to prove or disprove conclusively that vaccines 'do not impair health'. Until this study is done, mandates are farcical.

The poor are in this together: The rich are in this together: The only division is rich and poor. Oxfam told us we're not in this together! Inequality has worsened and the socioeconomic gap has widened, making it the world's largest megachasm. Bezos and Musk are flying to space and we can't fly to Marbella! The 'pandemic' has led to one of the greatest wealth transfers in history. Globally, workers lost US$3.7 trillion. The ruling class took it all and more. Supermarkets are the pandemic's winners and women workers are the pandemic's biggest losers. The people we call 'essential' or 'frontline' workers, the ones we clapped for and called heroes, saw their incomes stagnate or even fall (1479). Millions become millionaires during the pandemonium. While the poor got poorer, 5.2 million people became millionaires in 2020 and there are now 56.1 million millionaires globally (1480).

We are all carrying the same economic burden due to COVID-19 lockdowns. More lockdowns are coming unless we stand. Are you in the hospitality and tourism Sector? Tourism has been decimated by COVID-19 lockdowns. Irish Minister for Tourism Brendan Griffin said, *"In the space of a few short weeks, the Irish tourism sector has been decimated, and many tourist businesses were written off in 2020"* (1481). Do you want to fight to save your industry from further lockdowns? We are on your side. Stand with us! Do you work for the airlines? 195,000 jobs have been lost because of COVID-19 lockdowns. 100s of pilots, cabin crew and travel agents protested COVID-19 restrictions outside the Palace of Westminster (1482). Hospitality and tourism sector, we are on your side. Stand with us! Are you a musician or artist? Up to 100 demonstrators took part in a protest outside the Irish Dáil in June 2021 (1483). Musicians and artists, we are on your side. Stand with us!

Are you a new startup? The number of new Irish startup companies was decimated by COVID-19 lockdowns. There were 30% fewer startups in 2020 (1484). Do you want to fight to save your business? Business owners, we are on your side. Stand with us! Are you unemployed? Irish unemployment jumped to 25%! In 2020, 600,000 Irish were out of work (1485). Do you want to be employed? We are on your side. Stand with us! Have you had to use a food bank? Restrictions and job losses saw an unprecedented demand for food banks (1486). The UK saw a 47% increase in people needing food banks, and food banks found themselves being threatened with closure (1487). If you don't want to use a food bank or see them close, we are on your side. Stand with us! Do you work in the courthouse? You are threatened with mandatory vaccines. In July 2021 protestors were gathering outside the Dayton-Montgomery County Courthouse to speak out against mandatory vaccines. Workers, we are on your side. Stand with us! Are you a student? You are threatened with mandatory vaccines. 100s of colleges have already said the COVID-19 vaccine will be mandatory. Not all students plan to comply. They plan to march! There are swathes of students now protesting against mandatory vaccines in the US [(1488)]. Students, we are on your side. Stand with us!

We all carry the same mental health burden due to COVID-19 lockdowns. The demand for mental health and suicide prevention services soared during the pandemonium. Isolation, lack of social interaction, financial stress and fear drove a mental health crisis [(1489)]. A Health Service Executive (HSE) specialist said Ireland faces a "tsunami of mental health need...that will persist for months to years and be compounded by the economic impact of the pandemic" [(1490)]. Are you depressed, psychotic or suicidal or have a loved one who is? We are on your side. Stand with us!

We all carry the same physical health burdens due to COVID-19 lockdowns [(159)]. The pandemonium response created a 'cancer pandemic' with one million cancers in Europe having gone undiagnosed due to restrictions to screening services. The Irish public health chief said 2000 cancers have been missed as a result of COVID-19 lockdowns [(1491)]. Do you know someone who was misdiagnosed or had their cancer treatment affected because of COVID-19 lockdowns? We are on your side. Stand with us! Was your maternity care impacted because of COVID-19 lockdowns? Trinity College Dublin said COVID-19 lockdowns saw a rise in elective caesarean rates, caesareans in general and induced labours [(1492)]. If you don't want maternal services scaled back again, we are on your side. Stand with us!

We are all threatened with mandatory vaccines. The Health Information and Quality Authority (HIQA) recently told National Public Health Emergency Team (NPHET) that Irish healthcare workers (HCWs) who refuse the COVID-19 vaccine will be redeployed to a lower risk area, continually tested, and continually having to wear personal protective equipment (PPE) [(1493)]. 150 employees at a Houston, Texas hospital who refused the COVID-19 vaccine were fired or resigned [(1494)]. In October 2020, a Tallaght University Hospital (TUH) study found that 20% of HCWs had antibodies to

SARS-CoV-2 [1120]. A BioNTech poll found that 50% of German nurses and 25% of German doctors would refuse the COVID-19 vaccine [304]. Kaiser Family Foundation said that 50% of all US HCWS would refuse the COVID-19 vaccine [1495]. Are you a HCW threatened with mandatory vaccination even though you have been exposed and have natural immunity? Don't be coerced. We are on your side. Stand with us!

Emergency COVID laws are illegal and immoral: The Irish Human Rights and Equality Commission (IHREC) report says the government has persistently blurred the boundary between legal requirements and public guidance. We live under public health police powers. There has been no opportunity for the Oireachtas (Irish National Parliament) to scrutinise human rights and equality in this country. Garda enforcement of emergency COVID powers disproportionally affects the young, ethnic and racial minorities, and Traveller and Roma communities [1496]. If you stand for human rights and equality, we are on your side. Stand with us!

George Orwell said, *"There was truth and there was untruth, and if you clung to the truth even against the whole world, you were not mad"* [1497]. We're not mad as in cuckoo. We are mad as in we have had enough of being told what to do, what to say, how to think and how to live. If you've had enough of the fear-mongering, lying, cheating, finagling, bullying experts and authorities, we are on your side. Stand with us! Archbishop Desmond Tutu said, *"If you are neutral in situations of injustice, you have chosen the side of the oppressor"* [3]. Get off the fence! This is an attack on our civil liberties. It has been prewritten and forewarned. The ruling class have spelt it out in black and white. The Greta Reset says look forward to climate lockdowns. We need feet on the ground to stand against mandatory vaccination and to protect our personal freedoms.

Forceful public health policy should be an antiquated reminder of a bygone era. Again, the new era of public health is supposed to depend on good science, yet trial results are being withheld, and publication bias is a concern for leading health officials and government bodies and some members of our community [452]. In order for people to trust public health officials, we need all the information whilst having our personal liberty protected. The alternative is to harken back to old public health and hold people down and beat them into submission to accomplish the Global Health Security Agenda (GHSA) of universal vaccination [792].

The world is run by the ruling class, a global elite cabal of cajolers who have cajoled us into believing they care about us. It's no conspiracy. It's a GHSA for population control. Totalitarianism is already upon us. Any form of dissent is oppressed or removed from office. Anyone with an opinion opposing the agenda is labelled racist, homophobic or unable to reason. Our individual freedoms have been stripped under the guise of 'human rights', the fifth of which is the right to be protected from infectious disease whether we like it or not. Our oppressive government already exercises an extremely high degree of control over our public and private life. We haven't been able to shake hands, hug, or kiss. We couldn't meet in our homes. We couldn't sing 'Happy Birthday' or Christmas carols! Heaven knows when we can go to a gig, an art opening or a traditional Irish music session without a QR code (I have an IQ code). Our politicians do not represent us. Our politicians are paid puppets of big industry; paid actors in an all-encompassing fear campaign broadcast through the Gates-controlled mass media to generate interest in and increase uptake of vaccines. It really is as simple as turn off the television and the wireless. It was never about childhood vaccinations, that was a warm up. They are coming for every single man, woman, person and child on the planet with an ever-increasing schedule of yearly vaccines against infectious diseases that actually strengthen our immune systems to protect us from cancer and autoimmune disease under the guise of "Healthy Ageing 2030". Enough is enough! We have a right to choose not to poison ourselves! Bob Marley said (it is) "Better to die fighting for freedom than be a prisoner all the days of your life" [(1498)]. We are here. Listen to us! Stand! Hold the line, hold it, hold it, hold....FREEDOM!

*   *   *

Publisher's Note: *COVERT-19 contains approximately 1500 fully-referenced quotes from qualified sources. To keep the cost of production down in this paperback version, those references can be found in a free searchable online document on the CheckPoint Press website. The academic hardcover version contains all 80+ pages of references in full print format.*

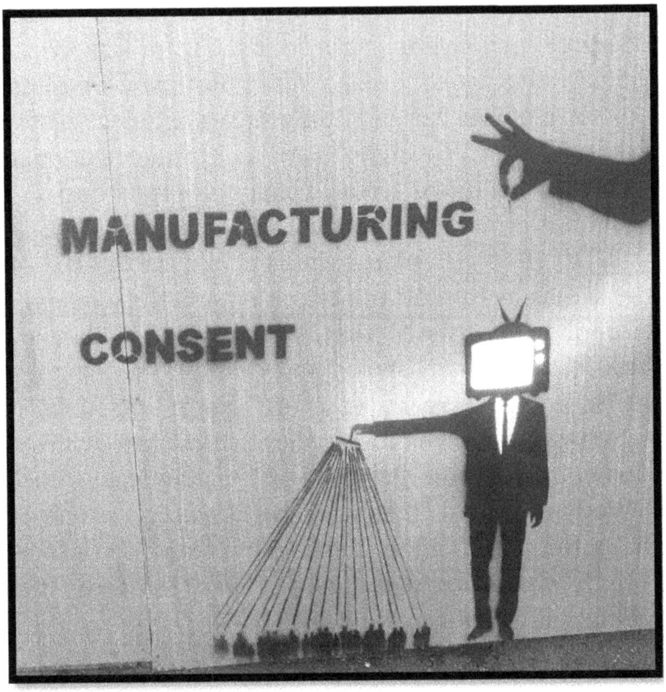
MANUFACTURING
CONSENT

About the Author

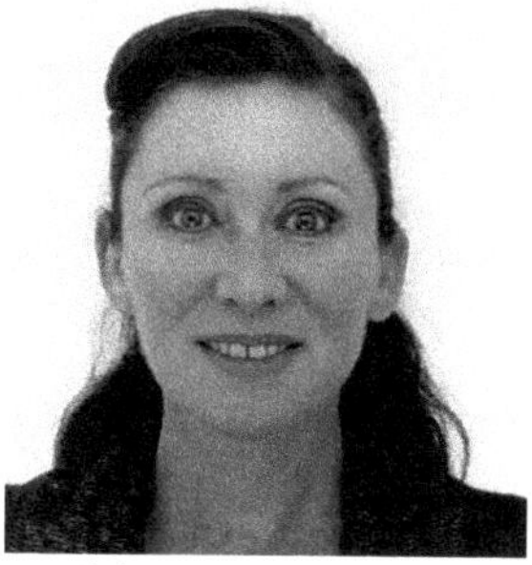

Carina Harkin holds three Honours Bachelor of Health Science Degrees in Complementary and Alternative Medicine (CAM), a Masters in Public Health and 22 years clinical experience. Before COVID (BC), Carina chaired, moderated and presented at international CAM conferences on topics including, 'Annual Influenza Vaccine Review of Current Attitudes, Effectiveness and Natural Evidence-Based Alternatives in the Likelihood of a Pandemic', 'Plastic Bioaccumulation, Health Implications and Enhancing Biotransformation using Herbal Medicine' and 'Heavy Metal Biotransform-ation using Plant Lignands Metallothioneins and Phytochelatins'. Carina worked in public health as an acupuncturist at the Northern Hospital Melbourne, where she conducted a world first trial, 'A Prospective, Randomised Control Trial of Acupuncture for Select Common Conditions within the Emergency Department', and in Box Hill Hospital's Drug and Alcohol Rehabilitation Unit.

Carina specialises in treating antimicrobial-resistant(AMR) disease, beyond the biomedical approach. Carina's dissertation was entitled 'Systematic Review and Meta-Analysis of Plant-derived antimicrobials (PDAms) in WHO Priority Pathogens'. BC, Carina's goal was to complete a PhD in Biomedicine to answer either, are the neuroprotective and neuroregenerative properties of Chinese herbal medicines, including their effects on stem cell biology, suitable to treat and control neurodegenerative diseases, or, are PDAms suitable to treat and control AMR pathogens causing healthcare-associated infections?

As a mother of seven, there is not a childhood infectious disease Carina has not seen nor treated using natural medicine. Her hobbies are gardening, cycling, fiddling, singing, dancing and having the craic. Carina's current goal is to stand for freedom and natural immunity. Carina has a practice and global herbal dispensary.

Carina Harkin MPH, BHSc Nat, BHSc Hom, BHSc Acu, Cert IV TAE
ORCID ID 0000-0001-6091-059X

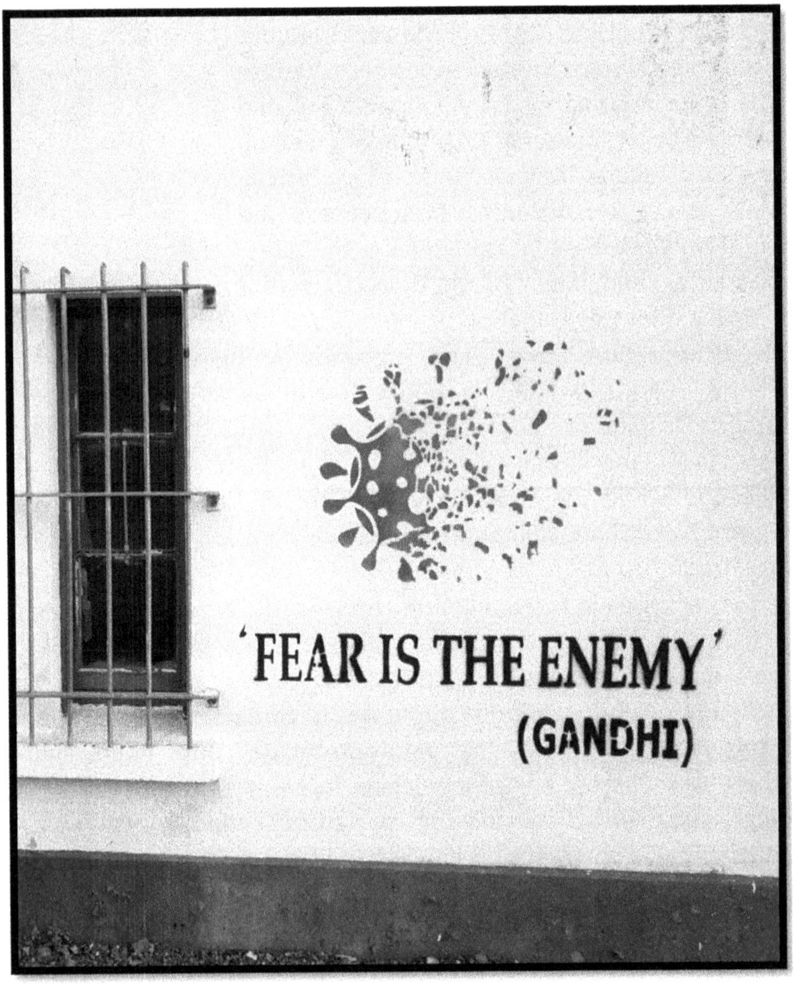
'FEAR IS THE ENEMY'
(GANDHI)

List of Abbreviations

A Absolute risk reduction (ARR)
Acceptable daily intake (ADI)
Accident & Emergency (A&E)
Acquired immune deficiency syndrome (AIDS)
Active pharmaceutical ingredients (API)
Acute disseminated encephalomyelitis (ADEM)
Adverse events following immunisation (AEFI)
Adverse reaction (ADR)
Advisory Committee on Immunisation Practices (ACIP)
Agency for Healthcare Research and Quality (AHRQ)
American College of Allergy, Asthma and Immunology (ACAAI)
American College of Obstetricians and Gynaecologists (ACOG)
American College of Rheumatology (ACR)
America's Frontline Doctors (AFD)
American Medical Association (AMA)
American Society of Nephrology (ASN)
Antibody-dependent enhancement (ADE)
Antibiotic-resistant (AR)
Antifa (anti-fascist)
Antimicrobial use (AMU)
Antimicrobial resistance (AMR)
Antiretroviral therapy (ART)
Army Medical Research Institute of Infectious Diseases (AMRIID)
Artificial intelligence (AI)
Attention deficit hyperactivity disorder (ADHD)
Australian Health Practitioner Regulation Agency (AHPRA)
Australian Technical Advisory Group on Immunisation (ATAGI)
Autism and Developmental Disabilities Monitoring (ADDM)
Autism spectrum disorder (ASD)
Autoimmune/auto-inflammatory syndrome induced by adjuvants (ASIA)
Autoimmune inflammatory rheumatic disease (AIRD)

B Bacillus Calmette-Guerin (BCG)
Before COVID (BC)
Biological and Toxins Weapons Convention (BTWC)
Biotechnology Innovation Organisation (BIO)
Binding antibody (bAb)

Black, Asian and Minority Ethnic (BAME)
Blood oxygen level (SpO2)
Body mass index (BMI)
Breakthrough infection (BI)

C Carbon dioxide (CO2)
Case fatality rate (CFR)
Central nervous system (CNS)
Central Statistics Office (CSO)
Centre for Biologics Evaluation and Research (CBER)
Centres for Disease Control and Prevention (CDC)
Centre for Evidence-Based Medicine (CEBM)
CEN Workshop Agreement (CWA)
Cerebral venous sinus thrombosis (CVST)
China Population Welfare Foundation (CPWF)
Chronic fatigue syndrome (CFS)
Coalition for Epidemic Preparedness Innovations (CEPI)
Community-acquired pneumonia (CAP)
Complement activation-related pseudoallergy (CARPA)
Complementary and Alternative Medicine (CAM)
Consolidated Standards of Reporting Trials (CONSORT)
Coronavirus disease 2019 (COVID-19)
Coronavirus Aid, Relief and Economic Security (CARES)
Countermeasures Injury Compensation Programme (CICP)
COvid-19 and high-dose VITamin D supplementation TRIAL (COVIT-TRIAL)
COVID-19 Vaccines Global Access (COVAX)
Cycle threshold (Ct)
Cytosine phosphoguanine (CpG)

D Defence Advanced Research Projects Agency (DARPA)
Deoxyribonucleic acid (DNA)
Department of Health and Human Services (HHS) Department of Health and Social Care (DHSC)
Developmental and Reproductive Toxicity (DART)
Diagnosis-related group (DRG)
Diphtheria-tetanus-pertussis (DTP)
Disease-modifying anti-rheumatic drug (DMARD)
Do-not-resuscitate (DNR)

Drug-drug interactions (DDIs)
Dual-use research of concern (DURC)

E Ebola Virus Disease (EVD)
Electric vehicles (EVs)
Emergency Use Authorisation (EUA)
Emerging infectious disease (EID)
Endogenous retrovirus (HERV)
European Centre for Disease Prevention and Control (ECDC)
European Committee for Standardisation (CEN)
European Information Centre for Complementary and Alternative Medicine (EICCAM)
European Medicines Agency (EMA)
European Union (EU)
Excess mortality rate (EMR)
Extensively drug-resistant TB (XDR TB)

F False positive rate (FPR)
False negative rate (FNR)
Family Tax Benefit (FTB)
Federal Aviation Administration (FAA)
Firefly luciferase (FLuc)
Follicle-stimulating hormone (FSH)
Food and Drug Administration (FDA)
Freedom of Information (FOI)
Front Line COVID-19 Critical Care Alliance (FLCCC)

G Gavi, the Vaccine Alliance (Gavi)
General Data Protection Regulation (GDPR)
General practitioner (GP)
General Medical Council (GMC)
Genetically modified organisms (GMOs)
GlaxoSmithKline (GSK)
Global Health Security Agenda (GHSA)
Global Influenza Surveillance and Response System (GISRS)
Global initiative on sharing all influenza data (GISAID)
Gonadotropin-releasing hormone (GnRH)
Government Communications Headquarters (GCHQ)
Greater Barrington Declaration (GBD)
Gross Domestic Product (GDP)

Guillain-Barré syndrome (GBS)

H Haemagglutinin (HA)
Haemophilus influenzae type b (Hib)
Haute Autorité de santé (HAS)
Health-care acquired infection (HAI)
Healthcare-associated infection (HCAI)
Healthcare workers (HCWs)
Health Information and Quality Authority (HIQA)
Health Products Regulatory Authority (HPRA)
Health Protection Surveillance Centre (HPSC)
Health Research Authority (HRA)
Health Resources and Services Administration (HRSA)
Health Service Executive (HSE)
Hepatitis B (HBV)
Herd immunity level (HIL)
Herd immunity threshold (HIT)
Human chorionic gonadotropin (hCG)
Human immunodeficiency virus (HIV)
Human papillomavirus (HPV)
Hydroxychloroquine (HCQS)

I In vitro diagnostic (IVD)
Immune thrombocytopenic purpura (ITP)
Immunisation Action Coalition (IAC)
Immunisation Safety Review Committee (ISR)
Immunoglobulin E (IgE)
Immunoglobulin G (IgG)
Inactivated polio vaccine (IPV)
Independent Scientific Advocacy Group (ISAG)
Indian Council of Medical Research (ICMR)
Infection fatality rate (IFR)
Infection prevention and control (IPC)
Inflammatory bowel disease (IBD)
Influenza-like illness (ILI)
Informed Consent Action Network (ICAN)
Initiative for Vaccine Research (IVR)
Inpatient prospective payment system (IPPS)
Institute for Health Metrics and Evaluation (IHME)

Instructions for use (IFU)
Intensive care unit (ICU)
Institute for Health Metrics and Evaluation (IHME)
Institute of Medicine (IOM)
International Air Transport Association (IATA)
International Bank for Reconstruction and Development (IBRD)
International Certificate of Vaccination or Prophylaxis (ICVP)
International Development Association (IDA)
International Federation of Pharmaceutical
International Monetary Fund (IMF)
In vitro diagnostic medical devices (IVDs)
Irish Human Rights and Equality Commission (IHREC)
Irish Medical Council (IMC)

J John Snow Memorandum (JSM)
Johnson & Johnson (J&J)
Joint Committee on Vaccination and Immunisation (JCVI)
Juvenile dermatomyositis (JDM)
Juvenile idiopathic arthritis (JIA)
Juvenile polymyositis (JPM)

K Klebsiella pneumoniae (K. pneumoniae)
Korea Food & Drug Administration (KFDA)

L Labcorp (Laboratory Corporation of America Holdings)
Least developed countries (LDCs)
Lipid nanoparticles (LNPs)
Low-to-middle-income countries (LMICs)
Luteinising hormone (LH)

M Major histocompatibility complex (MHC)
Major League Baseball (MLB)
Manufacturers Association (IFPMA)
Massachusetts Institute of Technology (MIT)
Measles-mumps-rubella (MMR)
Medicines and Healthcare Products Regulatory Agency (MHRA)
Messenger ribonucleuc acid (mRNA)
Methicillin-resistant Staphylococcus aureus (MRSA)
Metropolitan Atlanta Developmental Disabilities Surveillance Programme (MADDSP)

Microphysiological systems (MPS)
Middle East respiratory syndrome coronavirus (MERS-CoV)
Millennium Development Goals (MDGs)
Ministry of Food and Drug Safety (MFDS)
Morbidity and Mortality Weekly Report (MMWR)
Multidrug-resistant (MDR)
Multidrug-resistant tuberculosis (MDR-TB)
Multisystem inflammatory syndrome in children (MIS-C)
Myalgic encephalomyelitis (ME)

N National Academy of Medicine (NAM)
National Basketball Association (NBA)
National Centre for Biotechnology Information (NCBI)
National Centre for Health Statistics (NCHS)
National Childhood Vaccine Injury Act (NCVIA)
National Emergency Routine Immunisation Coordinating Centre (NERICC)
National Football League (NFL)
National Health and Nutrition Examination Survey (NHANES)
National Health Service (NHS)
National Immunisation Advisory Committee (NIAC)
National Immunisation Programme (NIP)
National Institute for Health and Care Excellence (NICE)
National Institute of Allergy and Infectious Diseases (NIAID)
National Institute of Health (NIH)
National Public Health Emergency Team (NPHET)
National Rugby League (NRL)
National Standards Authority of Ireland (NSAI)
National Vaccine Advisory Committee (NVAC)
National Vaccine Injury Compensation Programme (VICP)
National Virus Reference Laboratory (NVRL)
National Vital Statistics System (NVSS)
Natural killer cells (NK cells)
Near-infrared spectroscopy (NIR)
Neglected tropical diseases (NTDs)
Neisseria gonorrhoeae (N. gonorrhoeae)
Neuraminidase (NA)
Neurodevelopmental disorders (NDDs)
Neutralising antibody (nAb)

Non-communicable disease (NCD)
Non-governmental organisation (NGO)
Nonhuman primates (NHPs)
Notice of proposed rulemaking (NPRM)
Nucleic acid testing (NAT) Occupational Exposure Band (B-OEB)

O Office for National Statistics (ONS)
Oral poliovirus vaccine (OPV)
Ordinal Scale for Clinical Improvement (OSCI)
Organisation for the Prohibition of Chemical Weapons (OPCW)
Oxford-AstraZeneca (AZN)
Oxford University Hospitals (OUH)

P Paediatric autoimmune neuropsychiatric disease associated with strep infection (PANDAS)
Paediatric inflammatory multisystem syndrome (PIMS)
Particulate matter (PM)
Perfluorobutyrate (PFBA)
Persistent organic pollutants (POPs)
Personal protective equipment (PPE)
Pharmaceutical Research and Manufacturers of America (PhRMA)
Physical Containment Level 3 (PC3)
Pneumococcal conjugate vaccine (PCV)
Political action committees (PACs)
Polychlorinated biphenyls (PCBs)
Polyethylene glycol (PEG)
Polyfluoroalkyl substances (PFAS)
Polymerase chain reaction (PCR)
Porcine circovirus (PCV)
Postural orthostatic tachycardia syndrome with chronic fatigue syndrome (POTSCFS)
Prevention of Allergy-Risk Factors for Sensitisation in Children Related to Farming (PARSIFAL)
Pseudomonas aeruginosa (P. aeruginosa)
Public Health England (PHE)
Public Readiness and Emergency Preparedness Act (PREP Act)

Q Quantitative reverse transcription PCR (RT-qPCR)
Quantum dots (QDs)

R Randomised controlled trial (RCT)
Reignite Democracy Australia (RDA)
Relative risk reduction (RRR)
Research and development (R&D)
Research Ethics Service (RES)
Research use only (RUO)
Respiratory syncytial virus (RSV)
Reverse transcription-polymerase chain reaction (RT-PCR)
Ribonucleic acid (RNA)
Robert Koch Institute (RKI)
Rockefeller Foundation (RF)
Royal Australian and New Zealand College of Obstetricians and Gynaecologists (RANZCOG)

S SARS coronavirus (SCV)
Scientific Advisory Group for Emergencies (SAGE)
Scientific Pandemic Influenza Group on Modelling, Operational sub-group (SPI-M-O)
Selenoprotein P (SELENOP)
Serious adverse event (SAE)
Severe acute respiratory syndrome coronavirus (SARS-CoV)
Severe acute respiratory syndrome coronavirus 2 (SARS-CoV-2)
Shoulder injury related to vaccine administration (SIRVA)
Simian virus 40 (SV40)
Social determinants of health (SDH)
Socioeconomic status (SES)
Staphylococcus aureus (S. aureus)
Strategic Preparedness and Response Programme (SPRP)
Streptococcus pneumoniae (S. pneumoniae)
Sustainable Development Goals (SDGs)
Swine influenza (H1N1)
Syncytiotrophoblast (SynT)

T Teachta Dála (TD)
Tenders Electronic Daily (TED)
Thrombosis with thrombocytopenia syndrome (TTS)
Totally drug-resistant TB (TDR-TB)
Trihalomethanes (THMs)
Tuberculosis (TB)

Type 1 diabetes (T1D)United Nations (UN)

U Uppsala Monitoring Centre (UMC)
Under-vaccinated group (UVG)
United Kingdom (UK)
United States (US)
United Nations (UN)
United Nations Office for the Coordination of Humanitarian Affairs (UNOCHA)
United Nations Relief and Works Agency for Palestine Refugees in the Near East (UNRWA)
University College Dublin (UCD)
University College London (UCL)

V Vaccine Adverse Event Reporting System (VAERS)
Vaccines and Related Biological Products Advisory Committee (VRBPAC)
Vaccine-associated disease enhancement (VADE)
Vaccine Confidence Project (VCP)
Vaccine effectiveness (VE)
Vaccine escape mutant (VEM)
Vaccine-induced immune thrombotic thrombocytopenia (VITT)
Vaccine-induced prothrombotic immune thrombocytopenia (VIPIT)
Vaccine-induced serotype replacement (VISR)
Vaccine Injury Compensation Programme (VICP)
Vaccine-preventable disease (VPD)
Vaccine Supply Working Group (VSWG)
Variants of concern (VOC)
VST Enterprises (VSTE)

W World Bank Group (WBG)
World Doctors Alliance (WDA)
World Economic Forum (WEF)
World Health Organisation (WHO)
Wuhan Institute of Virology (WIV)
World Intellectual Property Organisation (WIPO)
World Trade Organisation (WTO)
WHO priority pathogen (WHO PP)

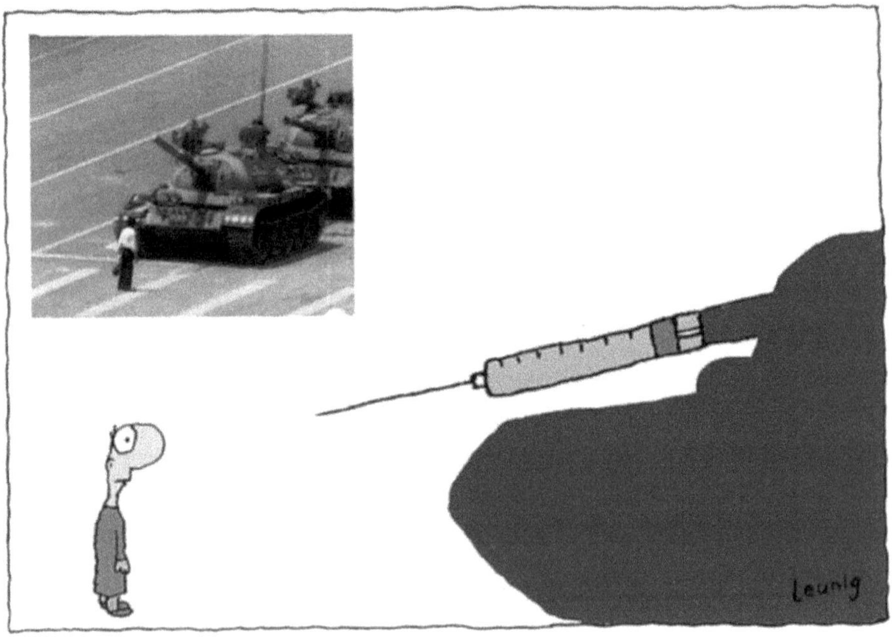

October 2021: "Newspaper cartoonist Michael Leunig has been axed from his prized position in *The Age* over an image comparing resistance to mandatory vaccination to the fight for democracy in Tiananmen Square.

In an image posted to his Instagram account, Leunig — whose career has spanned five decades — drew a lone protester standing in front of a loaded syringe, mimicking the iconic "tank man" image of protest in China. An inset of the 1989 photo also appears in Leunig's drawing.

The image was posted at the end of September and never made it to print in *The Age...*"

NEWS.COM.AU

" ...it has now been republished, with respect and gratitude to Michael's insight and courage, by Carina Harkin and CheckPoint Press."

CheckPoint Press

"Books With Something To Say!"

Lightning Source UK Ltd.
Milton Keynes UK
UKHW020637281221
396285UK00010B/717

9 781906 62879